AF443570

# Inflammatory Bowel Diseases:
## New Developments and Standards

FALK SYMPOSIUM 82

# Inflammatory Bowel Diseases:
# New Developments and Standards

EDITED BY

## W. E. Fleig

Klinik und Poliklinik für Innere Medizin I
Klinikum Kröllwitz der
Martin-Luther-Universität Halle-Wittenberg
D-06097 Halle/Saale
Germany

*Proceedings of the Falk Symposium No. 82, held in Halle/Saale, Germany,
November 18–19, 1994*

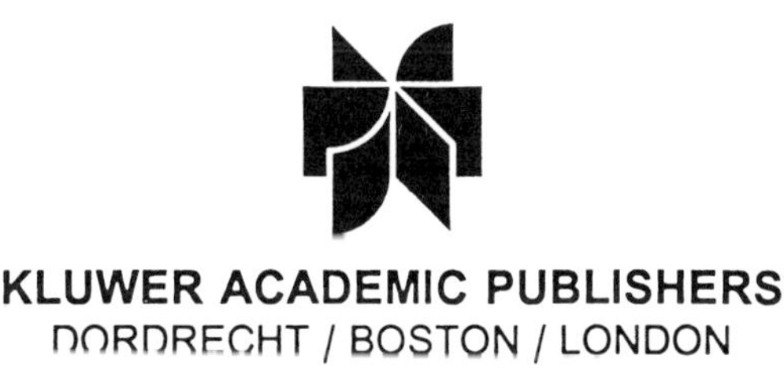

KLUWER ACADEMIC PUBLISHERS
DORDRECHT / BOSTON / LONDON

**Distributors**

---

*for the United States and Canada*: Kluwer Academic Publishers, PO Box 358, Accord Station, Hingham, MA 02018-0358, USA
*for all other countries*: Kluwer Academic Publishers Group, Distribution Center, PO Box 322, 3300 AH Dordrecht, The Netherlands

A catalogue record for this book is available from the British Library

ISBN 0–7923–8890–9

**Library of Congress Cataloging in Publication Data**

---

Falk Symposium (82nd : 1994 : Halle an der Saale, Germany)
    Inflammatory bowel diseases: new  developments and standards:
proceedings of the Falk symposium no. 82, held in Halle/Saale,
Germany, November 18–19, 1994. / Falk Symposium 82; edited by W. E.
Fleig.
        p.   cm.
    Includes bibliographical references and index.
    ISBN 0–7923–8890–9 (casebound)
    1. Inflammatory bowel diseases — Congresses.   I. Fleig, Wolfgang
E. II. Title.
    [DNLM: 1. Inflammatory Bowel Diseases — etiology — congresses.
2. Inflammatory Bowel Diseases — diagnosis — congresses.
3. Inflammatory Bowel Diseases — surgery — congresses. WI 420 F191ib
1995]
RC862. I53F35    1994b
616.3´44—dc20
DNLM/DLC
for Library of Congress                                           95–35526
                                                                       CIP

# Contents

CONTENTS

CONTENTS

# Preface

In the absence of a clear-cut aetiology and, thus, cause-related therapy, critical updates of the emerging knowledge on the pathophysiology of inflammatory bowel diseases and on their eventual therapeutic consequences are mandatory. From November 17 to 19, 1994, an international group of experts met in Halle (Saale) in an effort to exchange recent findings in the pathogenesis, clinical characteristics, diagnosis and treatment of these challenging diseases.

The most important and, sometimes, provocative new aspects of aetiology and pathogenesis were presented first. In a second session, information on extra-intestinal manifestations of IBD and on special problems such as pregnancy in IBD patients and the risk of cancer was updated. Then, measures of disease activity, prognosis and quality of life were discussed. Finally, established methods and new developments in diagnosis, medical and surgical treatment were reviewed. New original data related to the different topics were presented in a special poster session.

The meeting was successful in transmitting the current status of IBD mutually from the investigator in basic research to the clinician and vice versa. Furthermore, the special geographical location of Halle in the eastern part of Germany offered the unique opportunity to bring together experts and interested physicians from Eastern Europe with those from the West of the Continent, Scandinavia, Great Britain and America. More than 500 delegates from 22 different countries attended the meeting held in the year of the 300th anniversary of the foundation of Halle's Martin-Luther-University.

We are greatly indebted to the authors of the contributions, to the poster presenters and, last but not least, to Dr. Herbert Falk and the Falk Foundation for their generous support.

**W. E. Fleig**

# List of Principal Authors

**S. Bondesen**
Med. Dept. A,
Division of Gastroenterology
Rigshospitalet
National University of Denmark
Copenhagen
Denmark

**H.-J. Brambs**
Abteilung Röntgendiagnostik
Radiologische Klinik und Poliklinik
Steinhoevelstrasse 9
D-89075 Ulm
Germany

**G.-R. Burmester**
Department of Medicine III
Charité University Hospital
Humboldt University
Schumannstr. 20-21
D-10117 Berlin
Germany

**G.R. D'Haens**
Department of Gastroenterology
University Hospital Gasthuisberg
Herestraat 49
B-3000 Leuven
Belgium

**C. Ell**
Medizinische Klinik I mit Poliklinik der
  FAU Erlangen-Nürnberg
Krankenshausstr. 12
D-91054 Erlangen
Germany

**J. Emmrich**
Gastroenterologische Abteilung
Universitätsklinik für Innere Medizin
Ernst-Heydemann-Str. 6
D-18057 Rostock
Germany

**E. H. Farthmann**
Chirurgische Universitätsklinik
Hugstetter Str. 55
D-79106 Freiburg
Germany

**W. E. Fleig**
Klinik and Poliklin für Innere Medizin I
Martin-Luther-Universität
  Halle-Wittenberg
Ernst-Grube-Str. 40
D-06097 Halle/Saale
Germany

**H. Goebell**
Universitätsklinikum Essen
Medizinische Klinik und Poliklinik
Hufelandstr. 55
D-45122 Essen
Germany

**V. Gross**
Klinik und Poliklinik für Innere
  Medizin I
Klinikum der Universität Regensburg
D-93042 Regensburg
Germany

**M. R. B. Keighley**
University Department of Surgery
Queen Elizabeth Hospital
Edgbaston
Birmingham B15 2TH
UK

**W. Keller**
Abteilung Psychosomatik und
  Psychotherapie
Klinikum Steglitz der Freien
  Universität Berlin
D-12200 Berlin
Germany

**P. Layer**
Abteilung für Gastroenterologie
Medizinische Universitätsklinik
Hufelandstr. 55
D-45122 Essen
Germany

**H. Lorenz-Meyer**
Medizinische Klinik I
Städtisches Krankenhaus
Röntgenstr. 2
D-88048 Friedrichshafen
Germany

**W. C. Marsch**
Klinik und Poliklinik für Hautkrankheiten
Martin-Luther-Universität
Halle-Wittenberg
D-06097 Halle/Saale
Germany

**R. Modigliani**
Service Hépato-Gastro-Enterologie
Hôpital Saint-Louis
1 Avenue C. Vellefaux
F-75475 Paris Cedex 10
France

**G. Moser**
Clinic of Internal Medicine IV
Department of Gastroenterology and
    Hepatology
Währinger Gürtel 18–20
A-1090 Wien
Austria

**D. Rachmilewitz**
Department of Medicine
Hadassah University Hospital
Mount Scopus, PO Box 24035
IL-91240 Jerusalem
Israel

**R. B. Sartor**
Division of Digestive Diseases and
    Nutrition
CB#7080, 326 Burnett-Womack Bldg
University of North Carolina at Chapel
    Hill
Chapel Hill
NC 27599-7080
USA

**J. Schölmerich**
Klinik und Poliklinik für Innere Medizin I
Klinikum der Universität Regensburg
D-93042 Regensburg
Germany

**W.-B. Schwerk**
Abteilung für Innere Medizin
Philipps-Universität
Baldingerstr.
D-35033 Marburg
Germany

**A. Sonnenberg**
Section of Gastroenterology
VA Medical Center, 111F
2100 Ridgecrest Drive SE
Albuquerque
NM 87108
USA

**R. P. Spielmann**
Klinik und Poliklinik für Diagnostische
    Radiologie
Martin-Luther-Universität
D-06097 Halle
Germany

**E.-F. Stange**
Gastroenterologische Abteilung
Klinik für Innere Medizin der
    Universität zu Lübeck
D-23538 Lübeck
Germany

**M. Starlinger**
Chirurgische Universitätsklinik
Hoppe-Seyler-Str. 2
D-72076 Tübingen
Germany

**J. Stern**
Chirurgische Klinik der Universität
    Heidelberg
Im Neuenheimer Feld 110
D-69120 Heidelberg
Germany

**R. W. Summers**
Department of Internal Medicine,
    4545JCP
University of Iowa College of Medicine
200 Hawkins Drive
Iowa City
IA 52242
USA

**A. J. Wakefield**
University Department of Medicine
Royal Free Hospital School of
    Medicine
Rowland Hill Street
London NW3 2PF
UK

**W. D. Wong**
Department of Surgery
University of Minnesota Medical School
2550 University Avenue West
St Paul
MN 55114-1084
USA

**H. Yang**
UCLA School of Medicine
Division of Medical Genetics, SSB-3
Cedars-Sinai Medical Center
8700 Beverly Boulevard
Los Angeles
CA 90048
USA

**M. Zeitz**
Medizinische Klinik II
Klinikum der Universität des
  Saarlandes
D-66421 Homburg/Saar
Germany

# Section I
# New aspects in the pathogenesis of IBD

# 1
# Genetic susceptibilities – major aetiological risk factors for IBD

## H. YANG and J. I. ROTTER

## INTRODUCTION

The aetiologies of the chronic inflammatory bowel diseases (IBD) – ulcerative colitis (UC) and Crohn disease (CD) – are not clearly understood. Data from epidemiological and genetic epidemiological studies strongly suggest that genetic factors play an important role in the development of the disease(s). Such data include:

1. Consistent racial/ethnic differences in the incidence of disease, with Caucasians and especially those of Jewish origin at the highest population risk;
2. Significantly increased risks to family members;
3. An increased concordance rate in monozygotic twins compared with dizygotic twins;
4. Lack of increased risk in spouses of patients;
5. Significant genetic marker associations; and
6. Gene-targeted knock-out animal models.

Although environmental factors such as smoking may contribute to disease manifestation, the available evidence indicates that ulcerative colitis and Crohn disease are fundamentally genetic diseases with complex non-Mendelian patterns of inheritance.

Before we turn to reviewing this evidence, it is important to note two important implications of such a conclusion. First, given that various forms of IBD are due to specific genetic susceptibilities, we must identify those genes and understand how they act, since it is at that fundamental step that the disease process is presumably initiated. This is essential if we are ever to develop methods of disease prevention or fundamentally different therapies from those now available. Second, individual genetic susceptibility varies tremendously in the population, and thus we need genetic methods to identify those who are susceptible in order to initiate prevention strategies. The power of such a genetic approach has been seen not only in single Mendelian disorders, such as cystic fibrosis, but also in complex non-Mendelian diseases, such as insulin-dependent (type I) diabetes. In cystic fibrosis, the gene was localized, cloned and mutations identified[1,2]. This had led to new methods of carrier screening and prenatal diagnosis, and imminent prospects of new therapies which include replacement of the defective gene. In insulin-dependent diabetes, the locations of at least some of the responsible genes have been identified, and we can now identify at-risk individuals years before disease onset, as well as identify early preclinical stages in the disease process[3,4]. This has led to clinical trials of actual disease prevention[5]. For IBD, our goal should be no less than to understand the aetiology of UC and CD so completely that we can actually focus preventive measures on those individuals at highest risk for UC and CD.

## GENETIC EPIDEMIOLOGICAL EVIDENCE

It has become increasingly apparent that genetic factors play a major role in the development of the various forms of UC and CD[6,7]. The relevant genetic epidemiological evidence comes from ethnic differences, familial aggregation, and twin and spouse studies. The available data also suggest that IBD is not a single disease but a group of genetically different diseases with a common clinical endpoint.

### Consistent ethnic differences

There are large differences in IBD frequency between various racial/ethnic groups. It has generally been thought that UC and CD are more common in whites than in blacks, and rare in Asians[8]. While such observations can have both environmental and genetic explanations, an important finding is the repeated observation that the Jewish population has a consistently increased incidence/prevalence compared with other ethnic groups in the same geographical location (Figure 1). The fact that Jewish and non-Jewish differences occur across different time periods as well as across different geographical areas strongly suggests the existence of a genetic predisposition as the most likely explanation. Further analysis of the Jewish population indicates that IBD occurs in a non-random genetically predisposed subset of the Jewish population, with a higher risk among those of Middle European origin than those of Polish or Russian origin[9]. These latter data further support the concept of a genetic contribution to IBD. However, it should be noted that the fact that rates among Jews are variable, depending on geography, suggests that environmental factors may influence this inherited predisposition in important ways.

### Increased familial aggregation

Familial aggregation is clearly increased in UC and CD, although the data fit no simple Mendelian pattern of inheritance[6]. Several studies have shown that there is an approximate 10–30-fold increase in disease risk among siblings compared with the general population. Of note, the risk of having the other form of the two diseases is also increased. Thus the fact that the two diseases do exist in the same family with a higher frequency than just the co-occurrence by chance

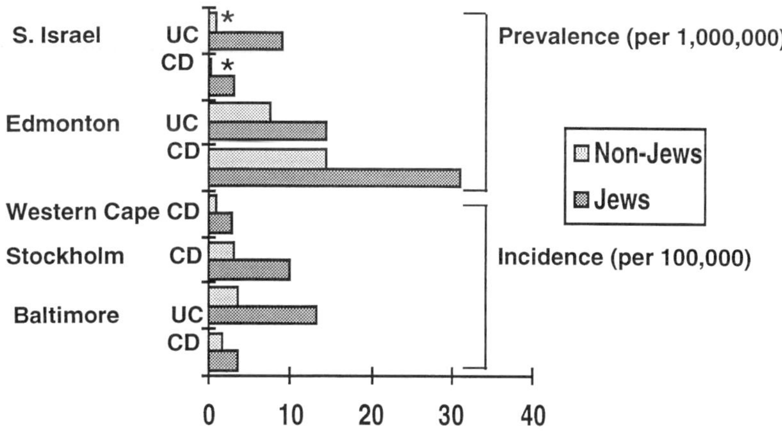


**Figure 1** Prevalence/incidence rates of UC and CD among Jewish and non-Jewish populations by areas. The Jewish population has a consistently increased prevalence/incidence compared with their non-Jewish neighbours (about 3-fold). (Adapted from Reference 6). *Israeli Arab

alone suggests an aetiological correlation between UC and CD (or at least some forms of UC and CD). Of interest, life-time risks for the relatives of non-Jewish patients were consistently lower than corresponding risks for relatives of Jewish patients from the same geographical area[10] (Table 1). Such family empirical risk data are useful, not only for genetic counselling, but also for inference regarding modes of inheritance. Regarding the latter, these data of significantly different empirical risks as a function of ethnicity are supportive for a genetic hetero-geneity model and argue strongly against a model of simple Mendelian inherit-

**Table 1** Empirical risks (%) for IBD in first-degree relatives of patients with IBD*

|  | Siblings | Parents | Offspring | Total |
|---|---|---|---|---|
| **Uncorrected empirical risks for the relatives of IBD probands** | | | | |
| Jewish probands affected with | | | | |
| CD | 8.0 | 3.0 | 1.8 | 4.5 |
| UC | 2.4 | 3.2 | 1.9 | 2.6 |
| Non-Jewish probands affected with | | | | |
| CD | 3.0 | 3.7 | 0 | 2.7 |
| UC | 0.4 | 0.9 | 2.3 | 0.9 |
| **Corrected empirical lifetime risk for relatives of IBD probands†** | | | | |
| Jewish probands affected with | | | | |
| CD | 16.8 | 3.8 | 7.4 | 7.8 |
| UC | 4.6 | 4.1 | 7.4 | 4.5 |
| Non-Jewish probands affected with | | | | |
| CD | 7.0 | 4.8 | 0 | 5.2 |
| UC | 0.9 | 1.2 | 11.0 | 1.6 |

*Data from Yang et al.[10]
†Corrected for age of at-risk relatives, using age-specific incidence data

ance (even with reduced penetrance). Another piece of information from this family study that supports the genetic heterogeneity model comes from the distribution of 'mixed families'[10]. It appears that, among the multiply affected IBD families, the proportion of families with both UC- and CD-affected individuals was greater in non-Jewish families than that in Jewish families (Figure 2). With the greater empirical risks in Jews, the converse would have been expected under the homogeneity model of UC and CD sharing identical or overlapping genetic determinants.

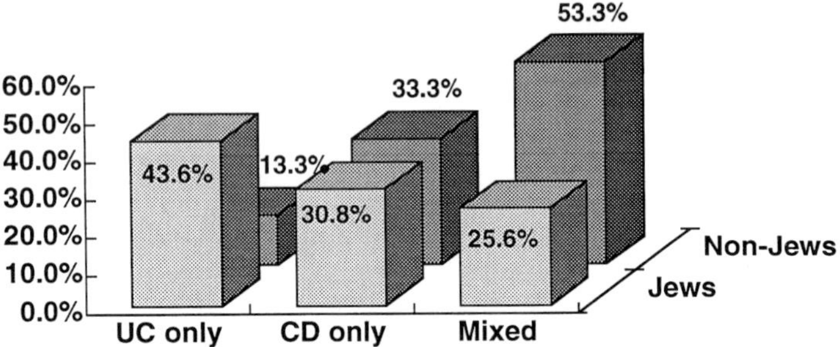


**Figure 2**   Relative frequencies of type of multiply-affected families (UC only, CD only, and mixed, i.e. both UC and CD in the same family) in Jewish and non-Jewish families with two or more affected individuals

## Increased monozygotic twin concordance rate and lack of increased risks for spouses

Observed familial aggregation may be due to shared genetic factors and/or shared environmental factors among family members. Aggregate twin data indicate that there is a higher concordance rate (i.e. both twins affected) for monozygotic twins than for dizygotic twins in both UC and CD[11], supporting the argument that genetic factors are an important component in the development of UC and CD. The observation that significantly less than 100% of monozygotic twins are concordant indicates that there is reduced penetrance for the UC and the CD genotype, presumably due to non-genetic factors. These non-genetic factors may be environmental or they may be due to random stochastic variation, such as occurs in the development of B cells and T cells of the immune system[12], which is especially relevant given the overwhelming data that the immune system is involved in the development of UC and CD.

From the limited number of family studies investigating the risk in spouses, the incidence of reported spouse concordance does not appear to be increased over population risks, and is dramatically less than the risk in siblings[13].

Such increased monozygotic twin concordance rates, the rarity of IBD concordance in spouses, and the numerous instances of affected relatives whose disease onset is separated geographically and temporally from other affected family members[14], argue for a major genetic component to disease susceptibility.

## GENETIC MARKER STUDIES

To identify the susceptibility genes for common disorders which exhibit familial aggregation but non-Mendelian inheritance, such as UC and CD, several approaches can be employed, including a candidate gene approach, a systematic linkage mapping approach, and an animal model approach. So far, such studies have been limited to candidate genes. Since a prominent role for the immune system in the pathogenesis of IBD has long been suspected[15,16], we and others have investigated genes in the MHC, immunoglobulin, and T-cell receptor regions. These might be termed immunospecific genes. Related genes might also be involved in the level of immune response, such as complement components, cytokines and cell adhesion molecules.

Both association studies and linkage analysis can be used to determine the importance of each gene or gene region examined in delineating the genetic basis of a complex trait[17]. If a disorder is found to be associated with a particular marker, this may suggest a causal  relationship (e.g. the association may be due to the effects of the associated gene, i.e. susceptibility gene) or suggest that the associated gene may be in linkage  disequilibrium (nearby on the same chromosome) with the disease susceptibility gene. Linkage studies are designed to examine whether a certain allele of a genetic marker locus is transmitted within a family with the disease of interest. Existence of a linkage between a given marker and a disease indicates that this marker is either the gene causing the disease or that it is located in close physical proximity to that gene. Association and linkage studies can each reveal the involvement of a gene in a disorder. Each of these methods has its own strengths and advantages. Association studies analyse a group of unrelated cases (e.g. UC patients) and a group of unrelated controls for specific genetic markers, e.g. DR2. Such studies are readily conducted but are quite susceptible to population stratification problems (i.e. controls may not come from the same genetic background as the cases). Linkage studies, which analyse families, have the major strength of being capable of detecting linkage, even when there is no population association. Utilizing both association and linkage analyses can distinguish whether the associated gene is a disease susceptibility gene itself or is simply a marker in linkage disequilibrium with a disease susceptibility gene[18]. Therefore, the two methods are complementary to each other and both are essential approaches in delineating the genetic determinants of a genetically complex disease, such as UC and CD.

### Immunospecific genes

By far, the MHC region on the short arm of chromosome 6 has been the most studied gene region. This is because genes at this complex are: (1) crucial in antigen recognition, (2) fundamental to the immune response, and (3) associated with various autoimmune diseases. In the HLA class I region, one intriguing observation as regards the few positive associations is that only alleles at the B locus were reported to be associated with either UC or CD, although with different alleles of the B locus in different studies[6,7]. But no definitive conclusions could be drawn from those markers alone. However, the situation was improved by studies of the class II region. DR2 has now been observed by ourselves and others to be associated with UC in the majority of studies (seven out of nine

**Table 2**  HLA-DR2 association with ulcerative colitis

| Authors | UC[†] | Controls[†] | Population/location |
|---|---|---|---|
| **Association observed** | | | |
| Smolen et al. 1982[19] | 37% (30) | 20% (125) | Caucasian/Vienna |
| Asakura et al. 1982[20] | 70% (40) | 31% (51) | Japanese/Japan |
| McConnell 1983[21] | 46% (31) | 30% (149) | Caucasian/Liverpool |
| Caruso et al. 1985[22] | 32% (41) | 17% (151) | Caucasian/Sicily |
| Kobayashi et al. 1990[23] | 85% (26) | 28% (54) | Japanese/Japan |
| Sugimura et al. 1993[24*] | 65% (37) | 30% (99) | Japanese/Japan |
| Toyoda et al. 1993[25*] | 41% (74) | 21% (77) | Caucasian/Los Angeles |
| **Association not observed** | | | |
| Burnham et al. 1981[26] | 24% (75) | 36% (500) | Unspecified/Nottingham |
| Cottone et al. 1985[27] | 23% (46) | 31% (169) | Caucasian/Oxford |

[†]Percentage of individuals with DR2 (total number of individuals)
*$p < 0.05$

published reports; Table 2). Besides our study, in which we carefully matched the ethnicity of the cases and controls, other studies which individually reported a statistically significant increase in DR2 allele in UC patients were from the Japanese population. It is interesting to note that the negative studies were from certain regions in England only. If there is indeed genetic aetiological heterogeneity within UC, then one would expect that heterogeneity to be minimized in a more homogeneous population such as the Japanese. For CD, a dramatic increase in DR4 has been reported in the Japanese population[28,29], and less dramatic increases in DR4 were observed in some Caucasian populations[19,30,31]. Most recently, using a combination of molecular and serological techniques, and carefully selected ethnically matched controls, we have observed that the DR1/DQ5 allele combination showed a positive association with CD[25]. This relationship was further observed in an independent study[32].

Although the lack of complete agreement at the HLA class II association data may be due to the limited sample size and inappropriate controls in some studies, at least two other potential explanations should be considered. One is that the HLA class II genes themselves are not primary disease susceptibility genes but are in linkage disequilibrium with one or more primary responsible genes located on the short arm of chromosome 6. This is supported by the finding that the strengths of the observed positive associations are only of moderate magnitude (odds ratio about 3). A recent observation of a potentially greater association of the tumour necrosis factor with CD is support for such an explanation[33]. Another explanation is that there may be genetic heterogeneity in the HLA class II allele  associations, as has been  demonstrated in another HLA-associated disease, insulin-dependent diabetes[3,34]. In support of this hypothesis, the authors have observed that the DR2–UC association was mainly contributed by UC patients who have serum antineutrophil cytoplasmic antibodies[35]. With different distributions of patients in different populations, the DR2 associations would be observed in some populations but not in others.

A strong genetic marker association may suggest potential aetiologies, but a spurious association could occur if both IBD and a specific marker are independently increased in frequency in a particular population. Thus, association studies should be contrasted and compared with family linkage studies. Parametric linkage analysis methods (LOD score method) are appropriate for diseases inherited with a Mendelian mode of inheritance because certain parameters are required for analysis, e.g. mode of inheritance, gene frequency and penetrance. In contrast, non-parametric methods (no parameters are assumed) are more appropriate for diseases that are not inherited in Mendelian fashion and the mode of inheritance is unknown, such as in UC and CD. The non-parametric methods basically utilize the information obtained from the affected individuals in the pedigree to assess linkage. The most common method is the sib-pair method and its various extensions.

While a limited number of linkage studies used non-parametric methods, four of nine studies demonstrated evidence for linkage of HLA with IBD[36–39] and the others did not show linkage[40–44]. It is possible that the inconclusive results in previous studies were due to the limitations in power utilizing sib-pairs only and/or may be a consequence of the heterogeneous nature of the IBD, i.e. HLA-linked and unlinked forms that differ in frequency in different populations. There is clearly a need to conduct linkage studies in a large number of multiplex families (families with more than one member affected) which are clinically and subclinically well characterized as homogeneous (i.e. appropriately sub-divided).

## Immunoregulatory genes

What characterizes the various forms of IBD is a failure to down regulate the normal self-limited inflammatory response of the gut. Thus, an alternative or complementary hypothesis to the immunospecific genes is that predisposing genes could be those that determine the level of the immune response along the inflammatory pathway, such as various cytokine genes and cell adhesion molecules.

In our initial investigations of some of these genes, preliminary data indicate that a rare allele which codes for a protein in the functionally important domain 3 of the intercellular adhesion molecule-1, is associated with subsets of UC and CD stratified by antineutrophil cytoplasmic antibodies[45]. In addition, we have recently developed data indicating that the highest risk marker yet identified to be associated with CD is a presumed tumour necrosis factor microsatellite defined haplotype[33]. Another positive report found that an allele of the cytokine interleukin-1 receptor antagonist gene was significantly increased in patients with UC but not CD[46]. These cumulative observations suggest that immunoregulatory genes may have a role in determining the genetic susceptibility to and pathogenesis of UC and/or CD or subsets of UC and CD. The importance of cytokine genes is also supported by recently reported animal models that showed that gene-targeted disruption of either one of two cytokine genes (IL-2 or IL-10) produced mice that develop intestinal lesions similar to those of human IBD[47,48].

## GENETIC HETEROGENEITY OF IBD

It is important to realize that the data now available strongly support the concept that IBD is not a single or even two diseases, but rather is several aetiologically and genetically distinct diseases presenting a similar clinical picture – the concept of genetic heterogeneity. Each of the individual component diseases could conceivably be inherited in a Mendelian, polygenic or multilocus mode of inheritance, and be influenced by environmental factors. Increasing evidence, from clinical differences, subclinical markers, genetic markers, and gene knock-out mice models, supports this heterogeneity concept[6,7].

Concurrence of UC and CD in the same family exceeds the expected frequency by chance alone, suggesting that these two disorders share some of their aetiology in common[10]. However, the clinical differences between UC and CD, and the differences observed in subclinical marker and genetic marker associations, argue strongly that UC and CD are also to a large extent genetically distinct[6,25,29,49]. Even within CD and within UC, further evidence for heterogeneity has been observed. Clinical characteristics of CD have been reported to be familial, including location of the inflammation, transmural aggressiveness, and age of onset[50]. A subset of antineutrophil cytoplasmic antibodies (ANCA) associated with UC with a high specificity (70% of UC patients have ANCA)[51,52] has been used as an indicator for heterogeneity within UC. At least two clinical phenotypes have been associated with the presence of ANCA, i.e. patients who have undergone a colectomy with ileal pouch–anal anastomosis and then developed pouchitis following surgery[53] and patients with treatment-resistant and left-sided UC[54]. Using ANCA, we and others have also provided evidence for heterogeneity within UC with family data[49,55] – the presence of ANCA has a familial distribution. This heterogeneity appears to have a genetic basis as demonstrated by the use of HLA class II genotyping[35] (the presence of ANCA in UC is associated with DR2 and the absence of ANCA in UC is associated with DR4) and the intercellular adhesion molecule-1 molecular polymorphisms[45].

The observation that IBD is associated with some well-defined genetic syndromes (e.g. Turner syndrome, the autosomal recessive Hermansky–Pudlak syndrome, and glycogen storage disease type Ib) is additional evidence for the genetic heterogeneity of IBD[6,7]. These associations also suggest that studies of elements of the immune pathways may be useful in understanding the aetiologies of at least some forms of IBD. Animal models with various knock-out genes that have similar clinical manifestations also support the genetic heterogeneity concept in IBD[47,48,56].

The importance of this genetic heterogeneity concept is that it will lead to identification of more aetiologically homogeneous groups based on clinical and subclinical characteristics for genetic studies. Such subclassification of the disease is essential for the understanding of aetiologies, and will eventually be a requirement for all therapeutic trials so that we can know which precise subgroups will respond to a given therapy.


## GENE–ENVIRONMENTAL INTERACTION

One issue regarding genetically mediated aetiology is the role of environmental factors. The two principal lines of evidence for the involvement of environmental factors are geographical differences and temporal changes in IBD frequencies. Even if environmental factors are involved, they appear to be so ubiquitous that, in any one population, only those genetically susceptible develop clinical disease. For example, although Jews from different geographical areas have very different disease frequencies, they always have increased frequencies compared with their non-Jewish neighbours. A further argument for the importance of environmental factors is often inferred from the lack of complete concordance in monozygotic twins. It is important to realize that these data by no means prove the importance of environmental factors since the stochastic model in the development of the immune system could also explain the reduced penetrance of UC and CD. In addition, the observation that the dizygotic twin concordance rate in IBD is of the same order of magnitude as the sibling recurrence risks[11] also argues that, if environmental factors are important, they are likely to be ubiquitous in the population without time and space aggregation. Community sanitation has been suggested and is supported by case–control data as one such ubiquitous environmental factor[6,7,57,58]. Thus, it is quite likely that it is gene(s), not the specific environment, that determines which members of a family or within a given population develop IBD.

## References


1. Kerem B-S, Rommens JM, Buchanan JA et al. Identification of the cystic fibrosis gene: Genetic analysis. Science. 1989;245:1073–80.
2. Rommens JM, Iannuzzi MC, Kerem B-S et al. Identification of the cystic fibrosis gene: chromosome walking and jumping. Science. 1989;245:1059–65.
3. Rotter JI, Vadheim CM, Rimoin DL. Diabetes mellitus. In: King RA, Rotter JI, Motulsky AG, eds. The genetic basis of common diseases. New York and Oxford: Oxford University Press; 1992:413–81.
4. Riley WJ, Maclaren NK, Krischer J et al. A prospective study of the development of diabetes in relatives of patients with insulin dependent diabetes. N Engl J Med. 1990;323:1167–72.
5. Eisenbarth GS, Verge CF, Allen H, Rewers MJ. Perspectives in diabetes: The design of trials for the prevention of IDDM. Diabetes. 1993;42:941–7.
6. Yang H, Rotter JI. The genetics of inflammatory bowel disease: genetic predispositions, disease markers, and genetic heterogeneity. In: Targan SR, Shanahan F, eds. Inflammatory bowel disease: From bench to bedside. Baltimore: Williams and Wilkins; 1994:32–64.
7. Yang H-Y, Rotter JI. Genetic aspects of idopathic inflammatory bowel disease. In: Kirsner JB, Shorter RG, eds. Inflammatory bowel disease, 4th edn. Baltimore: Williams & Wilkins; 1995:301–31.
8. Sandler RS. Epidemiology of inflammatory bowel disease. In: Targan SR, Shanahan F, eds. Inflammatory bowel disease: From bench to bedside. Baltimore: Williams and Wilkins; 1994:5–30.
9. Roth M-P, Petersen GM, McElree C, Feldman E, Rotter JI. Geographic origins of Jewish patients with inflammatory bowel disease. Gastroenterology. 1989;97:900–4.
10. Yang H, McElree C, Roth M-P, Shanahan F, Targan SR, Rotter JI. Familial empiric risks for inflammatory bowel disease. Differences between Jews and non-Jews. Gut. 1993;34:517–24.
11. Tysk C, Lindberg E, Jarnerot G, Floderus-Myrhed B. Ulcerative colitis and Crohn's disease in an unselected population of monozygotic and dizygotic twins. A study of heritability and the influence of smoking. Gut. 1988;29:990–6.
12. Hayward AR. Lymphoid cell development. In: Litwin SD, Scott DW, Reisfeld RA, Flaherty L, Marcus DM, eds. Human immunogenetics. New York and Basel: Marcel Dekker Inc.; 1989:145–62.
13. Mayberry JF, Rhodes J, Newcombe RG. Familial prevalence of inflammatory bowel disease in relatives of patients with Crohn's disease. Br Med J. 1980;280:84.
14. Kirsner JB. Genetic aspects of inflammatory bowel disease. Clin Gastroenterol. 1973;2:557–76.
15. Shanahan F. Pathogenesis of inflammatory bowel disease: A perspective. Autoimmun Forum Gastroenterol. 1989;1:1–4.
16. Snook J. Are the inflammatory bowel diseases autoimmune disorders? Gut. 1990;31:961–3.
17. Lander ES, Schork NJ. Genetic dissection of complex traits. Science. 1994;265:2037–48.

18. Hodge SE. Linkage analysis versus association analysis: distinguishing between two models that explain disease-marker associations. Am J Hum Genet. 1993;53:367–84.
19. Smolen JS, Gangl A, Polterauer P, Menzel EJ, Mayr WR. HLA antigens in inflammatory bowel disease. Gastroenterology. 1982;82:34–8.
20. Asakura H, Tsuchiya M, Aiso S et al. Association of human lymphocyte-DR2 antigen with Japanese ulcerative colitis. Gastroenterology. 1982;82:413–18.
21. McConnell RB. Ulcerative colitis – genetics features. Scand J Gastroenterol. 1983;18(Suppl 88):14–16.
22. Caruso C, Palmeri P, Oliva L, Orlando A, Cottone M. HLA antigens in ulcerative colitis: A study in the Sicilian population. Tissue Antigens. 1985;25:47–9.
23. Kobayashi K, Atoh M, Konoeda Y, Yagita H, Inoko H, Sekiguchi S. HLA-DR, DQ and T cell antigen receptor constant beta genes in Japanese patients with ulcerative colitis. Clin Exp Immunol. 1990;80:400–3.
24. Sugimura D, Asakura H, Mizuki N et al. Analysis of genes within the HLA region affecting susceptibility to ulcerative colitis. Hum Immunol. 1993;36:112–18.
25. Toyoda H, Wang S-J, Yang H et al. Distinct association of HLA class II genes with inflammatory bowel disease. Gastroenterology. 1993;104:741–8.
26. Burnham WR, Gelsthorpe K, Langman MJS. HLA-D related antigens in inflammatory bowel disease. In: Pena AS, Weterman IT, Booth CC, Strober W, eds. Recent advances in Crohn's disease. The Hague: Martinus Nijhoff; 1981:192–6.
27. Cottone M, Bunce M, Taylor CJ, Ting A, Jewell DP. Ulcerative colitis and HLA phenotype. Gut. 1985;26:952–4.
28. Fujita K, Naito S, Okabe N, Yao T. Immunological studies in Crohn's disease. I. Association with HLA systems in the Japanese. J Clin Lab Immunol. 1984;14:99–102.
29. Kobayashi K, Atoh M, Yagita A et al. Crohn's disease in the Japanese is associated with the HLA-DRw53. Exp Clin Immunogenet. 1990;7:101–8.
30. Purrmann J, Bertrams J, Knapp M et al. Gene and haplotype frequencies of HLA antigens in 269 patients with Crohn's disease. Scand J Gastroenterol. 1990;25:981–5.
31. Caruso C, Oliva L, Palmeri P, Cottone M. B cell alloantigens in Sicilian patients with Crohn's disease. Tissue Antigens. 1983;21:70–2.
32. Neigut D, Proujansky R, Trucco M et al. Association of an HLA-DQB-1 genotype with Crohn's disease in children. Gastroenterology. 1992;102:A671.
33. Plevy SE, Targan SR, Rotter JI, Toyoda H. Tumor necrosis factor (TNF) microsatellites associations within HLA-DR2+ patients define Crohn's disease (CD) and ulcerative colitis (UC)-specific genotypes. Gastroenterology. 1994;106:A794.
34. Pugliese A, Bugawan T, Moromisato R et al. Two subsets of HLA-DQA1 alleles mark phenotypic variation in levels of insulin autoantibodies in first degree relatives at risk for insulin-dependent diabetes. J Clin Invest. 1994;93:2447–52.
35. Yang H, Rotter JI, Toyoda H et al. Ulcerative colitis: a genetically heterogeneous disorder defined by genetic (HLA class II) and subclinical (anti-neutrophil cytoplasmic antibodies) markers. J Clin Invest. 1993;92:1080–4.
36. Kuhnl P, Sibrowski W, Bohm BO, Bender SW, Kalmar G, Loliger C. HLA antigen frequencies in familial Crohn's disease (CD). Beitrage zur Infusionstherapie. 1990;26:283–6.
37. Schwartz SE, Siegelbaum SP, Fazio TL, Hubbell C, Henry JB. Regional enteritis: Evidence for genetic transmission by HLA typing. Ann Intern Med. 1980;93:424–7.
38. Achord JF, Gunn GH, Jackson JF. Regional enteritis and HLA concordance in multiple siblings. Dig Dis Sci. 1982;27:330–2.
39. Shohat T, Cantor RM, Tyan D, McElree K, Rotter JI. Evidence for linkage to HLA in familial IBD. Am J Hum Genet. 1989;45:A218.
40. Kemler BJ, Glass D, Alpert E. HLA studies of families with multiple cases of inflammatory bowel disease (IBD). Gastroenterology. 1980;78:1194A.
41. Purmann J, Miller B, Lapsien B, Munch H, Reis HE, Strohmeyer C. HLA haplotype study in familial Crohn disease. Z Gastroenterol. 1985;23:432–7.
42. Eade OE, Moulton C, MacPherson BR, St. Andre-Ukena S, Albertini RJ, Beeken WL. Discordant HLA haplotype segregation in familial Crohn's disease. Gastroenterology. 1980;79:271–5.
43. Pena AS, Biemond I, Weterman IT, van Leewen A, Schreuder I, van Rood JJ. HLA antigen distribution and HLA haplotype segregation in Crohn's disease. Tissue Antigens. 1980;16:56–61.

44. Colombel JF, Guillemot F, Gossum AV et al. Familial Crohn's disease in multiple siblings: no linkage to the HLA system. Gastroenterol Clin Biol. 1989;13:676–8.
45. Yang H, Vora D, Targan SR, Toyoda H, Beaudet A, Rotter JI. Genetic heterogeneity within UC and Crohn's defined by antineutrophil cytoplasmic antibodies (ANCAs) and intercellular adhesion molecule-1 (ICAM-1) polymorphisms. Gastroenterology. 1994;106:A754.
46. Mansfield JC, Holden H, Tarlow JK et al. Novel genetic association between ulcerative colitis and the anti-inflammatory cytokine interleukin-1 receptor antagonist. Gastroenterology. 1994;106:637–42.
47. Sadlack B, Merz H, Schorle H, Schimpl A, Feller AC, Horak I. Ulcerative colitis-like disease in mice with a disrupted interleukin-2 gene. Cell. 1993;75:253–61.
48. Kühn R, Löhler J, Rennick D, Rajewsky K, Müller W. Interleukin-10-deficient mice develop chronic enterocolitis. Cell. 1993;75:263–74.
49. Shanahan F, Duerr RH, Rotter JI et al. Neutrophil autoantibodies in ulcerative colitis: familial aggregation and genetic heterogeneity. Gastroenterology. 1992;103:456–61.
50. Tokayer AZ, Reydel B, Bayless TM. Possible role of heredity in site and transmural aggressiveness of Crohn's disease. Gastroenterology. 1992;102:A705.
51. Saxon A, Shanahan F, Landers C, Ganz T, Targan S. A subset of antineutrophil anticytoplasmic antibodies is associated with inflammatory bowel disease. J Allergy Clin Immunol. 1990;86:202–10.
52. Duerr RH, Targan SR, Landers CJ, Sutherland LR, Shanahan F. Antineutrophil cytoplasmic antibodies in ulcerative colitis. Comparison with other colitides/diarrheal illnesses. Gastroenterology. 1991;100:1590–6.
53. Sandborn WJ, Tremaine WJ, Batts K, Pemberton JH, Phillips SF. Definition of pouchitis following ileal pouch–anal anastomosis (IPAA): a pouchitis disease activity index PDA1. Gastroenterology. 1992;104:A1774.
54. Vecchi M, Gionchetti P, Bianchi MB et al. p-ANCA reactivity in ulcerative colitis patients with and without pouchitis after protocolectomy. Gastroenterology. 1993;104:A796.
55. Seibold F, Slametschka D, Gregor M, Weber P. Neutrophil autoantibodies: a genetic marker in primary sclerosing cholangitis and ulcerative colitis. Gastroenterology. 1994;107:532–6.
56. Mombaerts P, Mizoguchi E, Grusby MJ, Glimcher LH, Bhan AK, Tonegawa S. Spontaneous development of inflammatory bowel disease in T cell receptor mutant mice. Cell. 1993;75:275–82.
57. Gent AE, Hellier MD, Grace RH, Swarbrick ET, Coggon D. Inflammatory bowel disease and domestic hygiene in infancy. Lancet 1994;343;766–7.
58. Rotter JI. Inflammatory bowel disease. Letter to the editor. Lancet. 1994;343;1360.

# 2
# Psychosocial factors

**G. MOSER**

---

## INTRODUCTION

Psychosocial factors in inflammatory bowel diseases (IBD) are often discussed in a controversal way, in particular the question of whether certain psychosocial factors predispose for the onset of the disease or whether these factors contribute to the disease activity. When considering psychosocial aspects of IBD it should be remembered that these are chronic disorders affecting young individuals. There are different approaches to assessment of psychological and social factors:

1. There is the question of the possible pathogenetic importance of psychosocial factors (predisposing/antecedental factors?).
2. We have to ask how psychosocial factors can influence the clinical course of IBD (modifying factors?).
3. We have to understand the psychosocial consequences and the impact of these chronic disorders (factors secondary to IBD).

## IBD AND PSYCHOLOGICAL DISTURBANCES

The early psychosocial approach to these diseases was characterized by the theory of psychosomatic specificity and it was assumed that specific personality profiles or conflicts may predispose for, or underlie, the disease[1,2]. Latimer[3] had already written in 1978 that it seems not to be possible to answer the question of 'psychogenesis' and 'too much effort has been spent on trying to answer ... probably unanswerable questions in this area'. The hypothesis of 'psychosomatic aetiology' cannot be verified or falsified in retrospective studies. Many investigators, who looked into the association of personality and intrapsychic conflicts with the disease and described psychosocial disturbances in patients with IBD, had not considered that the course of the disease changes the psychosocial situation of the patients[3,4].

Methodological limitations in most of these studies were: the bias of the investigators, retrospective design, small sample size, lack of control groups and failure to control for disease severity[3,5,6]. Most of these 'special personality features' of patients with IBD described in these studies seem to be a result and not a predisposing factor for the disease[4]. Disease-specific personalities have not been confirmed, but Engström and Lindquist[7] published a study which suggests that children and adolescents with IBD comprise a population at high risk for developing a psychiatric disorder. Psychological disturbances seem to be a component of the illness rather than being aetiological or specific to these disorders[5]. Patients with Crohn disease (CD) in particular seem to have slightly higher frequencies (up to 50%) of psychological disturbances compared with patients with other chronic disease[8,9]. Clouse and Alpers[10] reviewed a number of studies and concluded that CD patients – but not ulcerative colitis patients – are at a higher risk for major depression, compared with medically ill controls. The degree of psychological disturbances appears to correlate with the disease severity[3,11,12]. Other investigators suggest that the rate of psychiatric illness in IBD is not higher than in the general population[13–15]. It must be assumed that psychiatric treatment and psychotherapy will be as effective in IBD patients with a psychiatric disorder as in non-IBD subjects with psychological disturbances[4]. There are a very few studies published which have evaluated psychological treatments for patients with IBD[16–20]. Psychotherapy was reported to promote feelings of well-being and better capacity to cope with the illness[16,17,21]. However, until now, there is no study which has found any influence of psychotherapy on the (biological) course of the disease in the long run.

## IBD AND STRESSFUL EXPERIENCES

It appears that stress or emotional disturbances contribute to the clinical course of IBD. Stress is suggested to play an influential role in symptom exacerbation of patients not only with IBD but also with irritable bowel syndrome and other diseases[5,22–24]. For IBD, psychosocial stress may lead to dysregulation of the immune response, thereby affecting disease activity[25]. Immune effects may have a permissive role in disease activation in the predisposed individual[15]. Shanahan and Anton[26] reviewed the evidence for neuroendocrine regulation of the immune system. They suggested that the mechanisms of stress-induced immune alteration are multiple and complex and that the link between stress and the inflammatory process may be through the neuroendocrine–immune axis.

For influence of major life events on the biological disease activity, there are only a few prospective studies which have yielded contradictory results[27–30]. Riley et al.[28] and North et al.[29] found no association between life events and symptoms over a one- and two-year period, respectively. Using a larger sample of 124 IBD patients, Duffy et al.[30] found a strong relationship between major life events, particularly health-related events, and symptom exacerbation. Maybe these conflicting data reflect the methodological problems of studies dealing with major life events[31]. There might be an association between subjectively perceived stress regardless of whether the stress represents a major or minor life event. Interpretation of the events as stressful may be specific to the patient's own personality and history[24]. Garret et al.[22] found a significant relationship between daily stress and symptom experience: greater stress increased symptoms. Levenstein et al.[31] found a significant relation between perceived stress and rectal inflammation in asymptomatic patients with ulcerative colitis. Greene et al.[24] found, in eleven subjects, a positive concurrent relationship between both daily and monthly stress and IBD activity. Their investigations revealed a negative effect of the previous month's stress on IBD symptom severity. Therefore it is not surprising that the majority (59%) of IBD patients believed that psychosocial stress was the main reason for the onset and exacerbation of their disease when patients were asked for possible causes for the disease retrospectively[32,33] (Figure 1). Other factors, like genetic disposition, diet, environmental factors and infection, were considered important by less than 10% of IBD patients. The longer the disease had lasted, the more likely patients were to attribute the cause of their disease to psychological stress[33] (Table 1). Since it is known that the patient's belief about the aetiology of his or her disease is relevant for coping with the illness[34], it must be considered in clinical care.

## IBD AND SOCIAL IMPLICATIONS

Although several authors have reported on the social impact of inflammatory bowel diseases, the need for this type of information still abounds[35]. Interestingly, the first report of ulcerative colitis developing in Bedouin Arabs occurred in those who had moved from their nomadic life into government housing and the authors suggested that the stress of modern living or the change of lifestyle had influenced the development of the disorder[36]. For social factors,

**Table 1**  Disease related data and IBD patients' causal attribution

| | Psychosocial distress ($n = 59$) | Other causes ($n = 41$) | $p$ |
|---|---|---|---|
| Duration of illness: median (quartiles: 25%; 75%) | 5 (2; 9) years | 2 (1; 6) years | 0.01[*] |
| Disease activity at the time of interview | | | |
| Active | 27 (46%) | 17 (42%) | NS |
| Inactive | 32 (54%) | 24 (58%) | |
| Nutritional status | | | |
| Standard weight (± 3 kg) | 18 (31%) | 15 (37%) | NS |
| Chronically malnourished | 7 (12%) | 6 (15%) | NS |
| Disease severity | | | |
| Severe | 27 (46%) | 18 (44%) | NS |
| Mild | 32 (54%) | 23 (56%) | NS |
| Medication at the time of interview | 45 (76%) | 34 (83%) | NS |
| SASP or 5-ASA | 23 (39%) | 13 (32%) | NS |
| Corticosteroids | 19 (32%) | 19 (46%) | NS |
| Immunosuppressives | 3 (5%) | 2 (5%) | NS |
| Fistulae | 23 (39%) | 13 (32%) | NS |
| Any gastrointestinal surgery | 27 (46%) | 13 (32%) | NS |
| Location of disease: | | | |
| Small bowel | 2 (3%) | 3 (7%) | NS |
| Small bowel and colon | 33 (56%) | 20 (49%) | NS |
| Colon | 24 (41%) | 18 (44%) | NS |

[*]Wilcoxon test

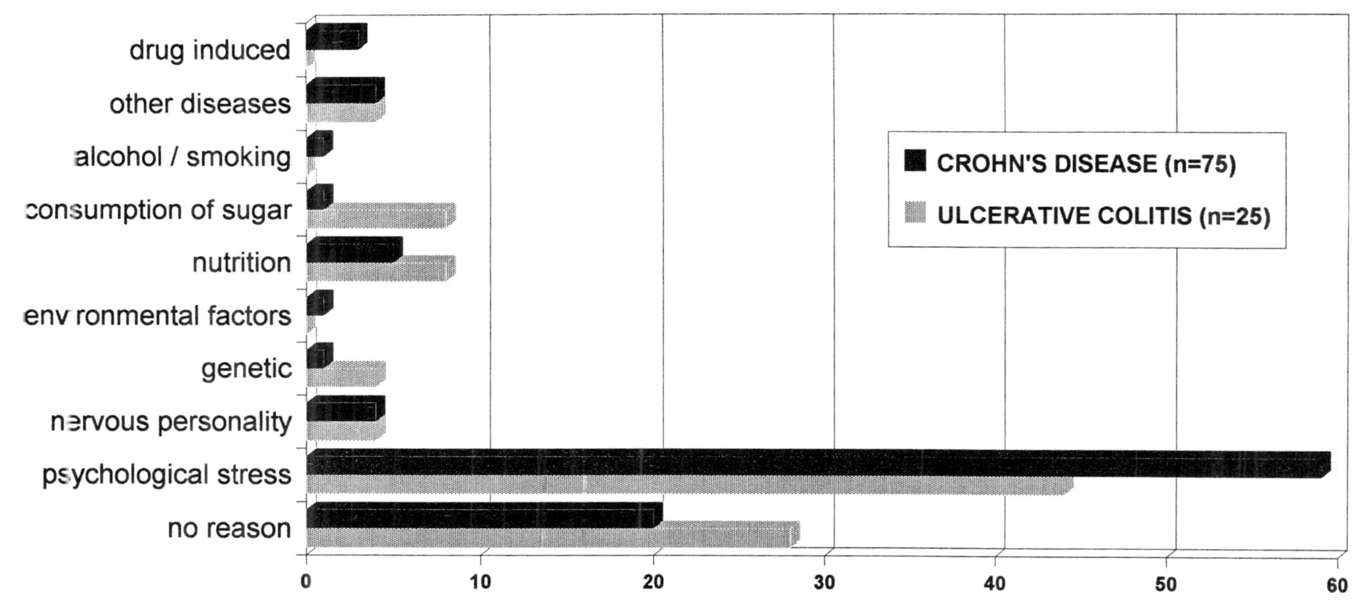


**Figure 1**   Patients' beliefs about different factors causing IBD ('main reason')

Sonnenberg[37] studied the occupational distribution of 12 014 patients who were granted rehabilitation as a result of IBD. He found that being exposed to air-conditioned artificial working conditions and extended or irregular shift working conferred a risk of contracting IBD. In 1992, Sonneberg published a study[35] which focussed on the actual social implications of these diseases. In his study, less than 5% of IBD patients became permanently disabled, and less than 10% were unemployed. Interestingly, for males and females alike, white-collar employees responded less to the rehabilitative measures than blue-collar workers. Similarly, Binder et al.[38] showed that the disablement rate in patients with CD amounted to 20% after 10 years against 4.4% in the normal Danish population. About 75% of the patients were able to maintain an almost normal life. Several other studies have shown that the majority of patients with IBD are able to remain within the work force and engage in gainful employment[39–42]. Most patients with IBD are able to lead a normal life in terms of social activities, family life and professional life[40,41,43–45].

Despite the fact that the occurrence of psychosocial problems seems to be no different among patients with CD and controls[41,46], Sorensen et al.[41] found that 54% of patients with CD felt that exacerbations of their disease strained their professional and personal life. Drossman et al.[12] found that patients with CD have more psychosocial difficulties which appear to be related to greater symptom severity. Mayberry et al.[47] reported that significantly more patients than controls had experienced long-term unemployment and, as a result of their experiences, up to 30% of patients with CD actively concealed their illness from employers. It should not be underestimated that patients coping with this chronic illness have many hidden worries and concerns related to their disease, and these worries are an important indicator of a patient's quality of life[48].

## PATIENT'S QUALITY OF LIFE AND COPING WITH IBD

It is obvious that patients' lives are more difficult during phases of high disease activity and that these diseases can lead to restrictions in social and professional life[35]. Physicians generally underestimate or fail to recognize the functional disabilities reported by patients[49]. Most clinical studies on patients with IBD have not considered the psychosocial impact of these chronic disorders. Patients with IBD often suffer from specific and socially difficult problems, including diarrhoea, (fear of) faecal incontinence, flatulence, abdominal pain, and disturbance of sexual life (especially in women with Crohn disease[50]). Some patients have frequent hospitalization with paintful procedures and disruption to family, school and workplace; some are malnourished and need potent pharmacotherapy, possibly resulting in systemic side-effects. All of this lowers the quality of life and level of psychosocial functioning. To assess this aspect of health-related quality of life, Drossman et al.[48] developed a questionnaire that rates 25 IBD-specific worries and concerns, the Rating Form of IBD Patient Concerns (RFIPC). Because Martin et al.[51] reported that more than 60% of patients with IBD consider themselves insufficiently informed about the disease, we recently studied the relationship between the information the patients have about IBD and their disease-related concerns. The issues of greatest concern of 105 con-

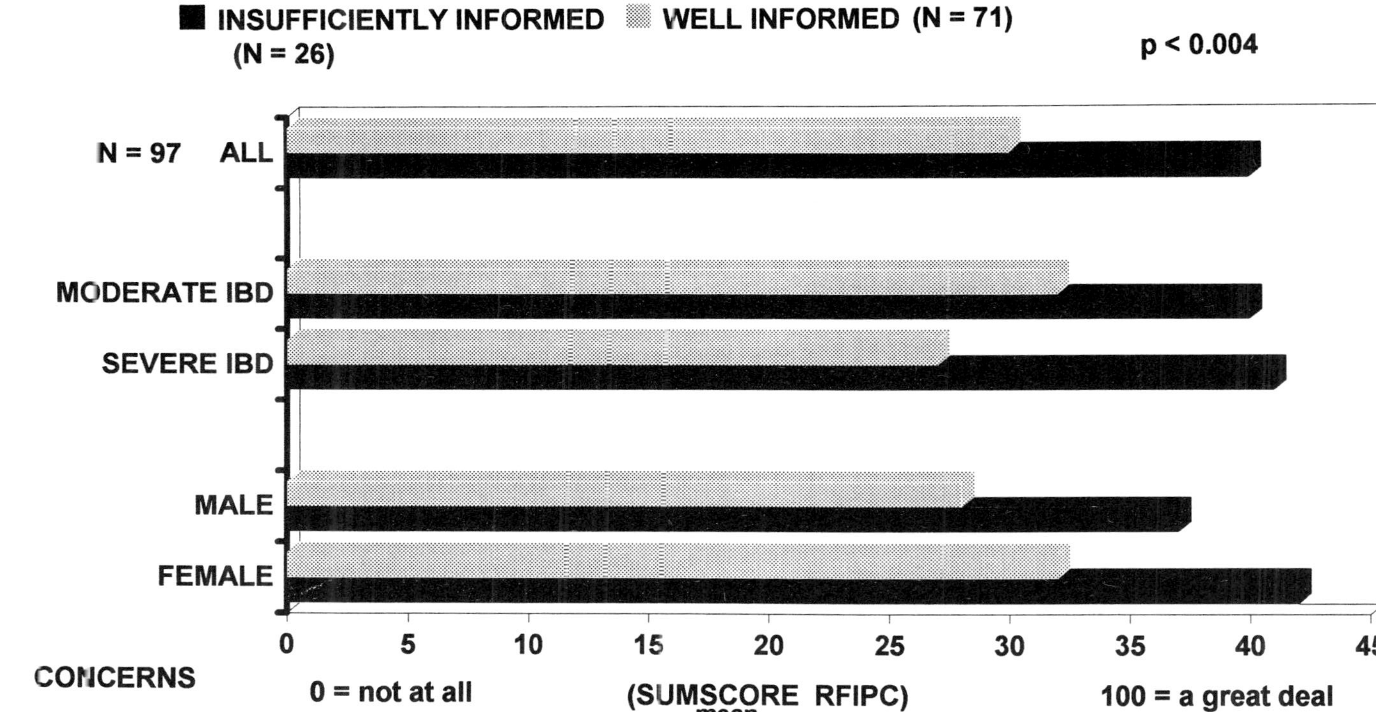


**Figure 2**   Comparison of RFIPC sumscore (concerns) between patients with different perceived information levels about IBD

secutive outpatients with IBD were as follows: having an ostomy bag, the side-effects of medication, surgery, the uncertain nature of the disease and energy level. These five greatest concerns found in our Austrian study population were similar to those in Drossman's study sample of the Crohn's and Colitis Foundation of America[48]. We found that there is a significant relationship between IBD patients' disease-related concerns and their information level about IBD. A lower information level was associated with greater concerns (Figure 2). Apart from disease duration, the perceived information level was not related to occupation, educational level, place of residence, sex, age or disease-related data. Patients are able to adjust to their disease much more readily when they are informed about its nature and effects. Better information about the disease to the patients and psychosomatic counselling for patients who show high levels of concern may improve both quality of life and clinical care.

## CLINICAL MANAGEMENT OF IBD TAKING INTO ACCOUNT PSYCHOSOCIAL FACTORS

Assessment of psychosocial factors in IBD is an essential part of treatment[52]. It is evident that current measures of disease activity are not sufficient to encompass the IBD illness experience[53]. Non-recognition of the psychological disorders may lead to unnecessary and aggressive interventions for IBD patients, such as medication changes or invasive procedures, especially when symptoms cannot be attributed to evident inflammatory bowel pathology[54]. We have to take into account that both psychosocial and physical health variables are related to the patient's well being and the number of physician visits. It was shown that physicians' rating of disease activity did not compare well with health-care utilization or patients' global rating of health[39]. Therefore biological and psychosocial factors cannot be separated. Psychosocial factors are a subsystem of the illness, which is influenced by multiple interacting biological, psychological and social factors[53]. Clinical care for the patient is insufficient if IBD-related psychosocial problems and quality of life are not considered in clinical practice. Patients are able to adjust to their disease much more readily when they know that they are free to discuss the problems with their physician. It makes sense to consider all these variables in diagnosis and treatment. Further studies are needed to provide a scientific basis for this comprehensive approach to IBD.

## References


1. Alexander F. Psychosomatic medicine: Its principles and applications. New York: Norton; 1950.
2. Alexander F, French TM, Pollack G. Psychosomatic specificity: Experimental study and results. Chicago: University of Chicago Press; 1968.
3. Latimer PR. Crohn's disease: A review of the psychological and social outcome. Psychol Med. 1978:8:649–56.
4. Vallis TM, Turnbull GK. Clinical management of inflammatory bowel disease: Beyond disease activity. Part I: Assessing psychosocial factors. Can J Gastroenterol. 1992;6:39–43.
5. Drossman DA. Psychosocial aspects of ulcerative colitis and Crohn's disease. In: Kirsner JB, Shorter RG, eds. Inflammatory bowel disease. Philadelphia: Lea and Febiger; 1988.
6. North CS, Clouse RE, Spitznagel EL, Alpers DH. The relation of ulcerative colitis to psychiatric factors: a review of findings and methods. Am J Psychiatry. 1990;147:974–81.

7. Engström I, Lindquist BL. Inflammatory bowel disease in children and adolescents: a somatic and psychiatric investigation. Acta Paediatr Scand. 1991;80:640–7.

8. Helzer JE, Chammas S, Norland CC, Stillings WA, Alpers DH. A study of the association between Crohn's disease and psychiatric illness. Gastroenterology. 1984;86:324–30.

9. Tarter RE, Switala J, Carra J et al. Inflammatory bowel disease: psychiatric status of patients before and after disease onset. Int J Psychiatr Med. 1987;17:173–81.

10. Clouse RE, Alpers DH. The relationship of psychiatric disorder to gastrointestinal illness. Annu Rev Med. 1986;37:283–95.

11. Andrews H, Barczak P, Allan RN. Psychiatric illness in patients with inflammatory bowel disease. Gut. 1987;28:1600–4.

12. Drossman DA, Leserman J, Mitchell CM, Li Z, Zagami EA, Patrick DL. Health status and health care use in persons with inflammatory bowel disease. A national sample. Dig Dis Sci. 1991;36:1746–55.

13. Whitehead WE, Bosmajian LS. Behaviourial medicine approaches to gastrointestinal disorders. J Consult Clin Psychol. 1982;50:972–83.

14. Blanchard EB, Scharff L, Schwarz SP, Suls JM, Barlow DH. The role of anxiety and depression in irritable bowel syndrome. Behav Res Ther. 1990;28:401–5.

15. Wells KB, Golding JM, Burnam MA. Psychiatric disorders in a sample of the general population with and without chronic medical conditions. Am J Psychiatry. 1988;145:976–81.

16. Milne B, Joachim G, Niedhardt J. A stress management program for inflammatory bowel disease patients. J Adv Nurs. 1986;11:561–7.

17. Künsebeck HW, Lempa W, Freyberger H. Kurz- und Langzeiteffekte ergänzender Psychotherapie bei Morbus Crohn. In: F. Lamprecht, ed. Spezialisierung und Integration in Psychosomatik und Psychotherapie. Berlin: Springer; 1987.

18. Schwarz SP, Blanchard EB. Evaluation of psychological treatment for inflammatory bowel disease. Behav Res Ther. 1991;29:167–77.

19. Jantschek G, Zeitz M, Feiereis H, Riecken EO, Klör HU, Rasenack J, German Study Group on Psychosocial Intervention in Crohn's Disease. Effect of psychotherapy on the somatic course of Crohn's disease. In: Abstract book of the 20th European Conference on Psychosomatic Research, Gent, Aug 24–27; 1994:FS82.

20. Zeitz M, Riecken EO, Pritsch M, Doppl W, Klör HU, Spahmer C, Rasenack J Jantschek G, Feiereis H und die Deutsche Studiengruppe. Psychosoziale Intervention bei M. Crohn. Z Gastroenterol. 1994;32:534.

21. Wietersheim J, Keller W, Scheib P, German Study Group on Psychosocial Intervention in Crohn's Disease. The effects of their psychotherapy in the view of Crohn's disease patients. In: Abstract book of the 20th European Conference on Psychosomatic Research, Gent, Aug 24–27; 1994:FS86.

22. Garrett VD, Brantley PJ, Jones GN, McNight CT. The relation between daily stress and Crohn's disease. J Behav Med. 1991;14:87–96.

23. Cohen S, Tyrrell DAJ, Smith AP. Psychological stress and susceptibility to the common cold. N Engl J Med. 1991;325:606–12.

24. Greene BR, Blanchard EB, Wan CK. Long-term monitoring of psychosocial stress and symptomatology in inflammatory bowel disease. Behav Res Ther. 1994;32:217–26.

25. Sternberg E, Chrousos GP, Wilder RL, Gold PW. The stress response and the regulation of inflammatory disease. Ann Intern Med. 1992;177:854–66.

26. Shanahan F, Anton P. Neuroendocrine modulation of the immune system: Possible implications for inflammatory bowel disease. Dig Dis Sci. 1988;33:41–9.

27. Campbell D, Shannon S, Collins SM. The relationship between personality, stress and disease activity in ulcerative colitis. Gastroenterology. 1986;90:A1363.

28. Riley SA, Mani V, Goodman MJ, Lucas S. Why do patients with ulcerative colitis relapse? Gut. 1990;31:179–83.

29. North CS, Alpers DH, Helzer JE, Spitznagel EL, Clouse RE. Do life events or depression exacerbate inflammatory bowel disease? A prospective study. Ann Intern Med. 1991;114:381–6.

30. Duffy LC, Zielezny MA, Marshall JR et al. Relevance of major stress events as an indicator of disease activity prevalence in inflammatory bowel disease. Behav Med. 1991;17:101–10.

31. Levenstein S, Varvo V, Berto E et al. Stress, rectal inflammation, and relapse in ulcerative colitis. Psychosom Med. 1993;55:A118.

32. Robertson DAF, Ray J, Diamond I, Edwards JG. Personality profile and affective state of patients with inflammatory bowel disease. Gut. 1989;30:623–6.

33. Moser G, Maier-Dobersberger Th, Vogelsang G, Lochs H. Inflammatory bowel disease (IBD): Patients' beliefs about the etiology of their disease – a controlled study. Psychosom Med. 1993;55:131.
34. Leventhal H, Zimmerman R, Gutmann M. Compliance. A self-regulation perspective. In: Gentry WD, ed. Handbook of behavioral medicine. New York: Guilford; 1984:369–436.
35. Sonnenberg A. Disability and need for rehabilitation among patients with inflammatory bowel disease. Digestion. 1992;51:168–78.
36. Salem SN, Shubair KS. Non-specific ulcerative colitis in Bedouin Arabs. Lancet. 1967;1:473–4.
37. Sonnenberg A. Occupational distribution of inflammatory bowel disease among German employees. Gut. 1990;31:1037–40.
38. Binder V, Hendriksen C, Kreiner S. Prognosis in Crohn's disease – based on results from a regional patient group from the county of Copenhagen. Gut. 1985;26:146–50.
39. Drossman DA, Patrick DL, Mitchell CM, Zagami EA, Appelbaum MI. Health-related quality of life in inflammatory bowel disease. Functional status and patient worries and concerns. Dig Dis Sci. 1989;34:1379–86.
40. Wyke RJ, Edwards FC, Allan RN. Employment problems and prospects for patients with inflammatory bowel disease. Gut. 1988;29:1229–35.
41. Sörensen VZ, Olsen BG, Binder V. Life prospects and quality of life in patients with Crohn's disease. Gut. 1987;28:382–5.
42. Tragone A, Lanfranchi GA. Quality of life and inflammatory bowel disease (correspondence). Gut. 1989;30:1798–9.
43. Hendriksen C, Binder V. Social prognosis in patients with ulcerative colitis. Br Med J. 1980;1:581–3.
44. Hendriksen C, Kreiner S, Binder V. Long term prognosis in ulcerative colitis – based on results from a regional patient group from the county of Copenhagen. Gut. 1985;26:158–63.
45. Sommer H, Hoenen H. Verlauf und soziale Auswirkungen von Morbus Crohn und 1994 Colitis ulcerosa. Med Klin. 1994;89:14–17.
46. Balzer K, Förster S, Goebell H, Seifert V, Köcker I. Demographische und soziale Charakteristik von Patienten mit Morbus Crohn in einer Großstadtregion. Eine Studie mit Nachbarschfts- und Krankenhauskontrollen. Z Gastroenterol. 1985;23:347–54.
47. Mayberry MK, Probert C, Srivastava E, Rhodes J, Mayberry JF. Perceived discrimination in education and employment by people with Crohn's disease: a case control study of educational achievement and employment. Gut. 1992;33:312–14.
48. Drossman DA, Leserman J, Li Z et al. The rating form of IBD patient concerns: A new measure of health status. Psychosom Med. 1991;53:701–12.
49. Calkins DR, Rubenstein LV, Cleary PD et al. Failure of physicians to recognize functional disability in ambulatory patients. Ann Intern Med. 1991;114:451–4.
50. Moody GA, Probert CSJ, Srivastava EM, Rhodes J, Mayberry JF. Sexual dysfunction amongst women with Crohn's disease: A hidden problem. Digestion. 1992;52:179–83.
51. Martin A, Leone L, Castagliuolo I, Di-Mario F, Naccarato R. What do patients want to know about their inflammatory bowel disease? Ital J Gastroenterol. 1992;24:477–80.
52. Vallis TM, Turnbull GK. Clinical management of inflammatory bowel disease: Beyond disease activity. Part II: Strategies for maximizing psychosocial health. Can J Gastroenterol. 1992;6:87–92.
53. Garret JW, Drossman DA. Health status in inflammatory bowel disease: Biological and behavioral considerations. Gastroenterology. 1990;99:90–6.
54. Walker EA, Gelfand AN, Gelfand MD, Katon WJ. Functional disability and psychological distress in patients with inflammatory bowel disease (IBD): a pilot study. Gastroenterology. 1994;106:A586.

# 3
# Microbial factors in the pathogenesis of IBD

R. B. SARTOR

Microbial agents can influence ulcerative colitis (UC) and Crohn disease (CD) in a number of ways[1–3]. Viral, bacterial and parasitic infections can reactivate and exacerbate these chronic disorders and have been shown to initiate typical inflammatory bowel disease (IBD) in a minority of cases. Moreover, extraluminal proliferation of intestinal bacteria is responsible for the frequent suppurative complications of CD, most notably abscesses and fistulae[2]. This brief review, however, will concentrate on the ability of persistent infections to cause IBD and the role of ubiquitous bacteria present in the lumen of the distal intestine in perpetuating IBD and experimental colitis. There are three primary theories for the aetiology of IBD (Table 1); intestinal microbial agents are prominently involved in each theory.

## PERSISTENT INFECTION

A specific persistent infection causing UC or CD is the most straightforward aetiological mechanism proposed and the one most amenable to therapeutic intervention. A number of pathogens have been advanced, particularly in CD[1,2], but only three are currently under active investigation.

**Table 1**  Current theories of IBD aetiology

Persistent infection
    CD: *Mycobacterium paratuberculosis*, paramyxovirus (measles), *Listeria monocytogenes*
    UC: altered pathogenicity of endogenous luminal bacteria

Defective mucosal barrier leading to enhanced uptake of luminal antigens and proinflammatory bacterial products

Abnormal host response to ubiquitous agents
    CD: luminal constituents
    UC: luminal constituents or epithelial antigens

## *Mycobacterium paratuberculosis*

CD closely resembles ileocaecal tuberculosis and Johne disease, which is a granulomatous enterocolitis of cattle and other ruminants that is caused by *M. paratuberculosis*[4]. Apparently identical *M. paratuberculosis* have been cultured from approximately 10 resected tissues from CD patients by at least 5 separate investigators, but no similar organisms have been recovered from UC or other control tissues[1,5]. *M. paratuberculosis* is an extremely slow-growing organism that is difficult to culture, even under optimal conditions. Therefore, more recent studies have concentrated on detection of *M. paratuberculosis* DNA in unidentified cultures and biopsies from IBD patients using sensitive molecular techniques, such as the polymerase chain reaction (PCR). A multi-copy genomic DNA insertion element (IS-900) specific for *M. paratuberculosis* has been found in approximately 25% of previously unidentified spheroplasts isolated from CD tissues compared with 0–17% of UC specimens[1,6]. Sanderson et al.[7] found IS-900 DNA in 65% of CD specimens, 4% of UC, and 15% of control tissues. However, other groups have reported variable results, with detection rates ranging from 0% to 72% in CD specimens and up to 29% in controls[1,2].

Of considerable public health concern, potential mechanisms of transmission of *M. paratuberculosis* have been reported. Viable *M. paratuberculosis* can be recovered from the milk of asymptomatic infected cows and routine pasteurization procedures may not kill this organism[8]. IS-900, but not viable organisms, has been detected in up 0% to 7% of commercially distributed milk samples in London[9]. Furthermore, high rates of CD in rivers draining areas inhabited by herds harbouring *M. paratuberculosis* suggest a water-borne transmission (J. Herman-Taylor, unpublished data).

While the *M. paratuberculosis* theory is plausible based on the above-mentioned data, this organism probably does not cause the majority of CD cases. There is no convincing epidemiological, immunological, histochemical or clinical support for this theory[1–3]. The incidence of CD is not increased in farm workers, their families, veterinarians associated with *M. paratuberculosis*-infected animals or people who drink unpasteurized milk. Acid-fast and immunohistochemical searches for this organism have been negative, although in-situ PCR has identified *M. paratuberculosis* DNA in intestinal tissue from one patient[10]. Most immunological studies have demonstrated non-specific humoral or cell-mediated immune responses to several mycobacterial species and normal bacteria, indicating frequent environmental exposure to these organisms[11,12]. Swift et al.[13] reported no benefit from prolonged treatment with ethambutol, rifampicin and INH, which is in agreement with several other studies (summarized in References 1 and 2) but in contrast to Prantera et al.[14]. Based on available data, it is impossible to determine whether *M. paratuberculosis* is an environmental contaminant that secondarily invades the ulcerated mucosa of CD patients to a greater extent than UC and inflammatory controls, or whether this organism causes CD in a small number of patients.

## Measles

Wakefield and colleagues have hypothesized that persistent measles infection of vascular endothelial cells causes a focal granulomatous vasculitis which leads to local ischaemia and ulceration in CD[15]. These authors identified paramyxovirus-like particles and measles RNA and protein within endothelial cells and granulomas in CD patients but not in inflammatory or normal controls. Moreover, an increased incidence of CD has been found in cohorts born following measles epidemics and in offspring of mothers infected with measles during pregnancy[16]. However, this provocative theory must be viewed as speculative because of the lack of independent confirmation. Knibbs et al.[17] were unable to demonstrate measles antigen in CD tissues by immunohistochemical staining, and Smith and colleagues[18] were unable to demonstrate a serological response to measles in children with CD.

## Altered pathogenicity of ubiquitous flora

Subtle alterations ('dysbiosis') in the composition or pathogenicity of the complex 'normal' bacterial components of the distal bowel lumen could lead to chronic inflammation by providing persistent antigenic stimuli or damaging epithelial barrier function[1–3]. Faecal concentrations of *Eubacteria, Peptostreptococci, Coprococcus* and *Bacteroides vulgatus* are specifically increased in CD, as are serum antibodies to these organisms[19,20]. Profiles of these anaerobic bacteria may be genetically determined and abnormalities may precede clinical symptoms of disease[21]. Although anaerobic bacterial concentrations appear to be normal in UC patients, a number of investigators have demonstrated functional abnormalities of aerobic bacteria in this disorder. Abnormal pathogenicity of *E. coli* from UC patients includes increased epithelial cell adherence and production of cytotoxins[22] (and reviewed in References 1–3). Furthermore, group D streptococci (enterococci) and *B. vulgatus* secrete mucin-degrading enzymes and hyaluronidase[1–3].

Luminal hydrogen sulphide, which is produced by anaerobic bacteria, is increased in UC patients, and sulphate-reducing bacteria (especially *Desulfovibrio* spp.) are found in 96% of patients with UC, in contrast to 50% of controls[23,24]. In addition to direct toxic effects on colonic epithelial cells and mucus[23,24], hydrogen sulphide selectively blocks epithelial butyrate metabolism with the greatest effects in the distal colon[25]. This could lead to epithelial cell starvation and impaired mucosal barrier function of the distal colon, as postulated by Roediger et al.[25].

## ENHANCED MUCOSAL PERMEABILITY

Mucosal permeability is increased in active CD as a consequence of local inflammation. However, some studies now suggest that mucosal permeability in CD may be an intrinsic defect, perhaps genetically determined[1–3,26]. Approximately 10% of family members of CD patients have demonstrable permeability defects[26] and a subset of IBD family members have enhanced responses to non-steroidal anti-inflammatory drugs[27]. Moreover, increased mucosal permeability in macroscopically normal jejunal segments of patients with active distal CD suggests an intrinsic global defect in barrier function[28]. The mechanisms of these permeability defects are unknown, but could be a result of specific alterations in mucin glycoprotein profiles, defective metabolism of short chain fatty acids due to hydrogen sulphide[25], or degradation of mucus by hydrogen sulphide or mucolytic bacterial enzymes[1-3]. The consequence of enhanced mucosal permeability is increased uptake of luminal bacterial components (Figure 1), which could continuously and overwhelmingly stimulate the mucosal immune system, leading to chronic inflammation of the distal ileum and colon.

## ABNORMAL HOST RESPONSE TO UBIQUITOUS CONSTITUENTS

The lumen of the distal ileum and colon contain high concentrations of predominantly anaerobic bacteria and bacterial products capable of inducing and perpetuating intestinal inflammation[1-3]. The distal ileum contains approximately $10^8$ viable bacteria per gram of luminal contents, whereas the colon contains $10^{11}-10^{12}$ anaerobic bacteria/g. In addition, normal luminal bacteria produce cell wall polymers, such as lipopolysaccharide (LPS, endotoxin) and peptidoglycan–polysaccharide (PG–PS), and chemotactic formylated oligopeptides, such as F-met-leu-phe (FMLP). These bacterial products are capable of inducing cytokine, arachidonic acid metabolites, oxygen radicals, and nitric oxide production by macrophages and neutrophils and of activating the complement and kallikrein–kinin cascades. Enhanced uptake of these phlogistic bacterial products across the 'leaky' mucosal barrier of the inflamed (and possibly noninflamed gut) and secondary invasion of mucosal ulcers and fistulae potentiate local inflammation and provide a continual stimulus of the intestinal inflammatory response. Systemic uptake of bacterial products via the lymphatics and portal vein could provide the stimulus for extraintestinal inflammation[29].

## CLINICAL EVIDENCE OF BACTERIAL INFLUENCES

There is abundant clinical evidence that normal luminal bacteria are involved in the pathogenesis of IBD, especially CD (Table 2). CD usually occurs in the distal ileum, right colon and perianal regions, which correspond with the highest luminal concentrations of bacteria in the small bowel and colon and represent areas of relative stasis where bacteria and their products maintain their most prolonged contact with the intestinal mucosa. The ileum is non-inflamed in UC except when anaerobic proliferation occurs within an ileal pouch following colectomy ('pouchitis').

The activity of CD reproducibly diminishes when jejunal bacterial concentrations are decreased by antibiotic treatment or by 'bowel rest' provided by total

**Table 2**　Clinical evidence that normal luminal bacteria are involved in the pathogenesis of IBD

Inflammation coincides with areas of highest luminal bacterial concentration
CD improves when luminal bacteria are decreased
Increased immune response to ubiquitous bacteria
Endogenous bacteria invade mucosal ulcers and translocate

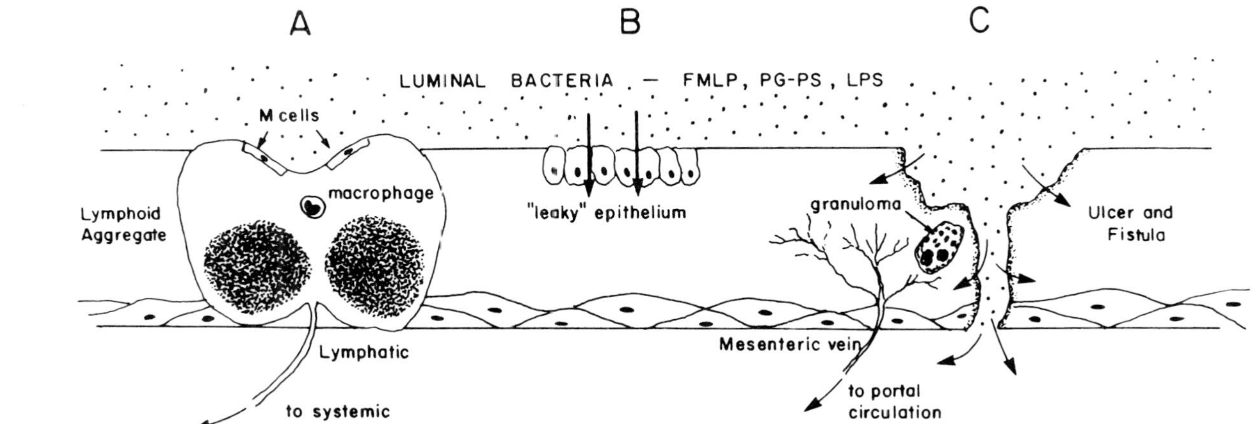


**Figure 1** Mechanisms of mucosal uptake of normal bacterial flora and bacterial products in intestinal inflammation. Luminal bacteria and bacterial products, such as chemotactic f-Met oligopeptides (FMLP), peptidoglycan–polysaccharide polymers (PG–PS) and lipopolysaccharide (LPS, endotoxin), are present in the distal ileum and colon. A: Specialized epithelial cells (M cells) over Peyer's patches and organized lymphoid follicles preferentially transport luminal macromolecules in the normal state, initiating a normal controlled mucosal immune response. **B**: Normally, the intact epithelium provides a relatively impenetrable barrier, but with non-ulcerative inflammation, NSAID exposure or perhaps subclinical CD, the epithelium is 'leaky', permitting enhanced uptake of luminal bacterial products. **C**: With intestinal ulceration, there is secondary invasion of viable bacteria and unrestricted uptake of bacterial products and antigens, further intensifying inflammation. Systemic uptake of bacterial products through the lymphatic and portal circulations leads to extraintestinal inflammation. Reprinted from: Sartor RB, Powell DW. Mechanisms of diarrhea in intestinal inflammation and hypersensitivity: Immune system modulation of intestinal transport. In: Field M., ed. *Controversies in gastroenterology, diarrheal diseases*. Norwalk, CT: Appleton and Lange. 1991:75–114, with permission of Appleton and Lange Publishing Co.

parenteral nutrition, elemental diet or surgical bypass. The influence of exposure to luminal contents on the activity of CD is graphically illustrated by the absence of inflammation following ileal division proximal to an ileocolonic anastomosis, with rapid recurrence of disease when bowel continuity is re-established[30]. Anaerobic bacteria are incriminated in postoperative recurrence of CD by attenuation of symptomatic relapses with metronidazole[31]. Metronidazole is equal to sulphasalazine[32] and superior to placebo[33] in the primary therapy of CD in well-controlled multicentre trials, further demonstrating a pathogenic role for luminal anaerobes in this order. Long-term metronidazole chronically suppresses *Bacteroides* spp. and luminal concentrations of these organisms correlate with therapeutic efficacy of metronidazole[34]. Other bacteria are also involved in the inflammatory response since local broad-spectrum antibiotics have been shown to be effective in uncontrolled trials[35]. Although most clinicians do not use antibiotics as primary therapy for UC a recent preliminary study demonstrates a benefit by chronic administration of antibiotics effective against aerobic Gram-negative organisms. Adjunctive treatment with ciprofloxacin in addition to standard anti-inflammatory drugs was significantly better than placebo in a 6-month trial[36].

Luminal bacteria cross the epithelial barrier in active CD and UC as indicated by enhanced immune responses to and uptake of ubiquitous bacteria and their products. In CD, secretory and serum antibodies are increased to many bacterial strains, especially ubiquitous anaerobic flora[1,20]. Pirzer and colleagues[11] demonstrated enhanced T-cell immune responses to a variety of normal flora as well as *Mycobacterium* spp. Increased humoral and cellular immune responses to heat shock proteins are evident in IBD[37,38], but microbial versus human origin of these antigens is not certain. Immunohistochemical evidence of *E. coli* and group D streptococcal antigen adjacent to mucosal ulcers and fistulae in CD[39], translocation of viable bacteria to the serosal surface, mesenteric lymph nodes, portal circulation, and frequent septic complications in patients with CD to a greater extent than UC patients clearly document secondary invasion of the mucosa during active inflammation[1,2].

## EVIDENCE OF BACTERIAL INVOLVEMENT IN EXPERIMENTAL INTESTINAL INFLAMMATION

Recent data in induced and spontaneous models convincingly document the ability of bacteria and bacterial products to induce and perpetuate chronic intestinal and systemic inflammation (Table 3). LPS and FMLP induce acute enterocolitis, whereas PG–PS from certain bacterial strains causes chronic spontaneously relapsing enterocolitis with systemic inflammation in genetically susceptible hosts[1,40]. In the PG–PS model, factors determining chronicity of inflammation include the source of the bacterial cell wall polymers, their fragment size, and the host genetic susceptibility. PG–PS from group A streptococci, certain *Eubacteria* strains, Mycobacteria, and group D streptococci (enterococci) and high-molecular-weight PG–PS fragments will induce chronic granulomatous infection due to their persistence within phagocytic cells[41]. In contrast, low-molecular-weight PG–PS polymers or PG–PS derived

**Table 3** Evidence of ubiquitous microbial flora in the pathogenesis of experimental intestinal and systemic inflammation

Induction and perpetuation of inflammation by purified bacterial products
Small bowel bacterial overgrowth induces and reactivates extraintestinal lesions
Antibiotics prevent and treat intestinal and systemic inflammation
Germ-free (sterile) environment attenuates acute injury and prevents chronic inflammation

from *Peptostreptococcus* spp. are rapidly biodegradable and will incite only transient acute inflammation. In addition to their ability to induce inflammation after intramural injection, luminal PG–PS can potentiate non-specific colitis and enteritis initiated by acetic acid and indomethacin, respectively, supporting the concept that sterile bacterial *products* mediate many of the inflammatory effects of intestinal bacteria[1,42].

The hypothesis that normal luminal bacteria can induce and perpetuate intestinal and systemic inflammation is further supported by the observation that altering luminal bacterial concentrations affects experimental enterocolitis and extraintestinal inflammation[1]. Broad-spectrum antibiotics or metronidazole attenuate acute enterocolitis in a number of models (indomethacin, carrageenan, dextran sodium sulphate, trinitrobenzene–sulphonic acid, HLA B27 transgenic and amoebiasis), whereas metronidazole almost totally prevents chronic small intestinal ulceration after subcutaneous injection[43]. Consistent with this theory, small bowel bacterial overgrowth of predominantly anaerobic bacteria induces local jejunal inflammation, hepatobiliary injury resembling sclerosing cholangitis, and reactivates arthritis[44,45]. Of interest, hepatobiliary inflammation following experimental jejunal bacterial overgrowth appears to be mediated by PG–PS polymers derived from luminal bacteria[46].

The influence of normal luminal flora in the pathogenesis of intestinal inflammation is convincingly documented by the failure of rodents raised in a germ-free (sterile) environment to develop chronic intestinal inflammation[1–3]. Lewis rats raised under conventional specific pathogen-free conditions develop chronic mid-small bowel ulceration with periportal hepatic inflammation, anaemia, and leukocytosis following subcutaneous indomethacin injection. In contrast, littermates raised in a sterile environment have attenuated acute inflammation and no evidence of chronic enterocolitis or systemic inflammation despite receiving identical indomethacin doses[47]. Similar results have been

**Table 4** Influence of normal luminal bacteria on spontaneous colitis in genetically engineered rodents

|  | Bacterial environment | | |
|  | Conventional | SPF[a] | Sterile |
|---|---|---|---|
| HLA-B$_{27}$/$\beta_{27}\mu$ transgenic rat | ++[b] | + | − |
| IL-2 knockout mouse | ++ | + | − |
| IL-10 knockout mouse | ++ | + | ? |

[a]SPF = specific pathogen-free
[b]Degree of colonic inflammation: ++ = aggresive, + = mild, ■ = none, ? = unknown

observed in genetically manipulated models of spontaneous colitis (Table 4). Human HLA-$B_{27}/\beta_2$ microglobulin transgenic rats raised under conventional conditions develop chronic colitis, gastritis, arthritis, dermatitis and epididymitis. However, germ-free transgenic rats have no evidence of colitis or arthritis, although they exhibit degrees of skin and testicular inflammation similar to those of conventional rats[48,49]. Mice deficient in interleukin-2 (IL-2 knockout mice) have active colitis with bloody diarrhoea in the conventional state, attenuated colitis (histological only) under specific pathogen-free conditions, and no colonic inflammation in the germ-free state[50]. The universal nature of these observations is further substantiated by the fact that IL-10 knockout mice have attenuated small intestinal inflammation in specific pathogen-free conditions compared with the normal environment[51].

The mechanisms by which normal luminal bacteria stimulate chronic intestinal inflammation are unknown. Attenuation of spontaneous colitis in HLA-$B_{27}$ transgenic rats with metronidazole[52] suggests a role for anaerobic bacteria. The determination of whether certain subsets of normal luminal flora have a predominant role in the inflammatory response will depend on reconstitution experiments in gnotobiotic rodents. The identification of the relative role of bacterial products (FMLP, LPS, PG–PS, etc.) in the inflammatory response can be accomplished by feeding sterile bacterial constituents to germ-free rodents and selective blockade of membrane receptors for these molecules. Induction of autoimmune responses to epithelial or other host antigens by 'molecular mimicry' or by adjuvant properties of luminal bacteria will need to be investigated.


## SUMMARY AND CONCLUSIONS

These clinical and experimental observations convincingly implicate ubiquitous luminal bacteria in the pathogenesis of chronic intestinal inflammation and its complications, including extraintestinal manifestations. In CD and experimental enterocolitis, endogenous anaerobic bacteria appear to be particularly involved, whereas functionally abnormal aerobic bacteria are more likely to mediate UC. Transient enteric pathogens may be important in initiating the inflammatory response and, in small subsets of CD patients, persistent mycobacterial, listerial or measles infections may perpetuate disease, although current data do not strongly support this aetiology in the majority of patients.

In view of the high concentrations of bacteria and bacterial products in the distal intestine which are capable of initiating and perpetuating an aggressive chronic inflammation, the critical question is why *everyone* doesn't develop IBD. In the normal host, these potentially phlogistic luminal constituents are efficiently excluded from uptake by a relatively impermeable mucosa, a mucus layer which traps macromolecules and secreted antibodies which complex luminal antigens (Figure 2). If these defences are breached, the mucosal immune response promptly downregulates inflammation via immunosuppressive T lymphocytes, cytokines, prostaglandins and neuropeptides. In the normal host, there is a net immunosuppression so that the lamina propria is in a state of 'controlled inflammation'. However, this delicate balance can be perturbed by genetic and environmental

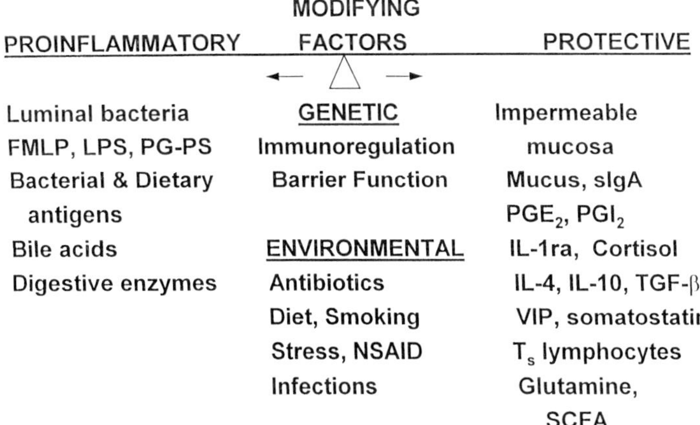


**Figure 2**  The balance between luminal proinflammatory factors and mucosal protective mechanisms. The genetically determined immune response to bacterial products and epithelial barrier function can influence host susceptibility to chronic inflammation while environmental factors can influence initial onset and spontaneous reactivation of inflammation. FMLP, *n*-formyl-methionyl-leucyl-phenylalanine; IL, interleukin; TGF-$\beta$, transforming growth factor-$\beta$; NSAID, non-steroidal anti-inflammatory drug; $T_S$, T suppressor lymphocytes; SCFA, short-chain fatty acids. Adapted from Sartor R. B. *Can J Gastroenterol*. 1990;4:271–7, and used with permission of Pulsus Group, Inc.

factors which shift the equation toward chronic inflammation. Recent data from animal models suggest that genetically determined immunoregulatory abnormalities, especially defective downregulation of inflammation, may be responsible for host susceptibility to chronic intestinal inflammation[3,40]. Environmental triggers, particularly intercurrent infections, stress and non-steroidal anti-inflammatory drugs, could profoundly influence inflammation by breaking the mucosal barrier and diminishing immunosuppressive mediators.

A better understanding of which bacteria and bacterial products have the greatest proinflammatory effects, how mucosal permeability can be diminished and how infectious triggers can be prevented will suggest novel and less-toxic therapeutic approaches to IBD. Although long-term elimination of all luminal bacteria is an unrealistic goal, the detrimental effects of selected bacterial species could be chronically suppressed by: specific antibiotics; blockade of bacterial adhesion to epithelial cells; immunization; encouraging the growth of organisms which compete for the same ecological niche; complexing, inactivating, or degrading secreted proinflammatory bacterial products; or inhibiting antigen-specific immune responses. Achieving these goals depends on identifying subsets of bacteria which preferentially induce and perpetuate chronic intestinal inflammation in genetically susceptible hosts.

## Acknowledgements

The author gratefully acknowledges the expert secretarial and editorial assistance of Brian Springer. Original research described in this review was supported by NIH grants DK 40249, DK 47700 and DK 34987, and the Crohn's and Colitis Foundation of America.

# References


1. Sartor RB. Microbial factors in the pathogenesis of Crohn's disease, ulcerative colitis and experimental intestinal inflammation. In: Kirsner JB, Shorter RJ, eds. Inflammatory bowel disease, 4th edn. Baltimore: Williams & Wilkins; 1995:96–124.
2. Sartor RB. Microbial agents in the pathogenesis, differential diagnosis and complications of inflammatory bowel disease. In: Blaser J, Smith PD, Ravdin JI et al., eds. Infections of the gastrointestinal tract. New York: Raven Press; 1995:435–58.
3. Sartor RB. Current concepts of the etiology and pathogenesis of Crohn's disease and ulcerative colitis. Gastroint Clin N Am. 1995;24:475–507.
4. Chiodini RJ. Crohn's disease and the mycobacterioses: A review and comparison of two disease entities. Clin Microbiol Rev. 1989;2:90–117.
5. Chiodini RJ, Van Kruiningen HJ, Thayer WR et al. Possible role of mycobacteria in inflammatory bowel disease. I. An unclassified mycobacterium species isolated from patients with Crohn's disease. Dig Dis Sci. 1984;29:1073–9.
6. Wall S, Kunze ZM, Saboor S et al. Identification of spheroplast-like agents isolated from tissues of patients with Crohn's disease and control tissues by polymerase chain reaction. J Clin Microbiol. 1993;31:1241–5.
7. Sanderson JD, Moss MT, Tizard ML et al. *Mycobacterium paratuberculosis* DNA in Crohn's disease tissue. Gut. 1992;33:890–6.
8. Chiodini RJ, Hermon-Taylor J. The thermal resistance of *Mycobacterium paratuberculosis* with Crohn's disease tissue sections.Gastroenterology. 1994;106:A680.
9. Millar DS, Ford J, Sanderson JD et al. IS900 PCR testing for *Mycobacterium paratuberculosis* in units of whole pasteurized cows milk widely obtained from retail outlets in England and Wales. In: Chiodini R, ed. Proceedings of the 4th International Colloquium on Paratuberculosis. International Association on Paratuberculosis. 1995:320.
10. Fidler HM, Woolford A, Ray R et al. Development of *in situ* polymerase chain reaction (PCR) to detect and localize *Mycobacterium paratuberculosis* within Crohn's disease tissue sections. Gastroenterology. 1994;106:A680.
11. Pirzer U, Schonhaar A, Fleischer B et al. Reactivity of infiltrating T lymphocytes with microbial antigens in Crohn's disease. Lancet. 1991;338:1238–9.
12. Stainsby KJ, Lowes JR, Allan RN et al. Antibodies to *Mycobacterium paratuberculosis* and nine species of environmental mycobacteria in Crohn's disease and control subjects. Gut. 1993;34:371–4.
13. Swift Gl, Srivastava ED, Stone R et al. Controlled trial of anti-tuberculosis chemotherapy for two years in Crohn's disease. Gut. 1994;35:363–8.
14. Prantera C, Kohn A, Mangiarotti R et al. Antimycobacterial therapy in Crohn's disease: Results of a controlled double-blind trial with a multiple antibiotic regimen. Am J Gastroenterol. 1994;89:513–18.
15. Wakefield AJ, Pittilo RM, Sim R et al. Evidence of persistent measles virus infection in Crohn's disease. J Med Virol. 1993;39:345–53.
16. Ekbom A, Wakefield AJ, Zack M et al. Perinatal measles infection and subsequent Crohn's disease. Lancet. 1994;344:508–10.
17. Knibbs DR, Van Kruiningen HJ, Colombe JF et al. Ultrastructural evidence of paramyxovirus in two French families with Crohn's disease. Gastroenterology. 1993;104:A725.
18. Smith MS, Khan K, Bradley NJ et al. IgG antibodies to measles virus in children with inflammatory bowel disease. Gastroenterology. 1994;106:A775.
19. Ruseler-van Embden JG, Both-Patoir HC. Anaerobic gram-negative faecal flora in patients with Crohn's diseases and healthy subjects. Antonie van Leeuwenhoek. 1983;49:125–32.
20. Auer IO, Roder A, Wensinck F et al. Selected bacterial antibodies in Crohn's disease and ulcerative colitis. Scand J Gastroenterol. 1983;189:217–23.
21. Van de Merwe JP, Schroder AM, Wensinck F et al. The obligate anaerobic faecal flora of patients with Crohn's disease and their first-degree relatives. Scand J Gastroenterol. 1988;23:1125–31.
22. Giaffer MH, Holdsworth CD, Duerden BI. Virulence properties of *Escherichia coli* strains isolated from patients with inflammatory bowel disease. Gut. 1992;33:646–50.
23. Pitcher MC, Gibson Gr, Neale G et al. Gentamicin kills multiple drug-resistant sulfate-reducing bacteria in patients with ulcerative colitis. Gastroenterology. 1994;106:A753.

24. Gibson GR, Cummings HJ, Macfarlane GT. Growth and activities of sulfate-reducing bacteria in gut contents of healthy subjects and patients with ulcerative colitis. FEMS Microbiol Ecol. 1991;86:103–11.
25. Roediger WE, Duncanb A, Kapaniris OK et al. Reducing sulfur compounds of the colon impair colonocyte nutrition: Implications for ulcerative colitis. Gastroenterology. 1993;104:802–9.
26. May GR, Sutherland LR, Meddings JB. Is small intestinal permeability really increased in relatives of patients with Crohn's disease? Gastroenterology. 1993;104:1627–32.
27. Pironi L, Miglioli M, Ruggeri E et al. Effect of non-steroidal anti-inflammatory drugs (NSAID) on intestinal permeability in first degree relatives of patients with Crohn's disease. Gastroenterology. 1992;103:A679.
28. Peeters M, Ghoos Y, Maes B et al. Increased permeability of macroscopically normal small bowel in Crohn's disease. Dig Dis Sci. 1994;39:2170–6.
29. Sartor RB, Lichtman SN. Mechanisms of systemic inflammation associated with intestinal injury. In: Targan S, Shanahan F eds. Inflammatory bowel disease: From bench to bedside. Baltimore: Williams & Wilkins; 1993:210–29.
30. Rutgeerts P, Goboes K, Peeters M et al. Effect of faecal stream diversion on recurrence of Crohn's disease in the neoterminal ileum. Lancet. 1991;338:771–4.
31. Rutgeerts P, Hiele M, Peeters M et al. Prevention of clinical recurrence after ileal resection for Crohn's disease with metronidazole: A placebo controlled study. Gastroenterology. 1994;106:A764.
32. Ursing B, Alm T, Barany F et al. A comparative study of metronidazole and sulfasalazine for active Crohn's disease: The cooperative Crohn's disease study in Sweden. Gastroenterology. 1982;83:550–62.
33. Sutherland L, Singleton J, Sessions J et al. Double-blind, placebo controlled trial of metronidazole in Crohn's disease. Gut. 1991;32:1071–5.
34. Krook A, Lindstrom B, Kjellander J et al. Relation between concentrations of metronidazole and *Bacteroides* sp. in faeces of patients with Crohn's disease and healthy individuals. J Clin Pathol. 1981;34:645–50.
35. Sartor RB. Antimicrobial agents in IBD: Implications for pathogenesis and management. Can J Gastroenterol. 1993;7:132–8.
36. Turunen U, Färkkilä M, Hakala K et al. A double-blind, placebo controlled six-month ciprofloxacin treatment improves prognosis in ulcerative colitis. Gastroenterology. 1994;106:A786.
37. Stevens TR, Winrow VR, Blake DR et al. Circulating antibodies to heat-shock protein 60 in Crohn's disease and ulcerative colitis. Clin Exp Immunol. 1992;90:271–4.
38. Szewczuk MR, Depew WT. Evidence for T lymphocyte reactivity to the 65 kilodalton heat shock protein of mycobacterium in active Crohn's disease. Clin Invest Med. 1992;15:494–505.
39. Cartun RW, Van Kruiningen HJ, Pedersen CA et al. An immunocytochemical search for infectious agents in Crohn's disease. Mod Pathol. 1993;6:212.
40. McCall RD, Haskill S, Zimmermann EM et al. Tissue interleukin-1 and interleukin-1 receptor antagonist expression in enterocolitis in resistant and susceptible rats. Gastroenterology. 1994;106:960–72.
41. Schwab JH. Phlogistic properties of peptidoglycan–polysaccharide polymers from cell walls of pathogenic and normal-flora bacteria which colonize humans. Infect Immun. 1993;61:4535–9.
42. Sartor RB, Bond TM, Schwab JH. Systemic uptake and intestinal inflammatory effects of luminal bacterial cell wall polymers in rats with acute colonic injury. Infect Immun. 1988;56:2101–8.
43. Yamada T, Deithch E, Specian RD et al. Mechanisms of acute and chronic intestinal inflammation induced by indomethacin. Inflammation. 1993;17:641–21.
44. Lichtman SN, Sartor RB, Keku J et al. Hepatic inflammation in rats with experimental small intestinal bacterial overgrowth. Gastroenterology. 1990;98:414–23.
45. Lichtman SN, Wang J, Sartor RB, Zhang C, Bender DE, Dalldorf FG, Schwab JH. Reactivation of arthritis induced by small bowel bacterial overgrowth in rats: Role of cytokines, luminal bacteria and bacterial polymers. Infect Immun. 1995;63:2295–301.
46. Lichtman SN, Okoruwa EE, Keku J et al. Degradation of endogenous bacterial cell wall polymers by the muralytic enzyme mutanolysin prevents hepatobiliary injury in genetically susceptible rats with experimental intestinal bacterial overgrowth. J Clin Invest. 1992;90:1313–22.
47. Sartor RB, Bender DE, Grenther T et al. Absolute requirement for ubiquitous luminal bacteria in the pathogenesis of chronic intestinal inflammation. Gastroenterology. 1994;106:A761.

48. Taurog JD, Hammer RE, Balish E et al. The germfree state prevents development of gut and joint inflammatory disease in HLA-B$_{27}$ transgenic rats. J Clin Microbiol. 1992;30:166–71.
49. Rath H, Grenther T, Bender DE et al. Influence of ubiquitous luminal bacteria in the pathogenesis of intestinal and systemic inflammation in HLA-B$_{27}$/$\beta_2$ microglobulin transgenic rats (abstract). Gastroenterology. 1995;108:A899.
50. Sadlack B, Merz H, Schorle H et al. Ulcerative colitis-like disease in mice with a disrupted interleukin-2 gene. Cell 1993;75:253–61.
51. Kuhn R, Lohler J, Rennick D et al. Interleukin-10-deficient mice develop chronic enterocolitis. Cell. 1993;75:263–74.
52. Rath HC, Bender DE, Holt LC et al. Metronidazole attenuates colitis in HLA-B$_{27}$/$\beta_2\mu$ trangenic (TG) rats: A pathogenic role for anaerobic bacteria. Clin Immunol Immunopathol. 1995;76:S45.

# 4
# Crohn disease: a virus-triggered vasculitis?

A. J. WAKEFIELD

## INTRODUCTION

This chapter describes research performed since 1989 at the Royal Free Hospital School of Medicine by the Inflammatory Bowel Disease Study Group. We tested the hypothesis that Crohn disease may be due to an abnormality of the mesenteric blood supply. This chapter describes a series of experiments which provide coherent evidence that the underlying pathogenetic abnormality in Crohn disease is a mesenteric granulomatous vasculitis in response to a persistent measles virus infection in the vascular endothelium.

## MULTIFOCAL GASTROINTESTINAL INFARCTION[1]

Crohn disease is characteristically a patchy inflammatory condition of the gastrointestinal tract. Many patients with Crohn disease require surgical resection of diseased bowel, with anastomosis between apparently healthy segments of intestine. Thus, the experimental pathologist is provided with an almost unique sample of tissue – that is, involving both diseased and apparently normal tissue, with a clearly defined mesenteric blood supply.

We studied resected tissue from patients with Crohn disease, where the vascular pedicle was divided at the final moment of excision of the bowel. Taken away from the patient, the mesenteric artery supplying the resected bowel was cannulated, and the bowel immediately perfused with heparinized saline. In the initial experiments (Table 1), the bowel was then perfused with a resin which

**Table 1** Identification of vasculitis – 1

- Vascular preservation
- Arterial cannulation
- Heparin–saline flush
- Perfusion fixation

formed a high-resolution cast of the mesenteric blood supply. After the resin had set, the bowel tissue was dissolved away using hydrochloric acid.

The corrosion casts of small and large intestine affected by Crohn disease revealed substantial damage to the mesenteric blood supply. Blood vessels in the submucosa were apparently blocked, with new capillary formation attempting to bypass areas of ischaemia. These changes were most severe in areas of macroscopic disease but there were also substantial abnormalities in bowel close to the resection margin which, to the naked eye, appeared normal.

Based on these experiments, it was suggested that Crohn disease was associated with substantial damage to the mesenteric blood supply, and that much of the tissue damage could be caused by blockage or obliteration of that blood supply. This would produce 'multifocal gastrointestinal infarction' – that is, multiple very small areas of ischaemic necrosis which, in turn, would result in inflammation, ulceration, fibrosis and fistula formation. The histopathological view of infarction – necrosis of tissue due to interruption of its blood supply (for example, in the myocardia or brain) – requires evidence of persisting necrotic tissue. Necrotic tissue is not evident in Crohn disease because the dead tissue is sloughed off or destroyed by secondary bacterial invasion. The intestine has immense powers of regeneration.

The major problem with corrosion casting of the mesenteric blood supply is that the intestinal tissue has been dissolved away by the hydrochloric acid.


## GRANULOMATOUS VASCULITIS IN CROHN DISEASE[2]

Perfusion fixation preserves resected specimens of small and large intestinal Crohn disease by arterial perfusion with formol saline at mean arterial pressure (100 mmHg). This perfusion fixation resulted in excellent preservation of the intestinal tissues, allowing histopathological examination of the blood vessels and bowel wall of the very highest standard. See Table 2.

**Table 2**  Identification of vasculitis – 2

- Multiple serial/step sections
- Immunostaining for vascular elements and macrophages
- Computerized 3-D reconstruction

Fifteen specimens of bowel wall contained granulomas on routine examination of haematoxylin- and eosin-stained sections. These 15 specimens were examined in detail using a range of immunohistochemical staining techniques to identify vascular structures and granulomas. A total of 485 granulomas were found, 85% of which were identified as being directly involved in vascular injury. Granulomas were usually in the walls of blood vessels, often extending into the lumen. The majority (77%) of granulomas were deep to the mucosa; they were found most frequently in the submucosa (42%). Perfusion fixation enhanced the recognition of granulomatous vasculitis. The results suggested that the majority of granulomas in Crohn disease form within walls of blood vessels – that is, Crohn disease is a granulomatous vasculitis (Table 3).

**Table 3**   Granulomatous vasculitis

| | |
|---|---|
| ● Focal | – Damage to vessel at one point may produce extensive injury |
| ● Destructive | – Effacement of vessel |
| ● Evanescent | – Lasts only as long as initiating stimulus persists? |
| ● Consequences | – Ischaemia<br>Ulceration<br>Fibrosis |

## Early mucosal changes in Crohn disease[3]

Aphthoid ulceration has been regarded as an early macroscopic feature of Crohn disease, yet the cause of this mucosal lesion is unknown. Examination of areas of apparently normal and non-inflamed bowel in Crohn disease allowed the identification of mucosal changes which occur before macroscopic or microscopic ulceration[3]. In Crohn disease, it was found that damage and rupture of small mucosal capillaries occurred before infiltration of the lamina propria by inflammatory cells. Loss of overlying epithelium, that is aphthoid ulceration, appears to follow this vascular damage.

## THROMBOTIC VASCULAR RISK FACTORS[4,5]

In the study of macroscopically normal bowel in Crohn disease, it was noted that loose accumulations of eosinophilic fibrillary material could be found in the superficial lamina propria[6]. This material formed 'fibrinoid' plugs partly occluding the lumen of damaged capillaries, particularly at the point of rupture. Immunohistochemistry identified that this material was Factor XIIIa. Factor XIIIa is the active subunit of plasma Factor XIII, responsible for cross-linking fibrin into a stable clot.

**Table 4**   Thrombosis and Crohn disease

| |
|---|
| ● Clotting is activated in Crohn disease |
| ● Mucosal and submucosal microthrombi are an early feature of the disease |
| ● Inherited abnormalities of coagulation appear to protect against development of Crohn disease |

It was demonstrated in 16 patients with Crohn disease that plasma Factor XIIIa concentrations are significantly lower in active disease (median 63 iu/dl) than in remission (median 90 iu/dl). In five patients with persistent aggressive Crohn disease, the Factor XIIIa concentration remained below the lower limit of normal despite apparent clinical improvement in response to medical treatment. Tissues from three patients who underwent surgical resection during the study were immunostained for Factor XIIIa: gut mucosal and submucosal macrophages stained strongly for Factor XIIIa. In one patient, capillary thrombi near superficial mucosal erosions immunostained for Factor XIIIa in macroscopically normal bowel mucosa. The demonstration of significantly low plasma

Factor XIIIa concentrations in active Crohn disease, and the immunostaining of Factor XIIIa capillary thrombi in the bowel wall, suggest that activation of coagulation may be involved in the pathogenesis of Crohn disease.

Another study investigated the prevalence of independent thrombotic risk factors (Factor VII coagulant activity, lipoprotein (a), fibrinogen, plasma triglycerides and smoking) in patients with Crohn disease and normal controls[5]. In Crohn disease ($n$ = 75), the mean plasma Factor VIIc, lipoprotein (a) and fibrinogen concentrations were significantly greater than in the normal population ($n$ = 85). Ninety-three per cent of patients with Crohn disease, compared with 61% of the normal population, had at least one risk factor for thrombotic vascular disease.

Thus, the clinical picture of Crohn disease may be due to the combination of granulomatous vasculitis and also a hypercoagulable state. To develop the full clinical picture of Crohn disease, it may be necessary to have these two defects. Together, they may cause intravascular thrombosis with resulting multifocal gastrointestinal infarction.

## A FERRET MODEL OF ACUTE MULTIFOCAL GASTROINTESTINAL INFARCTION[7]

The acute histological changes produced by interruption of the submucosal and mucosal microcirculation were investigation in the ferret mid-gut. Two techniques were used. Firstly, up to 30 adjacent vasa recta were ligated using microsurgical techniques; this produced no evidence of ischaemic damage. Secondly, interruption of the submucosal collateral plexus by the intra-arterial injection of styrene microspheres (27, 50 or 90 $\mu$m diameter) produced acute intestinal mucosal damage. A combination of 27 and 90 $\mu$m spheres resulted in focal mucosal inflammation, necrosis and ulceration. 'Summit' lesions with normal adjacent mucosa were observed 48 h after embolization, with evidence of regeneration of the mucosa overlying the occluded vessels at 72 h. Two weeks later, the tissue was both macroscopically and microscopically normal. This model showed that focal gastrointestinal infarction, with normal adjacent mucosa, can be produced by acute occlusion of submucosal and mucosal arteries.

**Table 5**  Effects produced by microembolization of the submucosa

- Patchy inflammation
- Summit ulceration
- Transmural inflammation

The tendency of Crohn disease to return at the site of intestinal anastomosis remains one of the most striking clinical features of Crohn disease. Indeed, recent colonoscopic surveillance of ileocolonic anastomoses suggests that recurrent disease is almost inevitable. The disease first returns as mucosal aphthous ulceration, gradually evolving into the deep ulceration, scarring and fibrosis that are characteristic of a recurrent stricture. Our early work, using the corrosion cast technique, indicated that macroscopically normal bowel in Crohn disease almost inevitably has substantial damage to the microvascular circulation. Similarly, the ferret intestine soon recovers from embolization resulting from the intra-arterial injection of styrene microspheres[7].

In the development of the ferret model, segments of ferret mid-gut were embolized with microspheres and allowed to recover[8]. The bowel was then re-explored surgically, the segment resected with the incision through the middle part of embolization. Normal bowel was anastomosed to bowel that had recovered from microembolization – the result was dramatic ulceration at the site of the anastomosis. Hence, it appears that the double ischaemic insult (microspheres plus surgical incision) results in macroscopic damage to the intestinal mucosa.

## EVIDENCE OF PERSISTENT MEASLES VIRUS INFECTION IN CROHN DISEASE[9]

**Table 6**  Hypothesis for the involvement of measles virus in Crohn disease

| |
| --- |
| • Crohn disease is caused by a cell-mediated immune response to persistent virus infection of the mesenteric microvascular endothelium |
| • This virus may be measles |

Based upon the ability of measles virus to infect the mesenteric vascular endothelium during acute disease, and its ability to persist with late sequelae, measles virus was proposed as the causative agent in this condition.

Transmission electron microscopy was used to examine the microvasculature of perfusion-fixed tissues from Crohn-disease and control patients. Paramyxovirus-like particles, and inclusions consisting of condensations of nucleocapsid, in giant cells and endothelium at the foci of vascular injury were identified in nine Crohn-disease patients. Tissues from patients with Crohn disease were also examined by either in-situ hybridization ($n = 10$) or immuno-histochemistry ($n = 15$), and compared with inflammatory and non-inflammatory controls ($n = 22$). Hybridization for measles virus N protein genomic RNA was positive in all cases of Crohn disease, localizing to foci of granulomatous vasculitis and lymphoid follicles. Positive immunohistochemical staining for measles virus nucleocapsid protein was positive in 13 of 15 patients with Crohn disease, localizing to foci of granulomatous inflammation.

**Table 7**  Methods of identification of measles virus in inflammatory foci in Crohn disease

| |
| --- |
| • Electronmicroscopy |
| • In-situ hybridization |
| • Immunohistochemistry |
| • Immunogold electronmicroscopy |

Persistent measles infection of the intestine has been confirmed recently by the technique of immunogold electronmicroscopy[10]. Gold particles colocalized with intranuclear structures that were consistent morphologically with paramyxovirus nucleocapsids. Positively staining cells were restricted to areas of granulomatous inflammation in Crohn disease and subacute sclerosing panencephalitis, a persistent cerebral measles infection[10].

These observations suggest that measles virus is capable of causing persistent infection of the intestine, and that Crohn disease may be caused by a granulomatous vasculitis in response to this virus.

## Epidemiological evidence of an association between measles virus and Crohn disease

- Perinatal viral infection is a strong risk factor (PR18) for the development of both Crohn disease and ulcerative colitis[11].

- Early exposure to measles virus appears to be a risk factor for the subsequent development of Crohn disease[12].

- Measles vaccination may be a risk factor for the later development of both Crohn disease and ulcerative colitis[13].

## CONCLUSIONS

Research by the Inflammatory Bowel Disease Study Group at the Royal Free Hospital[14] and others suggests that Crohn disease is initiated by a granulomatous vasculitis in response to a persisting measles virus infection within the mesenteric vascular endothelium. This type of inflammatory reaction may be an unusual host response to measles infection (which may well have a genetic basis) or it may be due to infection by an unusual measles virus. The granulomatous vasculitis results in vascular occlusion which in turn causes intestinal damage by multifocal gastrointestinal infarction. The tendency to thrombosis and ischaemia may be increased by either a hypercoagulable state or by surgical intervention – for example, at the site of a surgical anastomosis. This work raises a number of important questions – in particular the potential role of measles vaccination, the use of either antiviral drugs or anticoagulation for the management of patients with Crohn disease, and the need for further basic research.

## References


1. Wakefield AJ, Sawyerr AM, Dhillon AP et al. The pathogenesis of Crohn's disease: multifocal gastrointestinal infarction. Lancet. 1989;2:1057–62.
2. Wakefield AJ, Dhillon AP, Sawyerr AM et al. Granulomatous vasculitis in Crohn's disease. Gastroenterology. 1991;100:1279–87.
3. Sankey EA, Dhillon AP, Anthony A et al. Early mucosal changes in Crohn's disease. Gut. 1993;34:375–81.
4. Hudson M, Wakefield AJ, Hutton RA et al. Factor XIIIA subunit and Crohn's disease. Gut. 1993;34:75–9.
5. Hudson M, Chitolie A, Wakefield AJ, Hutton RA, Smith MSH, Pounder RE. Thrombotic vascular risk factors in inflammatory bowel disease. [In press].
6. Dhillon AP, Anthony A, Sim R et al. Mucosal capillary thrombi in rectal biopsies. Histopathology. 1992;21:127–33.
7. Hudson M, Piasecki C, Sankey EA. A ferret model of acute multifocal gastrointestinal infarction. Gastroenterology. 1992;102:1591–6.
8. Osborne MJ, Hudson M, Piasecki C et al. Crohn's disease: a vascular model of anastomotic recurrence. Br J Surg. 1993;80:226–9.

9. Wakefield AJ, Pittilo RM, Sim R et al. Evidence of persistent measles virus infection in Crohn's disease. J Med Virol. 1993;39:345–53.
10. Lewin J, Dhillon AP, Sim R, Mazure G, Pounder RE, Wakefield AJ. Persistent measles virus infection of the intestine: confirmation by immunogold electron microscopy. Gut. 1995;36:564–9.
11. Ekbom A, Adami HO, Hernick CG, Jonzon A, Zack MM. Perinatal risk factors for inflammatory bowel disease: A case control study. Am J Epidemiol. 1990;132:1111–19.
12. Ekbom A, Wakefield AJ, Zack M, Adami HO. Perinatal measles infection and subsequent Crohn's disease. Lancet. 1994;344:508–10.
13. Thompson NT, Montgomery SM, Pounder RE, Wakefield AJ. Is measles vaccination a risk factor for inflammatory bowel disease? Lancet. 1995;345:1071–4.
14. Miyamoto H, Tanaka T, Kitamoto N, Fukuda Y, Shimoyama T. Detection of immunoreactive antigen, with a monoclonal antibody to measles virus, in tissue from a patient with Crohn's disease. J Gastroenterol. 1995;30:28–33.

# 5
# The role of the cellular immune response in the pathogenesis of IBD

M. ZEITZ and A. STALLMACH

## INTRODUCTION

Despite the appearance of an enormous amount of data on the cause of the chronic destructive mucosal inflammation in inflammatory bowel disease (IBD), the aetiopathogenesis of Crohn disease and ulcerative colitis is still unknown. Most authors agree that immunological abnormalities in the local mucosa-associated immune system play a crucial role[1,2]. Physiologically, the intestinal mucosal immune system is in close contact with a large number of foreign antigens and mitogenic substances in the gut lumen. Adapted to its specific function, i.e. to protect the host against invasion of potential pathogens or an inappropriate immune response to the enormous number of antigens, a highly differentiated gut-associated lymphoid system (GALT) has developed[3-5]. Lymphocytes in the GALT are either localized in organized lymphoid structures such as the Peyer's patches and the lymphoid follicles in the colonic mucosa, or are disseminated diffusely in the intestinal lamina propria (lamina propria lymphocytes – LPL) and above the basement membrane between epithelial cells (intraepithelial lymphocytes – IEL). Antigens from the gut lumen are transported by a specialized epithelium (M cells) into the lymphoid follicles. Here the mucosal immune response is initiated by the uptake and processing of antigenic material by macrophages and follicular dendritic cells and its presentation to T and B cells (afferent limb of the GALT). Primed lymphocytes leave the mucosa, enter the circulation, and migrate back to mucosal surfaces ('homing'). These cells then are found in the lamina propria (LPL) or above the basement membrane (IEL) where they carry out specific effector functions (efferent limb of the GALT)[6,7]. Lymphocytes within the mucosal immune system differ in many respects from lymphocytes in other compartments of the body and there are indications that the tissue-specific differentiation of mucosal T cells is disturbed in IBD.

## PRINCIPLES OF INFLAMMATORY REACTIONS

Inflammation of the intestine, regardless of specific initiating events, shares common pathways of tissue injury and repair. The first step of an inflammatory reaction is usually a specific immune response which is highly regulated. The result of this specific response is the activation of immune, mesenchymal and parenchymal cells, recruitment of circulating effector cells, tissue damage, and/or healing. A complex array of soluble mediators released by activated cells determines the outcome of the immune response. These mediators include cytokines, arachidonic acid metabolites, reactive oxygen intermediates and growth factors. Over the past decade, increasing evidence has accumulated that cytokines play a central role in intestinal inflammation and damage[8]. Cytokines are a group of proteins which act locally at the site of inflammation. They have autocrine, paracrine and endocrine activities, which provide signals for the communication between different cell populations. Chronic inflammation of the intestine is thought to result from the failure of these regulatory mechanisms that normally serve to limit the immune response and to eliminate a pathogen[9]. Despite increasing knowledge of cytokine networks, the precise cellular and humoral immunological mechanisms that mediate intestinal injury remain poorly defined. In this review, general principles of the induction and regulation of immune responses will be discussed in view of their relevance for understanding mucosal inflammation and damage. Evidence will be given that the highly regulated mucosal T-cell immune response is disturbed in IBD.

## INDUCTIVE AND EFFECTOR PHASE OF AN IMMUNE RESPONSE

The initial step of immune response is uptake and presentation of antigens by specialized antigen-presenting cells. T-cell activation is initiated by the presentation of processed antigens in context with the major histocompatibility complex (MHC). The interaction of T cells and antigen-presenting cells requires the appropriate T-cell receptor (TCR) repertoire for recognition of the specific antigen. In addition, intercellular binding of adhesion molecules to their counter-receptor is necessary for appropriate activation. Presentation of antigens in association with MHC class I molecules results in activation of CD8-positive T cells, whereas presentation in association with MHC class II molecules induces CD4 T cell activation. In recent years, it has been shown by several groups that intestinal epithelial cells can serve as antigen-presenting cells. Antigen presentation by intestinal epithelial cells leads, under physiological conditions, to the stimulation of CD8-positive cells with suppressor function[10,11].

Analysis of the cellular immune response to infectious pathogens has indicated that the course of an infectious disease is fundamentally influenced by the selective activation of one of at least two CD4-positive T-cell subsets with distinct patterns of lymphokine production[12]. One subset, referred to as $T_h1$ cells, produces IL-2 and IFN-$\gamma$ upon activation and promotes cell-mediated effector responses. A second subset, type 2 helper T cells ($T_h2$), secretes IL-4, IL-5, IL-6 and IL-10 and supports antibody production by B cells. The initial events that induce the maturation of distinct $T_h$-cell subpopulations are unknown. Several different mechanisms have been proposed which determine differentiation of $T_h0$ cells either into $T_h1$ or $T_h2$ cells. These include locally present cytokines, type of the antigen-presenting cell, antigen characteristics and lymphoid tissue microenvironment.

The cytokine secretion pattern of stimulated T cells determines the effector mechanisms of an immune response. A $T_h1$-like response (delayed-typed hypersensitivity, DTH) is characterized by significant T-cell proliferation, induction of a cytotoxic T-cell response, induction of natural killer cells, macrophage activation and other effects of IFN-$\gamma$ production, e.g. enhanced MHC expression and direct antiviral effects. In contrast, a $T_h2$-like response mediates humoral immunity[12].

## $T_h$ SUBSET IMBALANCE, MUCOSAL IMMUNOLOGY AND DISEASE PATHOGENESIS

There are several indications that in both animal models and human diseases, the cytokine secretion profile of the relevant T cells determines the outcome of an infection, i.e. resistance and resolution or susceptibility and progression. One example is infection with *Leishmania major*. Most mouse strains control *Leishmania major* replication locally with resolution of the infection, while susceptible BALB/c mice infected with this agent develop a non-healing progressive disease[13]. Susceptibility to infection correlates with a predominance of $T_h2$ activation, whereas the ability to successfully resolve infection correlates with $T_h1$ activation and IFN-$\gamma$ secretion[14]. It is thought that, in HIV-infected human individuals, a $T_h1$ to $T_h2$ switch occurs with progression to AIDS[15]. This hypothesis is based on the finding that progression to AIDS is characterized by loss of IL-2 and INF-$\gamma$ production concomitant with increases in IL-4 and IL-10 synthesis. In addition, HIV infection results in B-cell activation and hyper-gamma-globulinaemia, including increase in IgE, which may be caused by $T_h2$ cytokines. Furthermore, in many seronegative HIV-exposed individuals, HIV envelope-specific synthetic peptides induce strong IL-2 synthesis in peripheral blood lymphocytes. This observation of HIV-specific $T_h1$ reactivity in the absence of HIV antibodies raises the possibility that cell-mediated immunity may protect against HIV infection[15].

The cytokine secretion profile of intestinal T cells is incompletely investigated. There is convincing evidence that both $T_h1$ and $T_h2$ cytokines are produced in the intestine and that both populations are necessary for the maintenance of the immunological barrier of the mucosa[8]. In recent years, studies in cytokine or T-cell receptor mutant mice ('gene knockout mice') have provided important unexpected results regarding the mechanisms of mucosal immunoregulation and inflammation: animals with non-functioning IL-2, IL-10 or T-cell receptor genes develop chronic intestinal inflammation resembling IBD in several respects[16–19]. Although IL-2 and IL-10 are completely different cytokines, a lack of one of these regulatory factors results in mucosal damage. These findings clearly indicate that any imbalance of the cytokine network in the highly regulated mucosal immune system may lead to disruption of the immune barrier and to uncontrolled inflammation[20]. Our understanding of the immunopathogenesis of IBD has gained in many respects by these animal models.

# CELLULAR IMMUNE RESPONSE IN IBD

## Mucosal T-cell activation in IBD

Phenotypic studies on lamina propria T-cell subpopulations in IBD using both immunohistology of frozen sections of intestinal tissue in IBD or cytofluorometric analysis of isolated intestinal lamina propria mononuclear cells did not reveal significant changes in the T-cell subpopulations, CD4 or CD8[21]. These studies correlate with the finding of an undisturbed helper and suppressor T-cell function of isolated lamina propria lymphocytes from IBD patients in pokeweed-mitogen-driven systems[22]. In studies investigating the state of activation of lamina propria mononuclear cells in patients with IBD, it has been shown that the number of mononuclear cells expressing CD25 or other activation markers is increased in involved areas in Crohn disease compared with involved areas or control tissue[23,24]. Another finding documenting increased activation of T cells in IBD is the demonstration of higher concentrations of circulating soluble IL-2 receptors in the serum of patients with active Crohn disease compared with controls. These studies demonstrate an increased state of T-cell activation in intestinal inflammatory lesions and are a first indication of an up-regulated mucosal immune response in patients with IBD[25,26].

Several experimental and clinical findings clearly indicate that activated T cells interact with intestinal epithelial cells and influence viability and proliferation of these cells. In investigations from our group and other laboratories, it has been shown that soluble factors of activated T cells inhibit proliferation and decrease viability of the colon cancer-derived human intestinal epithelial cell line, HT29[27,28]. The epithelial cell line, HT29, may differentiate in vitro and gain some characteristics of mature enterocytes. If this cell line is incubated in vitro with supernatants of anti-CD3-stimulated T cells, a decrease in viability occurs as measured by the MTT test or by vital propidium iodide staining. Applying cell cycle analysis by propidium iodide staining of fixed and permeable cells together with surface staining for MHC class II expression (HLA-DR), we were able to show that proliferation is inhibited and HLA-DR expression is increased by soluble T-cell factors[28].

## Disturbed differentiation of mucosal T cells in IBD

Under physiological conditions, the intestinal lamina propria contains T cells which have a distinctive phenotype and which are activated. Functionally, these T cells can be characterized as differentiated effector lymphocytes which respond to triggering the antigen-specific T-cell receptor by secreting helper factors for B cells[29,30]. Therefore, lamina propria T cells represent a subset of memory T cells with a unique maturational state adapted to the specific tasks in the intestinal mucosa. An antigen-specific response of intestinal lamina propria T cells, in the form of a down-regulation of proliferation and an increase in the secretion of regulatory factors, prevents potentially harmful clonal expansion of T cells in the mucosa and at the same time allows protective immune responses, e.g. immunoglobulin secretion[31],

There are limited data available on T-cell responsiveness of mucosal T cells in IBD. In one study[32] lamina propria T cells were isolated from involved and uninvolved intestinal mucosa of IBD patients as well as from the peripheral blood. These T-cell populations were stimulated in vitro with several recall antigens. As expected, T cells from uninvolved mucosa only had minimal proliferative responses. Interestingly, T cells from inflammatory intestinal lesions from IBD patients exhibited proliferation to antigenic stimulation comparable to, or even higher than peripheral blood T cells. A recent study by Qiao and coworkers confirmed these findings: lamina propria T cells from IBD patients had an increased responsiveness upon T-cell receptor stimulation compared with controls[33]. A high spontaneous proliferation to low doses of exogenous IL-2 was also observed in this study, indicating in-vivo preactivation of intestinal T cells in IBD[33]. Using antigens from the resident intestinal bacterial flora as stimulating antigens, an abnormal increase in the proliferative response of intestinal mononuclear cells from inflamed areas of IBD patients was shown in a preliminary study[34]. These data clearly show a different responsiveness of lamina propria T cells of IBD patients with an increased proliferation after stimulation of the antigen-specific T-cell receptor and support the hypothesis of a disturbed differentiation of intestinal T cells in IBD.

Another important finding in the context of the cellular immune response in IBD is that the antigen-presenting function of intestinal epithelial cells may also be changed. As discussed earlier, intestinal epithelial cells are able to present antigens to T cells which leads to a preferential stimulation of CD8-positive cells with suppressor function under normal conditions[11]. However, intestinal epithelial cells from patients with IBD stimulate CD4-positive cells with helper function under identical in-vitro conditions[35]. This induction of helper mechanisms might contribute to an overshooting immune response in the gut-associated lymphoid tissue in IBD.


## SUMMARY AND CONCLUSIONS

Antigen-specific immune responses are highly regulated and the outcome of an immune response is mainly determined by the kind of helper T cell which is activated and which produces a certain profile of cytokines. The balance of T-helper cells in a specific immune response is critical in the induction of an inflammatory reaction with tissue destruction. Especially at mucosal surfaces immunoregulatory mechanisms are highly specialized and disruption of these mechanisms is followed by mucosal inflammation. In IBD, an increased activation and a disturbed differentiation process of lamina propria T cells might lead to a different responsiveness of the T-cell receptor with an inappropriate expansion of mononuclear cells in the intestinal mucosa. Such altered T cells might also secrete a different pattern of cytokines with proinflammatory function thereby inducing inflammatory effector mechanisms. In addition, an imbalance between helper and suppressor mechanisms in the intestinal mucosa in IBD has been shown which could result in a sustained and overshooting inflammatory and immune reaction against antigens normally occurring in the intestinal lumen. This unchecked immune reaction in the mucosa could be responsible for

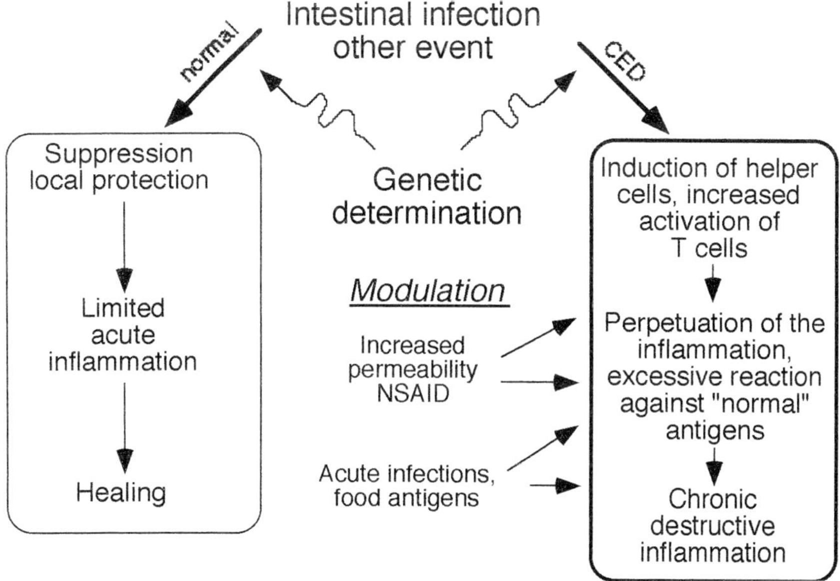


**Figure 1**  Model of the pathogenesis of inflammatory bowel diseases

the persisting and destructive nature of the inflammation in IBD patients (Figure 1). However, further studies on T-cell differentiation and function at the mucosal level in IBD are clearly needed to characterize the defects in mucosal immunoregulation and their role in the pathogenesis of IBD.

## Acknowledgements

Our own studies are supported by Grants from the German Research Council (DFG: Ze 188/3, Ze 188/4).

## References

1. Zeitz M. Immunoregulatory abnormalities in inflammatory bowel disease. Eur J Gastroenterol Hepatol. 1990;2:246–50.
2. Strober W, James SP. The immunologic basis of inflammatory bowel disease. J Clin Immunol. 1986;6:415–32.
3. Strober W, Jacobs D. Cellular differentiation, migration, and function in the mucosal immune system. In: Gallin JI, Fanci AS, ed. Advances in host defense mechanisms, Vol 4. New York: Raven Press; 1985:1–30.
4. Pabst R. The anatomical basis for the immune function of the gut. Anat Embryol. 1987;176:135–44.
5. Zeitz M, James SP, Strober W. Die Funktion des gastrointestinalen Immunsystems in der Abwehr enteropathogener Bakterien. Z Gastroenterol. 1986;24(Suppl. 3):43–52.
6. James SP, Zeitz M, Kanof ME, Kwan WC. Intestinal lymphocyte populations and mechanisms of cell-mediated immunity. In: Kagnoff M, ed. Immunology and allergy clinics of North America. Gut and intestinal immunology, Vol 8/3. Philadelphia. W B Saunders, 1988:369 91.
7. Zeitz M, Schieferdecker HL, James SP, Riecken EO. Special functional features of T-lymphocyte subpopulations in the effector compartment of the intestinal mucosa and their relation to mucosal transformation. Digestion. 1990;46(Suppl. 2).280–9.

8. James SP, Zeitz M, Mullin GE, Braun-Elwert L. Role of lymphokines in function of gastrointestinal mucosal T cells. In: Walker WA, Harmatz PR, Wershil BK, eds. Immunophysiology of the gut. San Diego: Academic Press Inc., 1993:129–43.

9. Focchi C. Cytokines and animal models: a combined path to inflammatory bowel disease pathogenesis. Gastroenterology. 1993;104:1202–19.

10. Bland PW, Warren LG. Antigen presentation by epithelial cells of the rat small intestine. II. Selective induction of suppressor T cells. Immunology. 1986;58:9–14.

11. Mayer L, Shlien R. Evidence for function of Ia molecules on gut epithelial cells in man. J Exp Med. 1987;166:1471–83.

12. Mosmann TR, Coffman RL. Th1 and Th2 cells: different patterns of lymphokine secretion lead to different functional properties. Annu Rev Immunol. 1989;7:145–73.

13. Scott P, Pearce E, Cheever AW, Coffman RL, Sher A. Role of cytokines and CD4+ T-cell subsets in the regulation of parasite immunity and disease. Immunol Rev. 1989;112:161–82.

14. Heinzel FP, Sadick MD, Holaday BJ, Coffman RL, Locksley RM. Reciprocal expression of interferon gamma or interleukin 4 during the resolution or progression of murine leishmaniasis. Evidence for expansion of distinct helper T cell subsets. J Exp Med. 1989;169:59–72.

15. Clerici M, Shearer GM. A Th1 → Th2 switch is a critical step in the etiology of HIV infection. Immunol Today. 1993;14:107–11.

16. Kühn R, Löhler J, Rennick D, Rajewsky K, Müller W. Interleukin-10-deficient mice develop chronic enterocolitis. Cell. 1993;75:263–74.

17. Sadlack B, Merz H, Schorle H, Schimpl A, Feller AC, Horak I. Ulcerative colitis-like disease in mice with a disrupted interleukin-2 gene. Cell. 1993;75:253–61.

18. Kündig TM, Schorle H, Bachmann MF, Hengartner H, Zinkernagel RM, Horak I. Immune responses in interleukin-2-deficient mice. Science. 1993;262:1059–61.

19. Mombaerts P, Mizoguchi E, Grusby MJ, Glimcher LH, Bhan AK, Tonegawa S. Spontaneous development of inflammatory bowel disease in T cell receptor mutant mice. Cell. 1993;75(2):274–82.

20. Strober W, Ehrhardt RO. Chronic intestinal inflammation: an unexpected outcome in cytokine or T cell receptor mutant mice. Cell. 1993;75(2):203–5.

21. James SP, Fiocchi C, Graeff AS, Strober W. Phenotypic analysis of lamina propria lymphocytes. Predominance of helper–inducer and cytolytic T-cell phenotypes and deficiency of suppressor–inducer phenotypes in Crohn's disease and control patients. Gastroenterology. 1986;91:1483–9.

22. James SP, Fiocchi C, Graeff AS, Strober W. Immunoregulatory function of lamina propria T cells in Crohn's disease. Gastroenterology. 1985;88:1143–50.

23. Zeitz M, Ullrich R, Schieferdecker HL, Weiss-Breckwoldt AN, James SP, Riecken EO. Characterization of T cell subpopulations in the intestinal lamina propria in inflammatory bowel disease. In: Goebell H, Ewe K, Malchow H, Koelbel C, eds. Inflammatory bowel diseases – Progress in basic research and clinical implications. Lancaster: Kluwer Academic Publishers; 1991:63–70.

24. Ullrich R, Zeitz M, Schieferdecker H, Brunn C, Riecken EO. Expression von aktivierungs – und proliferationsabhängigen Antigenen in der intestinalen Lamina propria (LP) von Kontrollpersonen und Patienten mit chronisch entzündlichen Darmerkrankungen (CED). Klin Wochenschr. 1989;67(Suppl.XVI):234.

25. Brynskov J, Tvede N. Plasma interleukin-2 and a soluble/shed interleukin-2 receptor in serum of patients with Crohn's disease. Effect of cyclosporin. Gut. 1990;31(7):795–9.

26. Mueller C, Knoflach P, Zielinski CC. T-cell activation in Crohn's disease. Increase levels of soluble interleukin-2 receptor in serum and in supernatants of stimulated peripheral blood mononuclear cells. Gastroenterology. 1990;98:639–46.

27. Deem RL, Shanahan F, Targan SR. Triggered mucosal T cells release tumour necrosis factor alpha and interferon-gamma which kill human colonic epithelial cells. Clin Exp Immunol. 1991;83:79–84.

28. Schmidt DC, Schieferdecker HL, Jahn HU, Hirseland H, Riecken EO, Zeitz M. Cytokines released by activated T cells decrease viability and proliferation, and increase MHC II expression of a colonic cancer cell line (HT29). FASEB J. 1992;6(5):A1993.

29. Zeitz M, Quinn TC, Graeff AS, James SP. Mucosal T cells provide helper function but do not proliferate when stimulated by specific antigen in lymphogranuloma venereum proctitis in non-human primates. Gastroenterology. 1988;94:353–66.

30. Qiao L, Schürmann G, Betzler M, Meuer SC. Activation and signaling status of human lamina propria T lymphocytes. Gastroenterology. 1991;101:1529–36.
31. Zeitz M, Schieferdecker HL, Ullrich R, James SP, Riecken EO. Phenotype and function of lamina propria T lymphocytes. Immunol Res. 1991;10:199–206.
32. Pirzer U, Schönhaar A, Fleischer B, Hermann E, Meyer zum Büschenfelde KH. Reactivity of infiltrating T lymphocytes with microbial antigens in Crohn's disease. Lancet. 1991;338:1238–9.
33. Qiao L, Golling M, Autschbach F, Schurmann G, Meuer SC. T cell receptor repertoire and mitotic responses of lamina propria T lymphocyctes in inflammatory bowel disease. Clin Exp Immunol. 1994;97(2):303–8.
34. Duchmann R, Kaiser I, Ewe K, Mayet W, Meyer-zum-Büschenfelde KH. Stimulation of IBD-LPMC from inflamed intestine by resident bacterial flora [Abstract]. Gastroenterology. 1994;106(2):A674.
35. Mayer L, Eisenhardt D. Lack of induction of suppressor T cells by intestinal epithelial cells from patients with inflammatory bowel disease. J Clin Invest. 1990;86:1255–60.

# 6
# Soluble inflammatory mediators

V. GROSS, T. ANDUS, R. DAIG, W. HANS, G. KOJOUHAROFF,
W. FALK and J. SCHÖLMERICH

## INTRODUCTION

The aetiology of Crohn disease and ulcerative colitis is still unknown. Epidemiological studies showed that genetic factors play an important role in their development. This is reflected by higher concordance rates of Crohn disease and ulcerative colitis in identical twins as compared with dizygotic twins[1] and increased incidence rates of inflammatory bowel disease in first-degree relatives of patients[2]. There exists, however, no simple Mendelian inheritance pattern. In addition to a genetic predisposition, environmental factors, bacteria and viruses have been proposed as aetiological factors. Concerning the pathophysiology of the chronic inflammatory process, an inadequate activation of the intestinal immune system seems to play an important role. This assumption is supported by the observation of an increased production of various cytokines and other soluble mediators (for a recent review, see Reference 3). The most abundant data are available for IL-1. There exists an increased number of activated colonic lamina propria mononuclear cells in inflammatory bowel disease as demonstrated by the increased in-vitro release of soluble IL-2 receptor[4]. Further support for the concept of an inadequate activation of the intestinal immune system comes from clinical studies demonstrating the effectiveness of immunosuppressive drugs in inflammatory bowel disease.

Among the soluble mediators orchestrating the functions of the specific and unspecific immune system, cytokines play a key role. They are early mediators rapidly secreted by inflammatory cells upon stimulation. On the other hand, they elicit a wide range of specific reactions; among others they induce the production of other inflammatory mediators like lipid mediators, nitric oxide and PAF.

In the course of inflammatory reactions, various functional groups of cytokines may be differentiated:

1. Proinflammatory cytokines which induce the recruitment and activation of inflammatory cells. Among these are IL-1, TNF, IL-8 and MCP-1.
2. A group of cytokines, which includes IL-6 as a typical species, induce protective mechanisms, like the synthesis of acute-phase proteins.

3.  A group of cytokines, which comprise IL-4, IL-10 and TGF, down-regulates
    the inflammatory process and promotes anabolic reactions.

The following overview will concentrate on the role of the proinflammatory
cytokines and some of their endogenous antagonists in inflammatory bowel
disease and will discuss the potential of a specific anticytokine therapy.

## IL-1 AND IL-1-RECEPTOR ANTAGONIST IN HUMAN INFLAMMATORY BOWEL DISEASE

IL-1 is produced by a variety of cells including monocytes and macrophages,
neutrophils, endothelial cells, keratinocytes, astrocytes and virally infected
B lymphocyctes or cell lines. IL-1 acts on multiple target cells to induce or
augment biological functions that are part of most immune and inflammatory
cell systems[5].

The effects of IL-1 are inhibited by a specific IL-1-receptor antagonist
(IL-1ra)[6–8]. IL-1ra has 19% and 26% homology with IL-1$\alpha$ and IL-1$\beta$, respectively. It competes with IL-1 for type 1 and type 2 IL-1 receptors without inducing signal transduction[9]. IL-1ra blocks the biological activity of IL-1 in vitro
and in vivo, e.g. it inhibits IL-1-induced hypertension in rabbits and baboons,
IL-1-induced fever in rabbits, IL-1-induced hepatic acute-phase protein synthesis, IL-1-induced increase in corticosterone in mice, IL-1-induced neutrophilia
in mice, IL-1-induced lymphocyte proliferation, IL-1-induced collagenase production by rabbit chondrocytes, IL-1-induced synthesis of IL-1, TNF, IL-6,
GM–CSF in monocytes, and IL-1-induced nitric oxide production in human
smooth muscle cells (reviewed in Reference 10).

IL-1 and IL-1ra have been determined in the systemic circulation as well as in
the colonic mucosa of patients with inflammatory bowel disease. Several studies
of systemic cytokine production have reported that peripheral blood mononuclear cells or monocytes from patients with Crohn disease are activated and
produce more IL-1 than those from patients with ulcerative colitis or normal
individuals. Using an ex-vivo whole-blood system, Andus et al.[11] measured IL-6
secretion with and without stimulation. Spontaneous IL-6 secretion in this
system was about 9 U/ml in patients with Crohn disease and below the detection
limit of 4 U/ml in healthy controls. Moderate stimulation of blood cells
(100 pg/ml lipopolysaccharide (LPS)) from patients with active Crohn disease
before and after treatment led to mean IL-6 concentrations of $1160 \pm 514$ and
$131 \pm 54$ U/ml, respectively. The peripheral blood mononuclear cells appear to
be activated in Crohn disease. Using the mouse thymocyte stimulation assay,
Satsangi et al.[12] reported spontaneous release of lymphocyte-activating factor
activity by peripheral blood mononuclear cells from 6/16 patients with Crohn
disease, 1/6 patients with ulcerative colitis and 1/10 healthy subjects. Suzuki et
al.[13] determined an increased synthesis of IL-1 by peripheral blood monocytes
from patients with Crohn disease. Increased circulatory levels of IL-1 in patients
with Crohn disease compared with patients with ulcerative colitis or healthy
controls were measured by Duclos et al.[14,15]. Similar results have been reported
for IL-6[16–18]. Mazlam and Hodgson[19] showed that resting levels of IL-1 production by peripheral blood mononuclear cells (PBMC) were not different

between controls and patients with Crohn disease or ulcerative colitis. After stimulation with LPS, however, PBMC from patients with active Crohn disease showed significantly increased IL-1 production compared with controls. LPS-stimulated PBMC from patients with active ulcerative colitis showed a trend towards an increased IL-1 production which did not reach statistical significance. Patients with inactive Crohn disease had higher levels of IL-1 production than controls, but lower levels than patients with active disease. Nakamura et al.[20] found that IL-1 production by PBMC stimulated with concanavalin A was increased in both active Crohn disease and ulcerative colitis. IL-1 levels appeared to be correlated with disease activity.

Increased concentrations of systemic levels of IL-1ra have recently been demonstrated by Hyams et al.[21].

We have measured blood levels of IL-1 and IL-1ra in patients with Crohn disease and in patients with ulcerative colitis, both during an active inflammatory episode and after successful therapeutic interventions in the same patients. We also included a group of control patients (Table 1). IL-1 was detectable in the circulation of only 2/21 patients with active Crohn disease and could not be detected in any of the other serum samples. IL-1ra, on the other hand, was detectable in control sera in a mean concentration of 0.23 ng/ml. In patients with active Crohn disease, circulatory IL-1ra levels were significantly increased, whereas patients with inactive Crohn disease had no increased levels. Patients with active ulcerative colitis also showed a tendency towards increased IL-1ra levels; however, the difference compared with controls was not statistically significant. Patients with inactive ulcerative colitis had IL-1ra levels in the same range as healthy controls. Systemic IL-1ra levels correlated with disease activity. This could also be demonstrated in individual patients (Figure 1).

**Table 1**  IL-1 and IL-1ra in serum of inflammatory bowel disease patients

|  | Control ($n = 50$) | CD active ($n = 21$) | CD inactive ($n = 21$) | UC active ($n = 12$) | UC inactive ($n = 12$) |
|---|---|---|---|---|---|
| IL-1β | ND | 2×det. | ND | ND | ND |
| IL-1ra (ng/ml) | 0.23 (0.15–0.30) | 0.61[*] (0.33–0.88) | 0.25 (0.14–0.37) | 0.51 (0.23–0.72) | 0.29 (0.17–0.42) |

IL-1ra correlates with Crohn disease activity index ($r = 0.48$, $p = 0.003$)
Values are given as mean (95% CI)
ND = not detectable; *$p < 0.05$; CD = Crohn disease; UC = ulcerative colitis

These data indicate that there is no systemic deficiency of IL-1ra in patients with inflammatory bowel disease. The increased IL-1ra levels during active episodes of inflammation may protect the body from the harmful effects of circulating IL-1.

Concerning mucosal IL-1 production, Mahida et al.[22] detected enhanced production of IL-1 by mononuclear cells isolated from mucosa of patients with active ulcerative colitis or Crohn disease. Similarly, an enhanced production during active inflammatory bowel disease was described by Ligumsky et al.[23]. Youngman et al.[24] localized the intestinal IL-1 activity and protein gene expres-

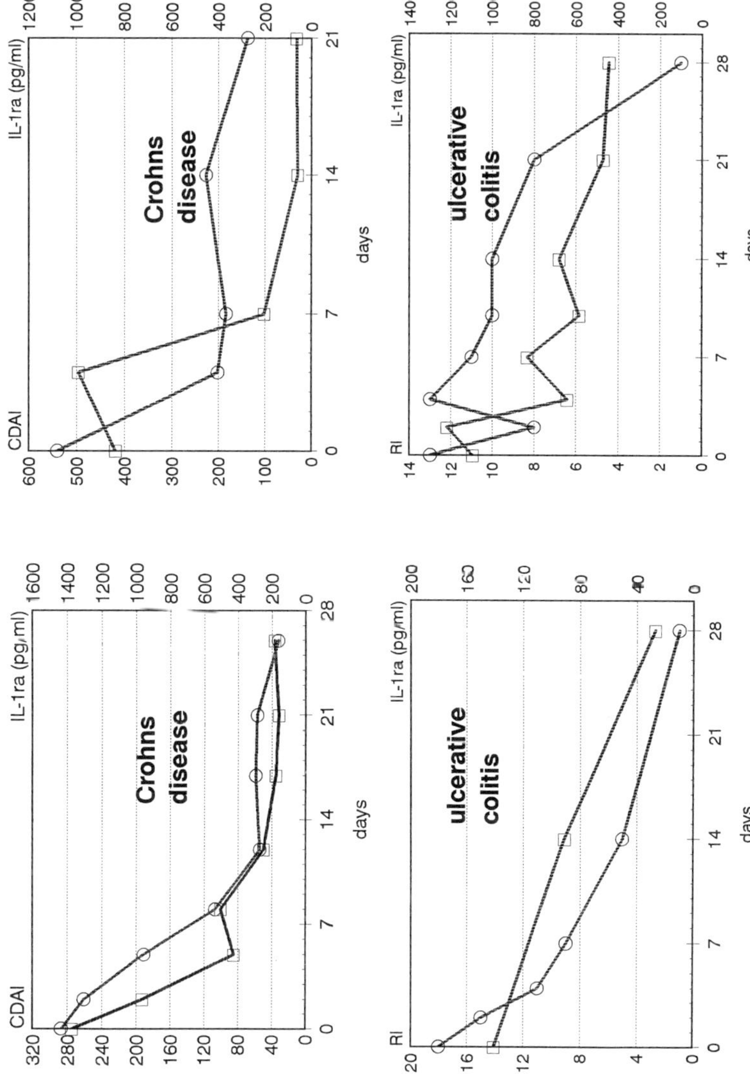

**Figure 1** IL-1ra levels in individual patients with Crohn disease or ulcerative colitis. CDAI (○), Rachmilewitz index (○) and circulatory IL-1ra levels (□) were repeatedly determined in individual patients with highly active Crohn disease (above) or high y active ulcerative colitis (below) during corticosteroid therapy

sion to lamina propria cells. Isaacs et al.[25] detected IL-1 mRNA in 7/8 specimens with active ulcerative colitis, 0/6 specimens with inactive ulcerative colitis, 4/6 specimens with active Crohn disease, 7/13 specimens with inactive Crohn disease, and in 2/12 specimens of non-inflammatory controls. These results were obtained by polymerase chain reaction amplification. The first indication that there might be an imbalance between IL-1 and IL-1ra in the mucosa of patients with inflammatory bowel disease came from findings of Cominelli et al.[26] who determined mRNA levels of IL-1$\alpha$, IL-1$\beta$, and IL-1ra in patients with inflammatory bowel disease. They found a decreased IL-1ra/(IL-1$\alpha$ + IL-1$\beta$) ratio in the mucosa of patients with inflammatory bowel disease.

We determined IL-1$\beta$ and IL-1ra in colonic biopsy specimens of 20 control persons, 14 patients with Crohn disease, and 9 patients with ulcerative colitis. Biopsy specimens of patients with inflammatory bowel disease were obtained both from macroscopically inflamed and uninflamed sites (Figure 2). Normal mucosa of control patients contained only very small amounts of IL-1$\beta$. IL-1$\beta$ was significantly elevated in inflammatory lesions of patients with Crohn disease or ulcerative colitis. Normal-appearing mucosa of patients with Crohn disease also contained increased amounts of IL-1; however, the difference compared with controls was not statistically significant. In contrast to IL-1, normal mucosa contained high levels of IL-1ra. The local concentrations of IL-1ra were increased in inflammatory lesions of patients with Crohn disease or ulcerative colitis. The increase in IL-1ra was, however, not as high as that of IL-1. This resulted in a decreased IL-1ra/IL-1$\beta$ ratio in inflammatory lesions of patients with Crohn disease or ulcerative colitis, as well as in the normal-appearing mucosa of patients with Crohn disease. The individual data are presented in Figure 3. There is thus an imbalance in the local mucosal IL-1ra/IL-1 system in patients with inflammatory bowel disease.

We were able to localize the sites of expression of IL-1$\beta$ mRNA in the mucosa by in-situ hybridization using a specific [$^{35}$S]UTP-labelled IL-1$\beta$ cRNA probe. As shown in Figure 4, IL-1-expressing cells were found within the mucosa presumably representing infiltrating mononuclear cells.

## TNF AND SOLUBLE TNF RECEPTORS IN HUMAN INFLAMMATORY BOWEL DISEASE

While there seems to be a general consensus in the literature concerning an increased expression of IL-1 in inflammatory bowel disease, the reported data about TNF are somewhat contradictory. Some groups were able to demonstrate increased levels of TNF, e.g. in the serum of patients with inflammatory bowel disease[27] or in the faeces of paediatric patients with intestinal inflammation[28]. In contrast to these findings, other groups were unable to demonstrate an increase in TNF levels in patients with inflammatory bowel disease, either at the mRNA or protein level[25,29].

Tumour necrosis factor is an important mediator of inflammation. It shares many proinflammatory activities with IL-1. The effects of TNF may be modulated by soluble TNF receptors which are derived from the membrane-bound receptors[30,31]. There are two distinct soluble TNF receptors with molecular

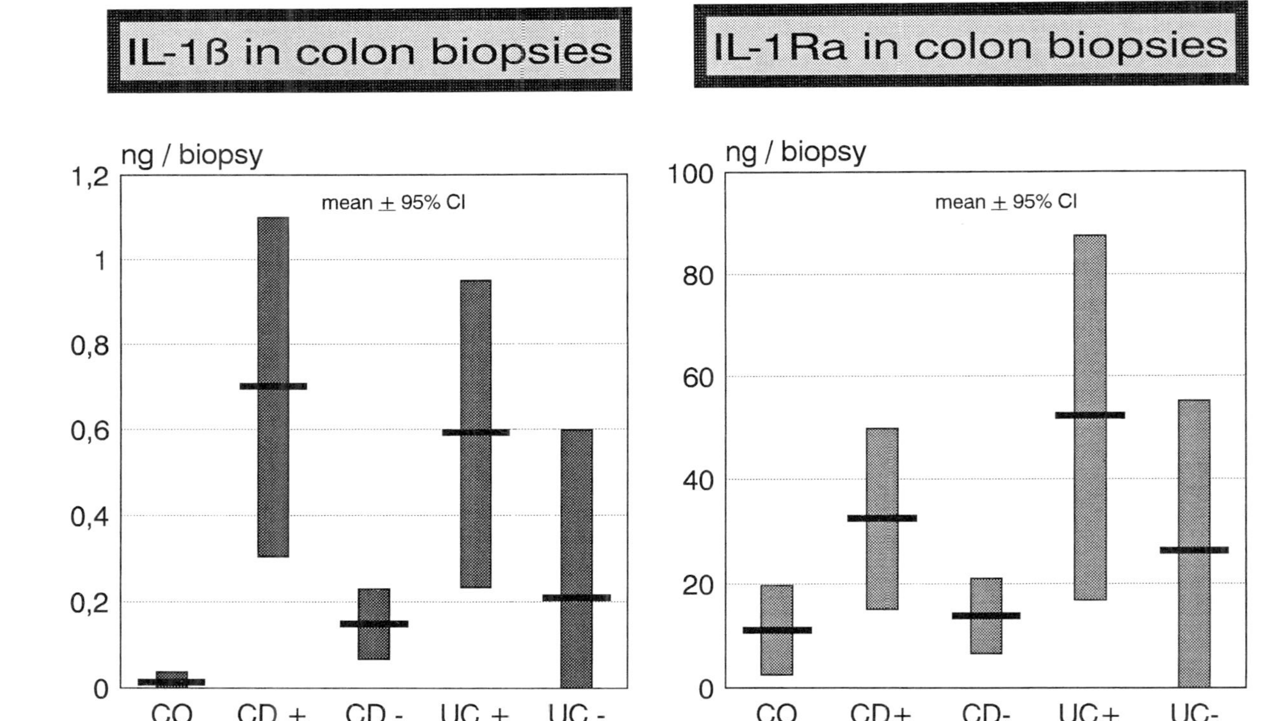


**Figure 2**   IL-1 and IL-1ra in the colonic mucosa of patients with inflammatory bowel disease.

IL-1 and IL-1ra were determined by ELISA in colonic biopsy specimens of 14 patients with Crohn disease (CD), 9 patients with ulcerative colitis (UC) and 20 controls (CO). Biopsies were taken from patients with inflammatory bowel disease both at macroscopically inflamed (+) and uninflamed (–) sites

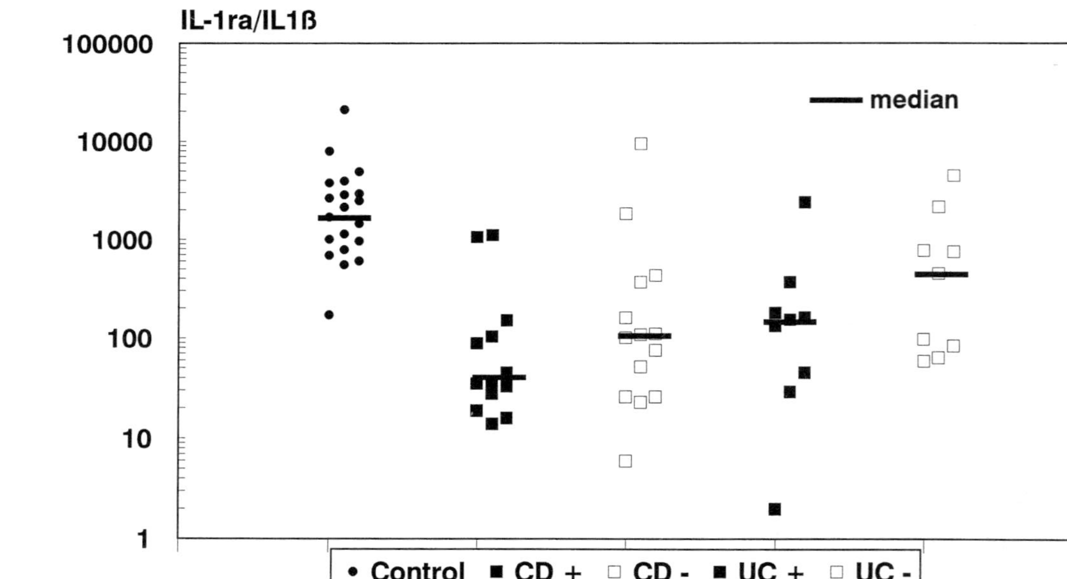


**Figure 3**   Ratio between IL-1ra and IL-1 in the colonic mucosa of controls and patients with inflammatory bowel disease.
The IL-1ra/IL-1$\beta$ ratio was calculated in colonic biopsy specimens from 20 controls, 14 patients with Crohn disease (CD), and 9 patients with ulcerative colitis (UC) both at inflamed (+) and uninflamed (–) sites

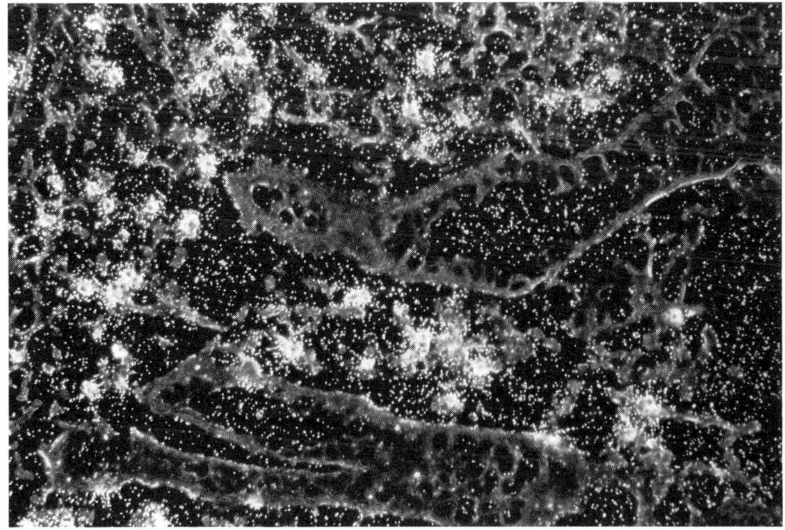

**Figure 4**  Detection of IL-1 mRNA by in-situ hybridization.

IL-1$\beta$ mRNA was detected in colonic biopsy specimens by in-situ hybridization using a [$^{35}$S]UTP-labelled cRNA probe. The figure shows IL-1$\beta$ mRNA in the mucosa of a patient with Crohn disease

masses of 55 000 Da (p55) and 75 000 Da (p75). Both soluble TNF receptors inhibit binding of TNF to its cellular receptors and reduce the biological effects of TNF in a dose-dependent manner[32]. To fully assess the balance of the TNF system in inflammatory bowel disease, we determined both TNF$\alpha$ and the soluble TNF receptors, p55 and p75, in the systemic circulation and in the colonic mucosa of patients with inflammatory bowel disease.

The serum levels of immunoreactive TNF$\alpha$ were significantly increased in patients with active Crohn disease but not in patients with ulcerative colitis or in patients with inactive Crohn disease (see Table 2). The serum levels of the soluble TNF receptors, p55 and p75, showed a significant increase only in

**Table 2**  TNF$\alpha$ and soluble TNF receptors in serum of inflammatory bowel disease patients

|  | Control ($n = 50$) | CD active ($n = 21$) | CD inactive ($n = 21$) | UC active ($n = 12$) | UC inactive ($n = 12$) |
|---|---|---|---|---|---|
| TNF$\alpha$ (pg/ml) | 3.7 (2.0–5.3) | 19.7* (0–43.2) | 9.4 (3.3–15.5) | 9.0 (4.1–13.9) | 8.3 (0.8–15.9) |
| p55 (ng/ml) | 1.02 (0.74–1.31) | 2.36* (1.34–3.18) | 1.78 (1.40–2.16) | 1.94 (0.87–3.07) | 1.80 (1.25–2.34) |
| p75 (ng/ml) | 3.50 (2.81–4.17) | 4.46 (3.55–5.62) | 3.20 (2.58–3.82) | 3.75 (2.35–5.14) | 4.22 (2.95–5.50) |

Values are given as mean (95% CI); *$p < 0.05$; CD = Crohn disease; UC = ulcerative colitis

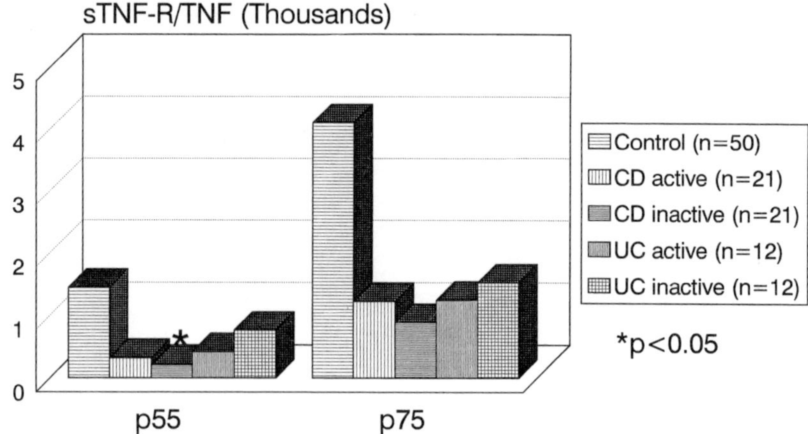


**Figure 5**  Soluble TNF receptor/TNFα ratios in serum of IBD patients.
Soluble TNF receptors, p55 and p75, and TNFα were determined by ELISA in the serum of 50 controls, 21 patients with Crohn disease (CD) with active and inactive disease, and 12 patients with ulcerative colitis (UC) with active and inactive disease

patients with active Crohn disease. When we calculated the ratios between the soluble TNF receptors and TNFα in the serum of IBD patients, we found a tendency towards decreased values in all samples obtained from patients with inflammatory bowel disease with most prominent decrease in patients with inactive Crohn disease ($p < 0.05$) (see Figure 5). This indicates that there is an imbalance in the TNF system in patients with inflammatory bowel disease at the systemic level.

When TNFα and the soluble TNF receptors, p55 and p75, were determined in colonic biopsy specimens of controls and patients with inflammatory bowel disease, there was a tendency towards increased local TNF concentrations in active Crohn disease and active ulcerative colitis. Due to a large variation of the individual data, there was, however, no statistically significant difference compared with controls. The same tendency could be observed for the soluble TNF receptors. With the exception of a significant increase of p75 in patients with Crohn disease, no significant differences could be observed in patients with inflammatory bowel disease compared with controls (Figure 6). Due to the large variation of the individual data, no significant alterations of the ratios between soluble TNF receptors and TNFα were detected in Crohn disease or ulcerative colitis mucosal biopsy specimens.

The expression of TNFα mRNA could be localized by in-situ hybridization with a specific TNFα cRNA probe. The distribution of TNFα-mRNA-expressing cells was similar to that of IL-1β-mRNA-expressing cells.

## IL-8 IN HUMAN INFLAMMATORY BOWEL DISEASE

IL-8 is a member of the chemokine family. It is a major chemotactic and activating peptide for neutrophils[33]. IL-8 is produced by various cells, e.g. mononu-

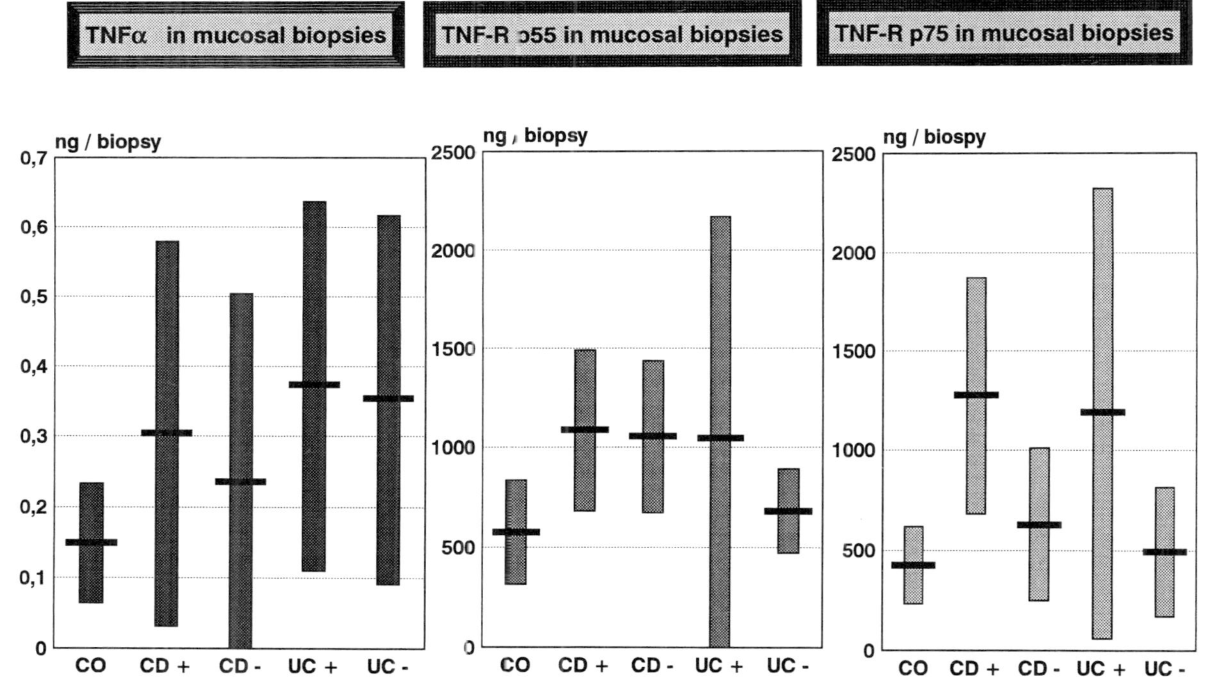



**Figure 5**   TNF and soluble TNF receptors, p55 and p75, in the colonic mucosa of patients with inflammatory bowel disease.
TNFα, p55 and p75 were determined by ELISA in colonic biopsy specimens of 20 controls, 14 patients with Crohn disease (CD) and 9 patients with ulcerative colitis (UC). Biopsies were taken from patients with inflammatory bowel disease both at macroscopically inflamed (+) and uninflamed (–) sites

clear phagocytes[34–36], endothelial cells[37], fibroblasts[38], and various epithelial cell types[39,40]. Recently, it has been demonstrated that IL-8 is synthesized by various colonic cancer cell lines[41–43]. Evidence has also been provided that isolated normal intestinal epithelial cells may synthesize IL-8[41].

An enhanced synthesis of IL-8 has been described in the mucosa of patients with inflammatory bowel disease. Whereas Mahida and coworkers[44] found enhanced mucosal tissue concentrations of IL-8 essentially only in patients with ulcerative colitis but not in patients with Crohn disease, Izzo et al.[45] also detected increased concentrations of IL-8 in the colonic mucosa from patients with Crohn disease.

We determined IL-8 by ELISA in colonic biopsy specimens of controls, patients with Crohn disease of various degrees of activity and patients with ulcerative colitis with various degrees of activity. IL-8 protein was significantly increased in macroscopically inflamed biopsy specimens of patients with Crohn disease and ulcerative colitis compared with controls. IL-8 was also increased in uninflamed biopsies of patients with Crohn disease, but not of patients with ulcerative colitis (Table 3). IL-8 protein in the mucosa correlated significantly with macroscopic inflammation in Crohn disease and in ulcerative colitis.

**Table 3**  Median IL-8 protein levels in the mucosa of inflammatory bowel disease patients

|  | IL-8 (pg/biopsy)* |
| --- | --- |
| Controls ($n = 15$) | 4.5 |
| Crohn disease (active) ($n = 32$) | 138 ($p < 0.0001$)[†] |
| Crohn disease (inactive) ($n = 14$) | 48 ($p = 0.0009$)[†] |
| Ulcerative colitis (active) ($n = 29$) | 113 ($p < 0.0001$)[†] |
| Ulcerative colitis (inactive) ($n = 11$) | 9 ($p = 0.7$)[†] |

*Mean biopsy weight $8.3 \pm 2.7$ mg with no significant difference between controls, Crohn disease and ulcerative colitis; [†] versus controls

Similar to IL-8 protein, IL-8 mRNA could be detected by in-situ hybridization. Inflammatory cells of the interstitium could be identified as sites of synthesis of IL-8, both in Crohn disease and in ulcerative colitis. IL-8 mRNA was not detected in mucosal epithelial cells, indicating that, in chronic inflammatory bowel disease, intestinal mucosal epithelial cells do not contribute considerably to IL-8 production. The measurements clearly demonstrate that IL-8 is an important mucosal inflammatory mediator in Crohn disease and in ulcerative colitis.

## CYTOKINES AS SPECIFIC TARGETS FOR INFLAMMATORY BOWEL DISEASE THERAPY

Based on the increased expression of proinflammatory cytokines in the mucosa of patients with inflammatory bowel disease, a rationale for a specific anticytokine therapy may be defined. Various groups have studied the effects of IL-1ra in experimental animal models of colitis. In the experimental immune-complex colitis in rabbits, IL-1ra decreased tissue injury[46]. Similar beneficial effects of IL-1ra were observed in the peptidoglycan/polysaccharide colitis of the rat[47], in the indomethacin colitis of the rat[47], and in the dextran sulphate colitis model of the mouse[48]. Thus far, no results of studies using IL-1ra in human inflammatory bowel disease have been reported.

Anti-TNF agents as well as anti-IL-8 agents have only rarely been studied in inflammatory bowel disease. Casini-Raggi et al.[49] recently reported that a specific monoclonal antibody against interleukin-8 suppresses inflammation in rabbit immune colitis, whereas recombinant human TNF-binding protein was not effective in this model. However, there has been a case report of successful treatment of paediatric refractory Crohn disease with monoclonal anti-TNF antibodies[50]. These results have recently been confirmed and extended by the same group[51]. The further confirmation of the beneficial effects of specific anti-TNF agents in refractory Crohn disease by controlled trials therefore seems desirable.

Although there is some enthusiasm concerning the use of specific inhibitors of proinflammatory cytokines, these agents may also produce disadvantageous effects, at least during certain conditions. In a mouse peritonitis model produced by caecal ligation and puncture, inhibition of TNF by anti-TNF antibodies resulted in a reduced survival rate of the animals[52]. If anti-TNF antibodies were administered at the time of induction of peritonitis, virtually all mice died within a short period, whereas survival was improved if anti-TNF antibodies were given 8 or 16 hours after the induction of peritonitis. Obviously, TNF seems to play an important protective role during the early phases of peritonitis. Therefore, various questions still have to be answered when we consider a specific anticytokine therapy in inflammatory bowel disease. We do not yet know whether the inhibition of a single cytokine is really effective since, due to their pleiotropic actions, various cytokines can replace the functions of others. We do not know which type of therapy is the best: cytokine antibodies, soluble cytokine receptors, cytokine receptor antagonists or receptor antibodies. Another important issue is the safety of this treatment approach.

In order to systematically address these questions, we have induced a chronic colitis in mice by the repeated administration of 5% dextran sulphate in their drinking water. After 4 cycles of dextran sulphate treatment, the mice developed a chronic colitis which persisted for several months. The colitis was characterized by a decreased weight gain of the animals, a shortening and thickening of the colonic wall and specific histopathological alterations, e.g. infiltration with inflammatory cells, development of large lymphocyte aggregates in the colonic mucosa, ulcers, intestinal dysplasias and occasionally development of carcinomas. The inflammatory alterations in the chronic dextran sulphate colitis are more pronounced in the distal than in the proximal colon. Figure 7 shows an example of the histological alterations in a mouse with chronic colitis.

When the animals were treated with dexamethasone during the chronic stage of inflammation, the inflammatory changes were rapidly attenuated. Figure 8 shows the effects of one week's treatment with dexamethasone. The inflammatory lesions were greatly reduced by dexamethasone. When the animals were treated with a specific monoclonal rat antibody against mouse TNF (V1q), the inflammatory lesions were decreased as well, but not to the same extent as after

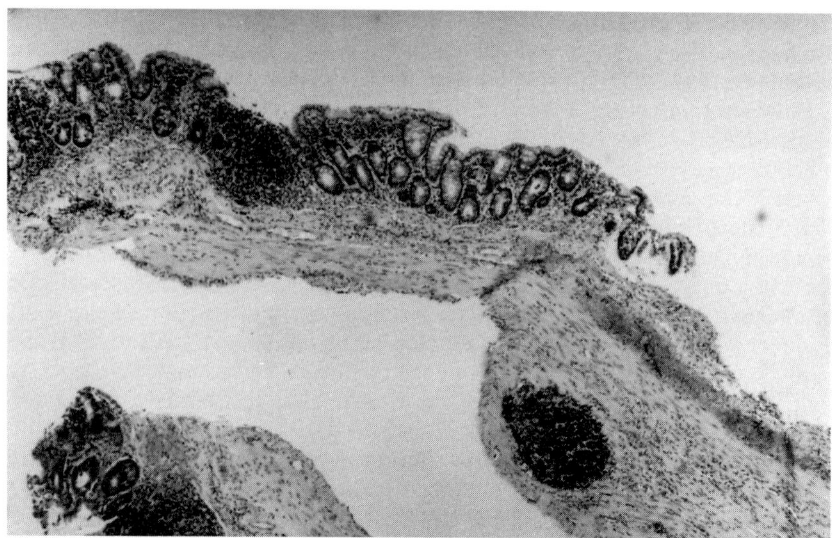

**Figure 7**    Chronic colitis induced in mice by repeated administration of dextran sulphate.

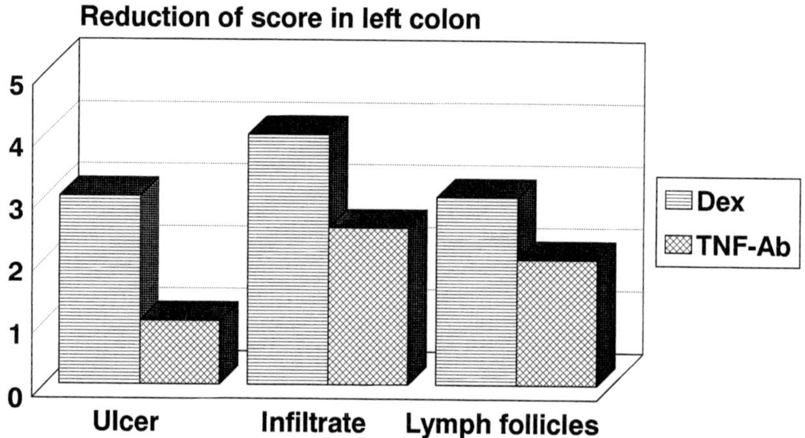


**Figure 8**    Treatment of chronic murine dextran sulphate colitis by dexamethasone or anti-TNF antibodies (TNF-Ab).

A chronic colitis was induced in BALB/c mice by four cycles of 5% dextran sulphate treatment. During the chronic stage (after 6 weeks), mice were treated with dexamethasone (3 $\mu$g/g body weight) for 1 week or with a specific monoclonal rat anti-mouse TNF antibody (V1q, 100 $\mu$g for 5 days). Mice were sacrificed on day 7. Ulcers, inflammatory infiltrates and lymph follicles were scored 1–4. Treatment effects were assessed 1 week after start of therapy

treatment with dexamethasone. No deterioration of the chronic intestinal inflammation was observed after administration of TNF antibodies. These results show that targeting TNF in chronic colitis might be a safe approach, at least in the chronic dextran sulphate colitis of the mouse. Targeting TNF alone is not as effective as treatment with corticosteroids. Further studies have to address the issue of whether a more efficient and long-term inhibition of TNF by the use of soluble TNF receptors is more beneficial. Furthermore, it must be investigated whether the combination of a broad-spectrum anti-inflammatory agent, e.g. a corticosteroid, with a specific anticytokine may produce a greater therapeutic benefit.

## CONCLUSIONS

There is an imbalance between pro- and anti-inflammatory cytokines in inflammatory bowel disease, both at the systemic level and at the mucosal level. This might be of pathogenetic relevance for the perpetuation of intestinal inflammation. It may provide a basis for alternative treatment approaches targeting specific proinflammatory cytokines.

## References


1. Tysk C, Lindberg E, Jarnero G, Floderus-Myrhed B. Ulcerative colitis and Crohn's disease in an unselected population of monozygotic and dizygotic twins. A study of heritability and the influence of smoking. Gut. 1988;29:990–6.
2. Mayberry JF, Rhodes J, Newcombe RG. Familial prevalence of inflammatory bowel disease in relatives of patients with Crohn's disease. Br Med J. 1980;280:84.
3. Stenson WF. Inflammatory mediators in inflammatory bowel disease. Curr Opin Gastroenterol. 1994;10:384–9.
4. Schreiber S, Raedler A, Conn AR, Rombeau JL, MacDermott RP. Increase in in vitro release of soluble interleukin-2 receptor by colonic lamina propria mononuclear cells in inflammatory bowel disease. Gut. 1992;33:236–41.
5. Dinarello CA. Biology of interleukin-1. FASEB J. 1988;2:108–15.
6. Mazzei GJ, Seckinger PL, Dayer JM, Shaw AR. Purification and characterisation of a 26 kDa competitive inhibitor of interleukin-1. Eur J Immunol. 1990;20:683–9.
7. Carter DB, Deibel MR, Dunn CJ et al. Purification, cloning, expression and biological characterisation of an interleukin-1 receptor antagonist protein. Nature. 1990;344:633–8.
8. Eisenberg SP, Evans RJ, Arend WP. Primary structure and functional expression from complementary DNA of a human interleukin-1 receptor antagonist. Nature. 1990;343:341–6.
9. Hannum CH, Wilcox CJ, Arend WP et al. Interleukin-1 receptor antagonist activity of a human interleukin-1 inhibitor. Nature. 1990;343:336–40.
10. Dinarello CA, Thompson RC. Block IL-1: interleukin-1 receptor antagonist in vivo and in vitro. Immunol Today. 1991;12:404–10.
11. Andus T, Gross V, Cäsar I et al. Activation of monocytes during inflammatory bowel disease. Pathobiology. 1991;59:166–70.
12. Satsangi J, Wolstencroft RA, Cason J, Ainley CC, Dumonde DC, Thompson RPH. Interleukin-1 in Crohn's disease. Clin Exp Immunol. 1987;67:594–605.
13. Suzuki K, Murata Y, Niida N et al. Increased synthesis of interleukin-1 (IL-1) by monocytes from patients with inflammatory bowel disease. Gastroenterology. 1991;100:A619.
14. Duclos B, Reimund JM, Dumont S et al. Discrepancy between tumor necrosis factor (TNF) and interleukin-1 (IL-1) blood levels and cytotoxic activity of blood monocytes in Crohn's disease (CD). Gastroenterology. 1991;100:A576.
15. Duclos B, Reimund JM, Lehr L et al. Interleukin-1 (IL-1), 6 (IL-6) and tumor necrosis factor (TNF) serum levels in Crohn's disease (CD). Gastroenterology. 1991;100:A576.
16. Gross V, Andus T, Caesar I, Roth M, Schölmerich J. Evidence for continuous stimulation of interleukin-6 production in Crohn's disease. Gastroenterology. 1992;102:514–19.
17. Gasché C, Reinisch W, Lochs H, Gangl A. Interleukin-6 production in Crohn's disease. Gastroenterology. 1992;103:1120–1.

18. Hyams JS, Fitzgerald JE, Treem WR, Wyzga N, Kreutzer DL. Relationship of functional and antigenic interleukin-6 to disease activity in inflammatory bowel disease. Gastroenterology. 1993;104:1285–92.
19. Mazlam MZ, Hodgson HJ. Peripheral blood monocyte cytokine production and acute phase response in inflammatory bowel disease. Gut. 1992;33:773–8.
20. Nakamura M, Saito H, Kasanuki J, Tamura Y, Yoshida S. Cytokine production in patients with inflammatory bowel disease. Gut. 1992;33:933–7.
21. Hyams JS, Fitzgerald JE, Wyzga N, Treem WR, Justinich CJ, Kreutzer DI. Characterization of circulating interleukin-1 receptor antagonist expression in children with inflammatory bowel disease. Dig Dis Sci. 1994;39:1893–9.
22. Mahida YR, Wu K, Jewell DP. Enhanced production of interleukin-1 by mononuclear cells isolated from mucosa with active ulcerative colitis on Crohn's disease. Gut. 1989;30:835–8.
23. Ligumsky M, Simon PL, Karmeli F, Rachmilewitz D. Role of interleukin-1 in inflammatory bowel disease – enhanced production during active disease. Gut. 1990;31:686–9.
24. Youngman KR, Simon PL, West GA et al. Localization of intestinal interleukin-1 activity and protein and gene expression to lamina propria cells. Gastroenterology. 1993;104:749–58.
25. Isaacs KL, Sartor RB, Haskill S. Cytokine messenger RNA profiles in inflammatory bowel disease mucosa detected by polymerase chain reaction amplification. Gastroenterology. 1992;103:1587–95.
26. Cominelli F, Fiocchi C, Eisenberg SP, Bortolami M. Imbalance of IL-1 and IL-1 receptor antagonist synthesis in the intestinal mucosa of Crohn's disease and ulcerative colitis patients. A novel pathogenetic mechanism. Gastroenterology. 1992;102:A603.
27. Maeda M, Watanabe N, Neda H et al. Serum tumor necrosis factor activity in inflammatory bowel disease. Immunopharmacol Immunotoxicol. 1992;14:451–61.
28. Braegger CP, Nicholis S, Murch SH, Stephens S, MacDonald TT. Tumor necrosis factor in stool as a marker of intestinal inflammation. Lancet. 1992;339:89–91.
29. Thies P, Jörres A, Müller C. Tumor necrosis factor in ulcerative colitis patients. Eur J Gastroenterol Hepatol. 1991;3:S60.
30. Loetscher H, Schlaeger EJ, Lahm HW, Pan Y-CE, Lesslauer W, Brockhaus M. Purification and partial amino acid sequence analysis of two distinct tumor necrosis factor receptors from HL60 cells. J Biol Chem. 1990:265:20131–8.
31. Seckinger P, Isaaz S, Dayer JM. Purification and biological characterization of a specific tumor necrosis factor inhibitor. J Biol Chem. 1989;265:11966–73.
32. Loetscher H, Gentz R, Zulauf M et al. Recombinant 55 kDa tumor necrosis factor (TNF) receptor. Stoichiometry of binding to TNF alpha and TNF beta and inhibition of TNF activity. J Biol Chem. 1991;266:18324–9.
33. Baggiolini M, Walz A, Kunkel SL. Neutrophil-activating peptide-1/interleukin-8, a novel cytokine that activates neutrophils. J Clin Invest. 1989;84:1045–9.
34. Yoshimura T, Matsushima K, Tanaka S et al. Purification of a human monocyte-derived neutrophil chemotactic factor that has peptide sequence similarity to other host defense cytokines. Proc Natl Acad Sci USA. 1987;84:9233–7.
35. Schroeder JM, Mrowietz U, Morita E, Christophers E. Purification and partial biochemical characterization of a human monocyte-derived, neutrophil-activating peptide that lacks interleukin-1 activity. J Immunol. 1987;139:3474–83.
36. Peveri P, Walz A, Dewald B, Baggiolini M. A novel neutrophil-activating factor produced by human mononuclear phagocytes. J Exp Med. 1988;167:1547–59.
37. Schroeder JM, Christophers E. Secretion of novel and homologous neutrophil-activating peptides by LPS-stimulated human endothelial cells. J Immunol. 1989;142:244–51.
38. Strieter RM, Phan SH, Showell HJ et al. Monokine-induced neutrophil chemotactic factor gene expression in human fibroblasts. J Biol Chem. 1989;264:10621–6.
39. Elner VM, Strieter RM, Elner SG, Baggiolini M, Linley I, Kunkel SL. Neutrophil chemotactic factor (IL-8) gene expression by cytokine treated retinal pigment epithelial cells. Am J Pathol. 1990;136:745–50.
40. Schmouder RL, Strieter RM, Wiggrins RC, Chensue SW, Kunkel SL. In vitro and in vivo interleukin-8 production in human renal cortical epithelia. Kidney Int. 1992;41:191–8.
41. Eckmann L, Jung HC, Schürer-Maly C, Panja A, Morzycka-Wroblewska E, Kagnoff MF. Differential cytokine expression by human intestinal epithelial cell lines: Regulated expression of interleukin-8. Gastroenterology. 1993;105:1689–97.

42. Nguyen HC, Ohno Y, Reinecker HC, Furth EE, MacDermott RP, Rombeau JC. CaCo-2 cells synthesize and secrete increased amounts of interleukin-8 after stimulation by PMA, IL-1$\alpha$, and IL-1$\beta$. Gastroenterology. 1993;104:A754.

43. Gross V, Andus T, Daig R, Aschenbrenner L, Falk W, Schölmerich J. Protein tyrosine kinase activation is required for induction of IL-8 by IL-1 or TNF in an intestinal epithelial cell line (HT-29). Gastroenterology. 1994;106:A694.

44. Mahida YR, Ceska M, Effenberger F, Kurlak L, Lindley I, Hawkey CJ. Enhanced synthesis of neutrophil-activating peptide-I/interleukin-8 in active ulcerative colitis. Clin Sci. 1992;82:273–5.

45. Izzo RS, Witkon K, Chen AI, Hadjiyane C, Weinstein MI, Pellecchia C. Neutrophil-activating peptide (interleukin-8) in colonic mucosa from patients with Crohn's disease. Scand J Gastroenterol. 1993;28:296–300.

46. Cominelli F, Nast CC, Clark BD et al. Interleukin-1 (IL-1) gene expression synthesis, and effect of specific IL-1 receptor blockade in rabbit immune complex colitis. J Clin Invest. 1990;86:972–80.

47. Sartor RB, Holt LC, Bender DE, Murphy ME, McCall RD, Thompson RC. Prevention and treatment of experimental enterocolitis with a recombinant interleukin-1 receptor antagonist. Gastroenterology. 1991;100:A613.

48. Murthy SN, Fondacaro JD, Murthy NS, Bolkenius F, Cooper HS. Effects of MDL 73404 (MDL) in experimental murine colitis. Gastroenterology. 1993;104:A752.

49. Casini-Raggi V, Herbert C, Monsacchi L, Cominelli F. A specific monoclonal antibody (MoAb) against interleukin-8 (IL-8) suppresses inflammation in rabbit immune colitis. Gastroenterology. 1994;106:A661.

50. Derkx B, Taminian J, Radema S, Stronkhorst A, Wortel C, Tytgat G, van Deventer S. Tumor-necrosis-factor antibody treatment in Crohn's disease. Lancet. 1993;342:173–4.

51. Van Dullemen HM, Hommes DW, Meenan J et al. Complete remissions of steroid-refractory Crohn's disease after administration of monoclonal anti-TNF antibody cA2. Gastroenterology. 1994;106:A1054.

52. Echtenacher B, Falk W, Männel DN, Krammer PH. Requirement of endogenous tumor necrosis factor/cachectin for recovery from experimental peritonitis. J Immunol. 1990;145:3762–6.

# 7
# Role of nitric oxide and free radicals in the pathogenesis of IBD

D. RACHMILEWITZ, J. S. STAMLER, F. KARMELI,
R. J. XAVIER, D. K. PODOLSKY and R. SAMUNI

## INTRODUCTION

The interaction of proinflammatory mediators, such as leukotriene $B_4$ ($LTB_4$) and platelet activating factor (PAF), with receptors on the plasma membrane of phagocytes activates NADPH oxidase to catalyse the reduction of $O_2$ to $O_2^-$ and $H_2O_2$. The interaction of $O_2^-$ and $H_2O_2$ with low-molecular-weight transition iron metals, such as Fe, yields the highly reactive radical $OH^\bullet$. Activated inflammatory cells secrete myeloperoxidase which catalyses the oxidation of halides, such as $Cl^-$ to yield the oxidizing agent, HOCl.

$$O_2 \xrightarrow{\text{NADPH}} O_2^- \rightarrow H_2O_2$$

$$O_2^- + H_2O_2 \xrightarrow{Fe^{3+}} O_2 + OH^- + OH^\bullet$$

$$H_2O_2 + Cl^- \xrightarrow{\text{MPO}} HOCl$$

Reactive oxygen metabolites induce lipid peroxidation, protein and sulphydryl oxidation and deoxyribose oxidation. HOCl also induces amino acid decarboxylation, protein degradation and chlorination of unsaturated fatty acids. All these processes alter membrane electrolyte transport because of their inability to maintain ionic gradients. The intracellular accumulation of calcium alters the cytoskeletal function and activates enzymes, such as phospholipase and protein kinase. These effects induce further changes in the chemical composition of cell membranes. Cell destruction is also induced by free-radical-mediated inactivation of essential enzymes, such as glycolytic enzymes. In addition, cytotoxicity and mutagenesis are induced by the free-radical-mediated degradation of DNA-associated deoxyribose which breaks the DNA backbone.

Nitric oxide (NO), in addition to its classical functions as neurotransmitter and vasodilator, has an important role in inflammatory processes, being a mediator of macrophage function[1]. NO is generated by the enzyme family, NO synthase (NOS), which is present in macrophages, granulocytes, neurons, endothelial cells and epithelial cells. NOS is present in several molecular isoforms: the two major subtypes encompass a constitutive form – calcium dependent, and an inducible form – calcium independent. The inducible isoform is the type expressed mainly in inflammatory cells[2]. Under basal conditions NOS activity in macrophages is negligible but stimulation with lipopolysaccharide or cytokines produces effective increases in NO generation. The inducible NOS activity is inhibited by glucocorticoids.

NO secreted by activated macrophages is an important cytotoxic molecule in the defence against various infectious agents, as well as in tumour cells[1,3]. However, high NO levels may be toxic and may damage healthy tissue. The coproduction of NO and superoxide by activated macrophages and inflammatory granulocytes, yields the highly cytotoxic species, peroxynitrite[4]:

$$O_2^{\cdot -} + NO^{\cdot} \rightarrow OONO^-$$

Peroxynitrite is stable only in alkaline solutions and, once protonated, it decays rapidly to the potent biological oxidants, $HO^{\cdot}$ and $NO_2^{\cdot}$.

$$OONO^- + H^+ \leftrightarrow OONOH \rightarrow OH^{\cdot} + NO_2^{\cdot} \rightarrow NO_3^{\cdot} + H^+$$

Peroxynitrite directly oxidizes sulphydryl groups at a rapid rate[5] and initiates lipid peroxidation without requirement for a transition metal[4].

In various pathological conditions, such as active inflammation, sepsis and reperfusion injury of ischaemic tissue, the simultaneous production of superoxide and NO, may lead to peroxynitrite formation[6]. Moreover, scavenging of superoxide, thereby limiting peroxynitrite formation, is one of the mechanisms to explain the reduction of tissue injury in experimental ischaemia by superoxide dismutase[7].

Experimental colitis and inflammatory bowel disease (IBD) are characterized by mucosal abundance of activated macrophages and granulocytes. Generation of high NO levels by these cells may lead to perpetuation and amplification of tissue injury, regardless of its trigger. In the present study, colonic mucosal $NO_x$ generation and NOS activity were determined in IBD patients and in two models of experimental colitis. In order to assess the potential deleterious effect of $NO^{\cdot}$, a model of peroxynitrite-induced colitis was established. In addition, the possible amelioration of colonic injury by potent scavengers of free radicals was evaluated.

## MATERIALS AND METHODS

### Trinitrobenzene sulphonic-acid-induced colitis

Inflammation of the colon was induced in male rats (200–250 g) under light ether anaesthesia by a single intracolonic administration of 0.25 ml of 50% ethanol containing 30 mg of trinitrobenzene sulphonic acid (TNB)[8]. The solution was introduced via a catheter placed 7 cm from the anus. The rats were killed 24 h after the induction of colonic injury. The colon was isolated and a 7-cm segment of distal colon was resected, its lumen rinsed with ice-cold saline and weighed. After obtaining tissue samples for organ culture, the remaining mucosa was scraped. Samples of the mucosal scrapings were processed for determination of NOS activity. Treated rats were given Tempol (0.5 g/kg) intragastrically immediately after induction of colonic damage and once daily thereafter until sacrifice. The control group was treated with saline.

## Acetic-acid-induced colitis

In male rats, under light ether anaesthesia, a midline abdominal incision was made and 2 ml of 5% acetic acid was injected into the lumen of the colon at its proximal part. The midline incision was closed and 24 h later the rats were killed and their colons removed and processed as in the TNB model. The treated rats received intragastric Tempol (0.5 g/kg) or 0.5 ml of saline immediately after damage induction.

## Determination of mucosal damage

Mucosal damage was quantitated as previously reported[9]. Both the macroscopic appearance and the lesion area were assessed and scored. In the scoring system, 0 = no damage; 1 = hyperaemia; 2 = linear ulceration without hyperaemia or bowel wall thickening; 3 = linear ulcer with inflammation; 4 = two or more sites of ulcers; 5 = two or more sites of major ulceration or one major site of damage >1 cm long; 6–10 = ulceration > 2 cm long.

## Induction of colitis with peroxynitrite

Under light ether anaesthesia, 0.165–3.3 mmol/L peroxynitrite, synthesized as previously described[4] in 0.4 ml of 0.15 mol/L NaCl, was introduced intrarectally via a catheter placed 5 cm from the anus. Control rats were treated with the vehicle, 0.1 ml of 0.1 mol/L NaOH and 0.4 ml of 0.15 mol/L NaCl. Rats were sacrificed 1, 3, 7, 14 and 21 days after the induction of colonic injury. The colon was isolated and a 7-cm long segment of the distal colon proximal to the anus was resected, its lumen rinsed with ice-cold saline and weighed. Cross-sections were obtained for histology. The remaining mucosa was scraped and processed for determination of myeloperoxidase activity.

## Human studies

Colonoscopic biopsies were obtained from inflamed and uninflamed sites of IBD patients and from normal controls. Colonic mucosal scrapings were obtained from surgical specimens of patients with active ulcerative colitis and from normal mucosa at the edge of colonic segments resected for colonic cancer.

## Organ culture

Human and rat colonic explants were cultured as previously described[9]. The tissue was weighed, oriented on metal grids and organ cultured for 24 h at 37°C, 95% $O_2$, 5% $CO_2$ in AIM-V medium (Gibco) containing penicillin and gentamicin. In several experiments, explants were organ cultured in the presence of calcium ionophore, lipopolysaccharide, $N^w$-nitro-L-arginine or interferon-$\gamma$.

## Measurement of NO production and NOS activity

NO, quantified by the accumulation of nitrite in the culture medium, was measured spectrophotometrically using the Greiss reaction[10] with sodium nitrite as a standard. NOS activity was monitored by the conversion of [$^3$H]L-arginine to citrulline, according to Bush et al.[11].

## Morphological studies

Sections of colon were fixed in phosphate-buffered formaldehyde, embedded in paraffin and routine 5-$\mu$m sections were prepared. Tissues were routinely stained with haematoxylin and eosin and were blindly evaluated by light microscopy.

## Statistical analysis

Data are expressed as the mean ($\pm$ SEM). Statistical analysis for significant differences was performed according to the Student's *t*-test for unpaired data and the Mann–Whitney U-test.

## RESULTS

Intracolonic administration of TNB/ethanol resulted in extensive haemorrhagic and ulcerative damage to the distal colon, as we have previously reported[8,9]. By 24 h, the damage was localized with a lesion score of $9.0 \pm 4.8$ and a lesion area of $616 \pm 54$ mm$^2$ ($n = 9$; mean $\pm$ SE). Twenty-four hours after administration of acetic acid, the colon was haemorrhagic and inflamed. The lesion score reached $5.8 \pm 0.6$ and the lesion area $213 \pm 46$ mm$^2$ ($n = 18$; mean $\pm$ SE). During 24 h of culture, NO$_x$ generation by inflamed colonic segments isolated from acetic-acid- and TNB-treated rats was 2- and 6-fold, respectively, higher than by explants isolated from control rats. In acetic-acid- and TNB-treated rats, colonic mucosal NOS activity was 1.5- and 4-fold, respectively, higher than in normal colonic mucosa (Table 1). Both in normal rats and in rats with experimental colitis, colonic NOS activity was significantly inhibited by N$^w$-nitro-L-arginine and was NADPH dependent.

NO$_x$ generation by cultured mucosal explants obtained from patients with active ulcerative colitis and Crohn colitis was 5- to 15-fold higher than by mucosal explants obtained from normal subjects (Table 1). In ulcerative colitis patients, NO$_x$ generation by explants obtained from healthy uninflamed mucosa was significantly lower than that from inflamed mucosa obtained from the same subjects.

Colonic NOS activity in patients with active ulcerative colitis was 2-fold higher than that in normal colonic mucosa (Table 1). Both in normal subjects and in patients with active ulcerative colitis, colonic NOS activity was significantly inhibited by the deletion of NADPH.

Tempol (0.5 g/kg body weight), given intragastrically immediately after TNB administration, decreased the lesion area by 43%. Co-administration of TNB and Tempol intrarectally did not significantly affect the extent of the damage induced by TNB, $503 \pm 115$ mm$^2$ ($n = 9$). In rats sacrificed 72 h after TNB

**Table 1** $NO_x$ generation in normal and inflamed colonic mucosa

| | $NO_x$ generation | | NO synthase | |
| --- | --- | --- | --- | --- |
| | $n$ | Basal ($\mu$mol/g) | $n$ | (nmol g$^{-1}$ min$^{-1}$) |
| Rats | | | | |
| Normal | 27 | $258 \pm 27$ | 8 | $2.0 \pm 0.2$ |
| Acetic acid colitis | 18 | $539 \pm 60^*$ | 12 | $3.0 \pm 0.4^*$ |
| TNB colitis | 12 | $1705 \pm 29^*$ | 7 | $8.7 \pm 0.2^*$ |
| Human | | | | |
| Normal | 26 | $172 \pm 33$ | 23 | $5.7 \pm 0.9$ |
| UC – inflamed | 19 | $1128 \pm 303^*$ | 13 | $10.0 \pm 2.1^*$ |
| UC – not inflamed | 4 | $281 \pm 96$ | | |
| CD – inflamed | 7 | $3358 \pm 1550^*$ | | |

Colonic explants and mucosal scrapings were obtained from normal, acetic acid- and TNB-treated rats, and from normal subjects and patients with ulcerative colitis (UC) and Crohn disease (CD). $NO_x$ generation during 24 h of organ culture and NOS activity were determined. Results are mean $\pm$SE. *Significantly different from normal, $p < 0.05$

administration and receiving Tempol, 0.5 g/kg body weight daily, the lesion area, $147 \pm 39$ mm$^2$ ($n = 10$) was reduced compared with that in rats treated with TNB only, $695 \pm 56$ mm$^2$ ($n = 17$) ($p < 0.05$). One week after the induction of damage by TNB, the lesion area was $826 \pm 125$ mm$^2$ ($n = 14$), while, in rats treated daily with Tempol, the lesion area averaged $217 \pm 142$ mm$^2$ ($n = 6$) ($p < 0.05$) (Table 2). Tempol prevented the increase in colonic weight observed 24 h and 72 h following TNB treatment.

One and three days after TNB administration, a section through the colonic wall showed widespread mucosal ulcerations with oedema and an acute inflammatory cell exudate in the lamina propria, extending also into the muscularis propria. Cross-sections through the intestinal wall of rats treated with TNB and Tempol showed similar findings, albeit with a slight decrease in the inflammatory infiltrate in the lamina propria and muscularis propria. Histological examination of colonic sections obtained from TNB-treated rats following one week of Tempol treatment revealed relative protection of the mucosa. The mucosal ulcerations were superficial and less extensive than those observed in rats treated with TNB.

Acetic acid induced extensive colitis. Twenty-four hours after its administration, the lesion area was $372 \pm 48$ mm$^2$ ($p < 0.05$; $n = 18$). Myeloperoxidase (MPO) activity increased from $1.5 \pm 0.5$ U/g in saline-treated rats to $3.5 \pm 0.7$ U/g in acetic-acid-treated rats.

In rats treated with Tempol immediately after induction of damage with acetic acid, there was significant (87%) reduction in the lesion area. The protection provided by Tempol was accompanied by a two-fold decrease in mucosal MPO activity (Table 2). Administration of five doses of tempol to acetic-acid-treated rats before and after damage induction did not provide further protection compared with administration of a single dose of Tempol. Intragastric administration of BSA also did not protect against acetic-acid-induced colonic damage (results not shown).

**Table 2** Effect of Tempol on TNB/ethanol- and acetic-acid-induced colitis

| | None | 24 hours | | 72 hours | | 7 days | | 24 hours | |
|---|---|---|---|---|---|---|---|---|---|
| | | TNB | TNB + Tempol | TNB | TNB + Tempol | TNB | TNB + Tempol | Acetic acid | Acetic acid + Tempol |
| No. of rats | 20 | 9 | 10 | 14–17 | 10 | 14 | 6 | 10–18 | 8–20 |
| Lesion area ($mm^2$) | — | $616 \pm 54$ | $354 \pm 111$** | $695 \pm 56$* | $147 \pm 39$** | $826 \pm 125$* | $217 \pm 142$** | — | — |
| Weight (g/10 cm) | $0.69 \pm 0.02$ | $5.30 \pm 0.09$* | $1.40 \pm 0.15$ | $2.00 \pm 0.10$* | $1.60 \pm 0.08$* | $2.21 \pm 0.20$* | $2.10 \pm 0.30$ | $0.92 \pm 0.05$* | $0.90 \pm 0.05$ |
| MPO activity (U/g) | $1.5 \pm 0.5$ (0.1–5.3) | — | — | — | — | — | — | $3.5 \pm 0.7$ (0.8–7.7) | $1.4 \pm 0.2$** (0.4–3.1) |

Colitis was induced by the intracolonic administration of 0.25 ml of 50% ethanol containing 30 mg TNB, or by intrarectal injection of 5% acetic acid, as described in Methods. Treated rats were given tempol (0.5 g/kg) intragastrically, once daily. Rats were sacrificed 24 h, 72 h or one week after damage induction with TNB or 24 h after acetic-acid treatment, and their colons processed as described in Methods. Results are mean $\pm$ SE.

* Significantly different from control rats (Mann–Whitney and Student's $t$ test), $p < 0.05$.

** Significantly different from TNB- or acetic-acid-treated rats only (Mann–Whitney and Student's $t$ test), $p < 0.05$

Histological section of colonic segments obtained from acetic-acid-treated rats revealed widespread deep ulcerations with an extensive acute inflammatory cell exudate. There was marked oedema with haemorrhages in the submucosa with an extension of the infiltrate into the muscularis propria. In contrast, the colonic wall of rats treated with tempol (0.5 g/kg body weight) showed an intact mucosa with only a mild inflammatory infiltrate confined to the mucosa.

Intrarectal administration of peroxynitrite induced mucosal inflammation and injury, which were time and dose dependent. Treatment with the vehicle did not induce any damage, indicating that mucosal injury induced by peroxynitrite is specific.

Maximal injury was observed 24 h after treatment. Macroscopically, the lesions progressed from congestion, erythema and patchy haemorrhage to overt ulceration. Mucosal oedema with occasional haemorrhagic ulceration was apparent following 24-h administration of 3.3 mmol/L peroxynitrite. The damage induced by 3.3 mmol/L was followed for up to 21 days after treatment. At three days, the bowel wall was thick and oedematous. On day 7, the lumen was narrow and on day 21 there were signs of stenosis.

Transmucosal necrosis was maximal 24 h post-treatment with 3.3 mmol/L. The injury was characterized predominantly by haemorrhage, exudative oedema and inflammatory cell infiltration (Figure 1). The muscularis mucosa was

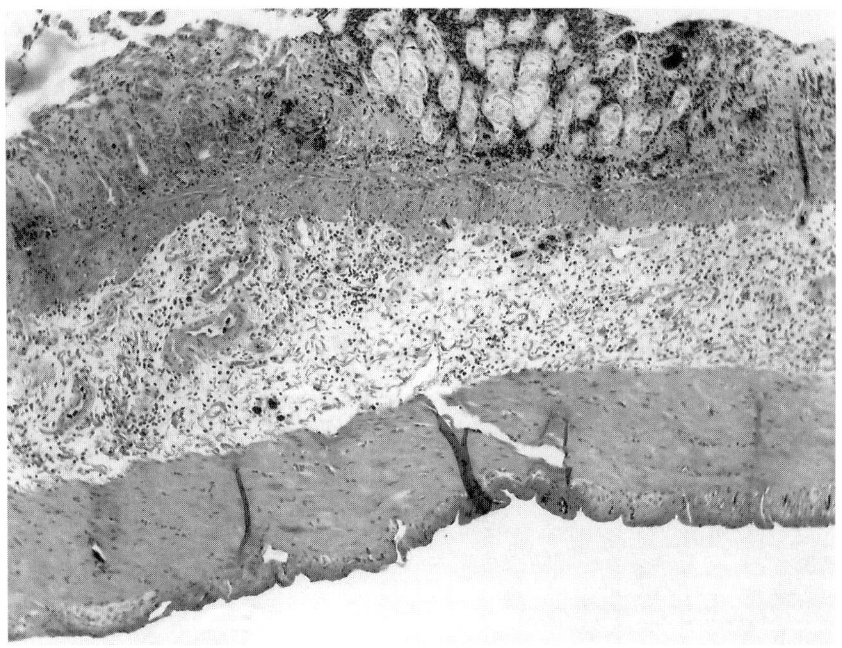

**Figure 1** Cross-section of colon obtained 24 h after exposure to peroxynitrite (3.3 mmol/L). Extensive transmucosal haemorrhagic necrosis with mild inflammatory cell infiltrate is present, together with extensive submucosal oedema. The muscularis mucosa is necrotic. H&E, magnification × 4

necrotic and increased inflammatory cellularity was noted in the lamina propria and submucosa. Expansion of the distance between the mucosa and external muscular layer was due to formation of exudative oedema.

There was progressive increase in neutrophilic infiltration in the lamina propria and submucosa three days and one week post-treatment with peroxynitrite (3.3 mmol/L). Attempts at surface re-epithelialization and viable muscularis mucosa were observed at one week. Two weeks post-treatment, the acute inflammation had completely resolved and the epithelial mucin distribution was normal. At three weeks there was increased fibrosis within the lamina propria and the muscularis mucosa and propria appeared markedly thickened (Figure 2).

## DISCUSSION

Activated inflammatory cells present in inflamed colonic mucosa synthesize and release cytokines and inflammatory mediators, as well as reactive oxygen metabolites[12]. Macrophages and inflammatory neutrophils also contain an inducible NOS that is activated by cytokines and bacterial products[1,2]. NO is generated from L-arginine. NO is a mediator of immunoregulatory[13], bactericidal, tumoristatic and tumoricidal activity of macrophages[1,3]. These latter properties are ascribed to the simultaneous generation of peroxynitrite from $O_2^-$ and

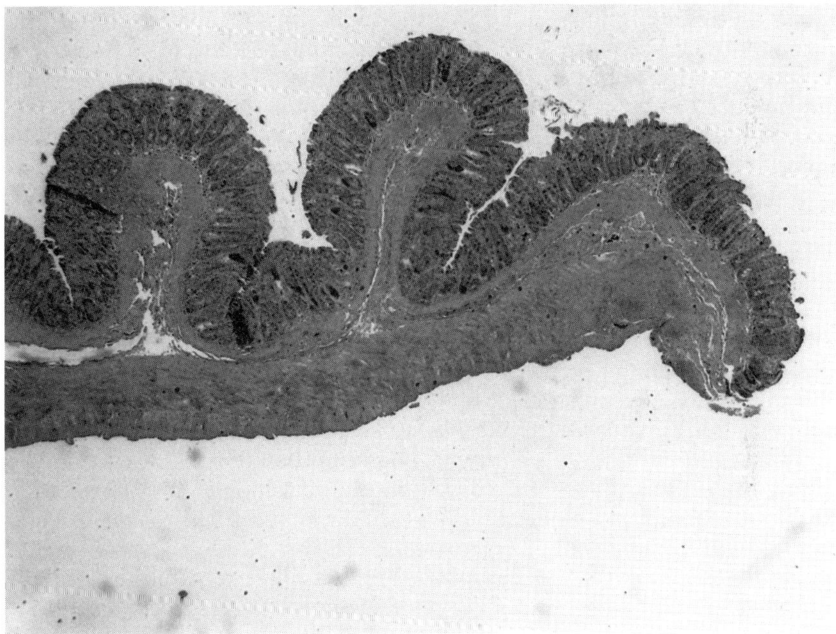

**Figure 2**  Cross section of colon obtained 21 days after exposure to peroxynitrite (3.3 mmol/L). Complete epithelial restitution is seen. There is marked thickening of muscularis mucosa and propria, together with mild fibrosis in the lamina propria (H&E, magnification × 4)

NO, which decompose to OH$^\cdot$ and NO$_2^\cdot$, two of the strongest biological oxidants. Peroxynitrite may be involved in the pathogenesis of tissue damage and inflammation, irrespective of its aetiology. The very short half-life of peroxynitrite prevents its direct detection in biological systems. In this study, peroxynitrite, in doses which may be locally produced[6], was shown to induce tissue injury and inflammation. The extent and severity of the damage induced were verified macroscopically and histologically.

Both in two models of experimental colitis and in patients with active ulcerative colitis and Crohn disease, colonic generation of nitrites reflecting NO$_x$ generation and colonic NOS activity are significantly increased when compared with the respective NO$_x$ generation and NOS activity of normal colonic mucosa. In both the two models of experimental colitis and in patients with active ulcerative colitis, the magnitude of stimulation of NOS activity correlates with the respective increase in NO$_x$ generation by colonic explants during 24 h of culture. Moreover, in experimental colitis, the magnitudes of the increases in colonic NO$_x$ generation and NOS activity were found to correlate with severity of tissue damage. The stimulation of colonic NO$_x$ generation in inflamed colonic segments is probably derived from macrophages and inflammatory neutrophils in which NO$_x$ generation is inducible[1].

NO is important for organ defence. It possesses bactericidal and cytostatic properties. However, in extreme excess it may have deleterious effects. The enhanced NO$_x$ generation by the inflamed colonic mucosa may amplify the extent of tissue inflammation and injury. Enhanced generation of free NO radical species by stimulated NOS of macrophages, inflammatory neutrophils and possibly other inflammatory cells may determine the extent and severity of the inflammatory response. Moreover, the enhanced colonic NO$_x$ generation may produce carcinogenic nitrosamines known to be generated by neutrophils during active intestinal inflammation[14]. Formation of nitrosamines may contribute to the increased risk of malignancy in chronic inflammatory bowel disease patients. The results obtained in this study encourage evaluation of modulation of NOS activity in order to develop possible therapeutic modalities in patients with inflammatory bowel disease.

Reactive oxygen metabolites mediate cell injury. Oxygen-derived free radicals are generated by several sources, including stimulated polymorphonuclear cells, eosinophils, xanthine oxidase, colonic bacteria and epithelial lipoxygenase, all of which are present in the inflamed bowel of inflammatory bowel disease patients. Several strategies for drug intervention specifically directed at the attenuation of oxidative stress have been considered. These include blocking of O$_2^-$ formation by phagocytes, scavenging of O$_2^-$ before it can react with iron, binding iron so that it does not redox cycle and scavenging $^\cdot$OH or HOCl. The primary defence against oxidative insult to tissue includes superoxide dismutase (SOD), catalase and glutathione peroxidase[5]. SOD and catalase were shown, in rats, to reduce intestinal damage induced by ischaemia reperfusion[24] and also experimental colitis[5,15–18,25]. They were also shown to be effective in uncontrolled clinical trials in human inflammatory bowel disease[19,20]. However, the short half-life of exogenously administered SOD and its inability to penetrate into cells where superoxide is formed have limited the potential of this treatment and led to a search for cell-permeable compounds possessing SOD-mimicking activity[21,22].

Tempol is a non-toxic cyclic-nitroxide stable radical that blocks biological damage by breaking chain reactions through selective termination reactions with deleterious free radicals[23]. In the present study, intragastric administration of tempol immediately after the induction of colitis by acetic acid provided significant and impressive protection. Tempol provides less-remarkable protection against injury induced by TNB/ethanol. In this model of experimental colitis, the protection reflected by a decrease in the lesion area was not correlated with histological appearance. The different type of insult in two models might be responsible for the different protective effects of Tempol. The injury induced by the acetic acid is superficial, affecting the mucosa, whereas, in the TNB model, the damage is more extensive and extends also to the muscularis propria.

Several mechanisms, all of which involve an interception of paramagnetic species, underlie the protection provided by nitroxides: both the nitroxide and its respective hydroxylamine can react with $O_2^-$, yielding oxygen and $H_2O_2$. Recently, the nitroxide and its respective oxoammonium cation are shown[24] to act also as a SOD-mimic, rapidly reacting with $O_2^-$, yielding oxygen and $H_2O_2$. Unlike SOD, nitroxides can remove both intra- and extracellular radicals.

The physiological function of SOD, which is present in cells of all aerobes, is to dismutate $O_2^-$, converting it to oxygen and $H_2O_2$. Yet, SOD cannot protect against $H_2O_2$-induced damage. Nitroxides also protect cells by reacting with reduced metal ions which usually, in aerated systems, react with $H_2O_2$, yielding a peroxo complex. Nitroxides compete with $H_2O_2$, oxidizing the reduced metal ions, such as iron[23], and protecting hypoxic cells where ROS are practically absent. Nitroxides protect hypoxic Chinese hamster cells against t-BuOOH-induced toxicity, which is catalysed by transition metals[23] and also against mitomycin C-induced toxicity[25].

The present study shows that both the acetic acid and TNB/ethanol models of colitis can be manipulated by Tempol, a non-toxic cell-permeable cycle nitroxide. The protection afforded by Tempol further implicates oxygen-derived free radicals in the pathogenesis of experimental colitis and provides a new approach towards the possible treatment and/or prevention of inflammatory bowel disease.

## References


1. Nathan C. Nitric oxide as a secretory product of mammalian cells. FASEB J. 1992;6:3051–64.
2. Xie Q, Cho HJ, Calaycay J et al. Cloning and characterization of inducible nitric oxide synthase from mouse macrophages. Science. 1992;256:225–8.
3. Ignarro LJ. Biosynthesis and metabolism of endothelium derived nitric oxide. Annu Rev Pharmacol Toxicol. 1990;30:535–60.
4. Beckman JS, Beckman TW, Chen J, Marshall PA, Freeman BA. Apparent hydroxyl radical production by peroxynitrite: Implications for endothelial injury from nitric oxide and superoxide. Proc Natl Acad Sci USA. 1990;87:1620–4.
5. Radi, R, Beckman TW, Bush KM, Freeman BA. Peroxynitrite oxidation of sulfhydryls. J Biol Chem. 1991;266:4244–50.
6. Ischiropoulos H, Zhu I, Beckman JS. Peroxynitrite formation from macrophage derived nitric oxide. Arch Biochem Biophys. 1992; 298:446–51.

7. Gryglewski RJ, Palmer RMJ, Moncada S. Superoxide anion is involved in the breakdown of endothelium derived vascular relaxing factor. Nature. 1986;320:454–6.
8. Rachmilewitz D, Simon PL, Schwartz LW, Griswold DE, Fondacaro JD, Wasserman MA. Inflammatory mediators of experimental colitis in rats. Gastroenterology. 1989;97:326–37.
9. Sharon P, Ligumsky M, Rachmilewitz D, Zor U. Role of prostaglandins in ulcerative colitis: Enhanced production during active disease and inhibition by sulphasalazine. Gastroenterology. 1978;65:638–40.
10. Stuehr DJ, Marletta MA. Mammalian nitrite biosynthesis: Mouse macrophages produce nitrite and nitrate in response to Escherichia coli lipopolysaccharide. Proc Natl Acad Sci USA. 1985;82:7738–42.
11. Bush PA, Gonzalez NE, Griscavage JM, Ignarro LJ. Nitric oxide synthase from cerebellum catalyzes the formation of equimolar quantities of nitric oxide and citrulline from L-arginine. Biochem Biophys Res Commun. 1992;185:960–6.
12. Skaleric U, Allen JB, Smith PD, Mergenhagen SE, Wahl SM. Inhibitors of reactive oxygen intermediates suppress bacterial cell wall-induced arthritis. J Immunol. 1991;147:259–264.
13. Albina JE, Abate JA, Henry WL. Nitric oxide production is required for murine resident peritoneal macrophages to suppress mitogen-stimulated T-cell proliferation: Role of INF-$\gamma$ in the induction of the nitric oxide synthesizing pathway. J Immunol. 1991;197:144–8.
14. Pallapies D, Peskar BA, Peskar BM. 5-Aminosalicylic acid (5-ASA) inhibits the activity of nitric oxide (NO): Contribution to its anti-inflammatory effects. Gastroenterology. 1992;102:A677 (abstract).
15. Babbs CF. Oxygen radicals in ulcerative colitis. Free Rad Biol Med. 1992;13:169–81.
16. Fretland DJ, Widomski DL, Anglin CP. Superoxide dismutase (SOD) modulates acetic acid-induced colitis in rodents. Gastroenterology. 1991;100:A581 (abstract).
17. Burakoff R, Zhao L, Joseph I, Kor H, Rosenfeld W. SOD prevents colitis and attenuates eicosanoid release and motility changes in trinitrobenzene sulfonic acid rabbit colitis. Gastroenterology. 1991;100:A565 (abstract).
18. Keshavarzian A, Haydeck J, Zabihi R, Doria M, D'Astice M, Sorenson JRJ. Agents capable of eliminating reactive oxygen species, catalase, WR-2721, or Cu(II) 2(3,5OIPS)4 decrease experimental colitis. Dig Dis Sci. 1992;37:1866–73.
19. Emerit J, Pelletier S, Tosoni-Verlignue D, Mollet M. Phase II trial of copper zinc superoxide dismutase (CuZnSOD) in the treatment of Crohn's disease. Free Rad Biol Med. 1989;7:145–9.
20. Emerit J, Pelletier S, Likforman J, Pasquier C, Thuillier A. Phase II trial of copper zinc superoxide dismutase (CuZnSOD) in the treatment of Crohn's disease. Free Rad Res Commun. 1991;12–13:565–9.
21. Brigelius R, Spottl R, Bors W, Lengfelder E, Saran M, Weser U. Superoxide dismutase activity of low molecular weight Cu2′ chelates studied by pulse radiolysis. FEBS Lett. 1974;47:72–5.
22. Koppenol WH, Levine F, Hatmaker TL, Epp J, Rush JD. Catalysis of superoxide dismutation by manganese aminopolycarboxylate complexes. Arch Biochem Biophys. 1986;251:595–9.
23. Mitchell JB, Samuni A, Krishna MC et al. Biologically active metal-independent superoxide dismutase mimics. Biochemistry. 1990;29:2802–7.
24. Krishna MC, Graham DA, Samuni A, Mitchell JB, Russo A. Oxoammonium cation intermediates in the nitroxide catalyzed dismutation of superoxide. Proc Natl Acad Sci USA. 1992;89:5537–41.
25. Krishna MC, de Graff W, Tamura S et al. Mechanisms on hypoxic and aerobic cytotoxicity of mitomycin C in Chinese hamster V-79 cells. Cancer Res. 1991;51:G622–8.

# Section II
# Extraintestinal manifestations and special problems in IBD

# 8
# Enterogenic arthropathy

## A. STROEHMANN, A. KRAUSE and G.-R. BURMESTER

## INTRODUCTION

Besides rheumatoid arthritis and ankylosing spondylitis, reactive arthritis is one of the most frequent inflammatory joint disorders. Reactive arthritis is characterized by a sterile synovitis after a previous extra-articular infection, mostly of the gastrointestinal or genitourinary tract. Gastrointestinal disorders like Crohn disease, ulcerative colitis and, less frequently, Whipple disease may also cause a joint inflammation called enteropathic arthritis; therefore, a more generalized terminology for these diseases is enterogenic arthropathy.

## PATHOGENESIS

Regardless of the underlying mechanism, such as bacterial infection with *Yersinia*, *Shigella*, *Salmonella*, *Campylobacter* or chronic inflammatory gastrointestinal diseases, including Crohn disease, ulcerative colitis, Whipple disease, or intestinal bypass surgery, the involvement of the synovia as matrix of inflammation is characteristic for enterogenic arthritis. The synovial tissue consists only of the synovial lining cells; the basement membrane is missing. Therefore, a variety of inflammatory substrates may pass into the joint space, where they induce and maintain inflammatory processes. Finally, hyperplastic synovial lining cells and large lymphocytic infiltrates appear. Table 1 shows the pathogenic mechanisms hypothesized.

One postulated mechanism leading to inflammation is the direct attack of synoviotropic micro-organisms and a consecutive exaggerated host defence. Another possibility would be the formation of immune complexes composed of microbacterial products combined with specific antibodies which initiate inflammation on the synovial site. Activation of the complement cascade, especially the alternative pathway, may then induce a hypersensitivity reaction type III (Arthus reaction). In addition, approximately 80% of the affected patients bear the HLA-B27 phenotype, while the frequency of this gene usually is only 8% in the general Caucasian population. HLA-B27 is an allele of the

**Table 1**   Hypothesized pathogenesis of reactive joint lesions and pathogenetic role of HLA-B27 in reactive arthritis

---

**Hypothesized pathogenesis of reactive joint lesions**

Direct attack of synovia by micro-organisms and exaggerated host defence

Bacterial products, specific antibodies by genetically predisposed individuals (e.g. HLA-B27-positive) causing immune complexes, consecutive complement activation and Arthus (type III) reaction

Molecular mimicry of bacterial products and hiscompatibility antigens inducing
    Autoimmune phenomena or
    Specific non-responsiveness against certain micro-organisms

**Pathogenetic role of HLA-B27 in reactive arthritis**
    Molecular mimicry
        Cross-reactive antibodies recognizing both HLA-B27 antigen and bacterial antigen (due to amino acid sequence homologies between HLA-B27 and certain bacterial antigenic epitopes) initiate an autoimmune response

    HLA-B27 modifying factors
        Some bacteria secrete factors which bind to HLA-B27 and modify it, resulting in cross-reactive antibodies to HLA-B27

    Defective first-line defence
        HLA-B27 facilitates the invasion of pathogens at the mucosal surface in a non-immunological fashion

    Arthritogenic peptide
        Bacterial or self antigen is presented by HLA-B27, stimulates cytotoxic T lymphocytes (CTL) which then mediate the arthritis

---

Adapted from Hermann E et al., Akt Rheumatol. 1994;19:77–83.

human leukocyte antigen B locus belonging to the major histocompatibility (MHC) gene complex. The role of HLA-B27 in seronegative arthritis has still not been clarified completely. Recently, a transgenic animal model with inbred Lewis and Fisher 344 rat strains has been established[17]. These rats exhibited the human HLA-B27 and interestingly developed HLA-B27-associated diseases like arthritis after inflammatory bowel disease, skin changes, cardiac and genital inflammation. Still the exact mechanisms remain unclear. A hypothesized similarity of the histocompatibility antigen HLA-B27 and certain bacterial products would induce tolerance to the infectant; thus, the immune system cannot discriminate between self and non-self. There are hints of an antigenic similarity of the HLA-B27 molecule and certain *Klebsiella* types, but others were unable to reproduce these experimental findings. HLA-B27-positive individuals would be unable to eliminate the infection in an appropriate way leading to persistent infection, the products of which then induce synovitis. In the affected joints, no other bacterial products have been found with the exception of chlamydial DNA detected by PCR techniques or *Yersinia* proteins. Likewise, in inflammatory bowel disease, the integrity of the intestinal barrier is affected by inflammation of the bowel; antigenic material is able to pass more easily into the circulation and may be enriched at the synovial site of the membrane.

# WORK-UP OF THE PATIENT WITH ENTEROGENIC ARTHROPATHY

A thorough patient history is of great importance to establish the exact diagnosis. Swelling, elevated temperature, pain and tenderness of joints occur, but previous events, such as fever, diarrhoea, abdominal pain, dysuria or genital infections and conjunctivitis, need to be asked for. Other important aspects are manifestations of the skin, e.g. erythema nodosum, localized lesions like the aphthosis in Behçet disease, or more generalized erythemas in virus infections. Finally, previous episodes of bowel affections, prior therapeutic interventions and the family history have to be noted. Table 2 condenses the important anamnestic features.

The physical examination should include a general examination and a specific examination of the gastrointestinal, genitourinary and skeletal system. The necessary clinical pathology is listed in Table 3.

To differentiate between inflammatory and non-inflammatory joint affections, ESR and/or CRP are reliable parameters; CBC excludes anaemia and/or leukocytosis and haematological disorders (e.g. leukaemia) sometimes occurring with arthritic lesions. The electrophoresis is important to differentiate between acute inflammation ($\alpha$-2-fraction increased) and chronic inflammation ($\gamma$-fraction increased).

**Table 2**  Important anamnestic features in enterogenic arthropathy

Pain and swelling of joints
    Lower extremities usually affected
    Asymmetrical
    Number of joints involved (oligoarthritic)

Back pain
    Increasing after midnight
    Increasing on motion

Chronological occurrence of arthritis and other symptoms
    Diarrhoea, abdominal pain
    Fever
    Ocular manifestations (conjunctivitis, uveitis)
    Swelling of lymph nodes
    Neurological manifestations

Skin eruptions
    Generalized (maculous rash)
    Erythema nodosum
    Aphthosis (oral, genital)

Previous therapeutic interventions
    Arthrocentesis and intra-articular injections
    Antibiotics

History
    Similar episodes in the past
    Chronic inflammatory diseases

Family history
    Similar cases
    Other rheumatic diseases

**Table 3**   Important laboratory parameters to be determined in enteropathic arthritis

---

ESR
CBC and differential count
Serum electrophoresis
Uric acid and serum creatinine
HLA-B27
Rheumatoid factor
Infection serology
Microbiology
Synovial fluid analysis

---

The presence of the HLA-B27 antigen is another step towards the diagnosis. This is rather a statistical than an absolute proof of the diagnosis, keeping in mind that approximately 20% of affected patients are negative with respect to this genetic marker. Reactive arthritis is likely when a bacterial infection of the gastrointestinal tract is detected. Microbiological proof is often impossible since the arthritic symptoms usually start 7–21 days after the acute infection of the bowel. Still, microbiological work-up is necessary, especially if diarrhoea persists. Agglutinating antibodies against *Yersinia*, *Salmonella*, *Shigella* and *Campylobacter* are an appropriate instrument to detect a possible bacterial infection; unfortunately, cross-reactions may occur (Table 4).

Synovial fluid analysis is helpful in addressing the arthritis, where wbc often exceeds 10 000 cells/$\mu$l (Table 5).

Other specific rheumatological tests, such as RF, ANA and immune complexes in serum, might be added if other rheumatic diseases need to be ruled out.

**Table 4**   Possible cross-reactivities of enteropathic bacteria

---

*Yersinia enterocolitica* O-group V and *Brucella abortus*, *B. meltensis* and *B. suis*

*Y. pseudotuberculosis* type II and *Salmonella* B-group (e.g. *S. typhimurium*, *S. paratyphi* B and others of this group)

*Y. pseudotuberculosis* type IV and *Salmonella* D-group (e.g. *S. enteritidis*, *S. typhi* and others in this group)

---

Modified from Knapp W et al. Infect Immun. 1973;2:113.

**Table 5**   Characteristics of synovial fluid in reactive arthritis

---

| | |
|---|---|
| Colour: | Yellow |
| Gross appearance: | Clear, sometimes cloudy |
| Viscosity: | Decreased |
| Total protein: | Comparable to serum or only a little less |
| Enzyme activities (e.g. LDH): | Increased |
| Leukocyte count: | > 5000/$\mu$l |
| Lymphocytes: | < 25% |
| Crystals: | Not detectable |
| Bacteria: | Not detectable by culture |
| Complement: | Comparable to serum or slightly reduced |

---

Apart from anamnestic, physical and laboratory–chemical examination, other diagnostic procedures have only secondary character. Radiological examinations usually do not show direct signs of arthritis except for collateral phenomena in phases of acute inflammation. Radiology of the sacroiliac joints might detect sacroiliitis in prolonged cases; scintigraphic imaging is more sensitive in early disease.

## SPECIAL FEATURES

Many gastrointestinal disorders may cause arthritic symptoms, including reactive arthritis after an acute infection with *Yersinia, Shigella, Salmonella* or *Campylobacter*, chronic intestinal disorders like Crohn disease, Whipple disease and other chronic diseases of the bowel, or bypass surgery common in Anglo-Saxon countries. Each of these enteropathic arthropathies exhibits its characteristic features.

### Reactive arthritis following acute bowel disease

#### *Yersinia*

*Yersinia* is a Gram-negative bacterium that has been well characterized. Two subspecies are important in terms of joint disease: *Yersinia enterocolitica* and *Yersinia pseudotuberculosis*, with *Yersinia enterocolitica* causing about 70% of the infections.

Infections with *Yersinia* are mostly characterized by gastroenteritis and may be endemic (e.g. by contaminated milk) or sporadic. The abdominal pain, often mistaken for appendicitis when appearing in the right lower abdominal quadrant, is a typical symptom. Enlarged mesenteric lymph nodes or acute terminal ileitis will often be detected by eventual laparotomy findings, which might lead to the false diagnosis of acute Crohn disease. High fever, pharyngitis, carditis and erythema nodosum, characterized by painful nodular red-and-blue-coloured infiltrations of the skin of the calves and/or lower arms are common signs of *Yersinia* infection. The period of time between enteritis and the onset of arthritis varies from 7 to 30 days with an average of 10–14 days. Almost all symptoms mentioned above may be missing, even the diarrhoea. Usually the arthritis is an oligoarthritis of two to four small or large joints, mostly of the lower extremities, especially of the knees and ankles. A minority of patients already show sacroiliitis initially. Ocular involvement with conjunctivitis and iridocyclitis may be found frequently. Our data show that about 30–50% of the *Yersinia*-induced arthropathies have a prolonged course, lasting for at least 6 months.

Laboratory data show an elevated ESR, a moderate leukocytosis with possible left shift; anaemia is rare, indicating a rather long-lasting disease. Approximately 80% of patients are HLA-B27 positive. Positive *Yersinia* serology by agglutination is a strong hint for the diagnosis.

For the therapeutic approach, NSAIDs (indomethacin, diclofenac, etc.) are the drugs of choice at the beginning. Except for rare cases of severe arthritis, corticosteroids are not necessary. Persisting diarrhoea or septic manifestations of *Yersinia* require tetracycline, while penicillin usually has no effect. Subsiding diarrhoea and no indication of sepsis should lead to a withdrawal of antibiotics.

## Salmonella

*Salmonella* are also Gram-negative bacteria. Reactive arthritis occurs after gastroenteritis, mostly caused by *Salmonella typhimurium* or *Salmonella enteritidis*. In contrast to *Yersinia* infection, *Salmonella* leads to massive gastroenteritis. Reactive arthritis appears in approximately 3% of the patients, equally for male and female, and at any age. Usually, 1–2 weeks after the initial infection, arthritis starts preferentially in the knees, ankles, and, occasionally, in small peripheral joints. Apart from oligoarthritic manifestations, migrating arthritis may occur; in this case, symmetrical involvement of the joints might mimic rheumatoid arthritis. In contrast to rheumatoid arthritis, all patients recover, and functional or structural lesions have not been reported. Conjunctivitis occurs in 20–30% of the patients, and iritis is rare. Skin manifestations and other extra-articular symptoms do not appear in *Salmonella*-induced arthritis.

General laboratory findings are similar to those seen in *Yersinia* arthritis; leukopenia may be present. The microbiological analysis of the synovial fluid is important because septic arthritis is possible. Besides direct proof of *Salmonella*, complement consumption is a valuable diagnostic hint in these cases. Half of the reactive arthritis cases after *Salmonella* infection exhibit a negative serological agglutination test and in positive cases cross-reactivities may occur. Cultivation of *Salmonella* from the patients' faeces, therefore, is the optimal test for *Salmonella*. The HLA-B27 antigen is expressed in 60–80% of patients.

Therapeutic strategies are basically the same as in *Yersinia*-induced arthritis: antibiotics are generally not necessary except for septic *Salmonella* arthritis. Corticosteroids are not necessary.

## Campylobacter

Recently, driven by intensive research, the Gram-negative *Campylobacter* has become more and more important. *Campylobacter jejuni* is responsible for 5–15% of all acute manifestations of diarrhoea, as demonstrated by several studies.

There is no typical clinical feature to differentiate *Campylobacter*-induced diarrhoea from other gastroenteritides. The clinical spectrum ranges from acute diarrhoea to recurring colitis, often similar to Crohn disease or ulcerative colitis. Diarrhoea, abdominal pain, fever, nausea, vomiting and malaise are the initial symptoms. Bloody diarrhoea, up to eight times a day, is common; fever is seen in 50% of patients. Sometimes the disease looks like an acute appendicitis. The pattern of joints affected is similar to that of *Yersinia*- and *Salmonella*-induced arthritis, again HLA-B27 is positive in 80% of cases.

Microbiology remains difficult; the cultivation of *Campylobacter* from faeces will be successful only if selective techniques, suppressing competitive microorganisms, are used. Therefore, only specialized laboratories are able to detect agglutinating antibodies against *Campylobacter*.

As in *Yersinia*-induced arthritis, tetracycline is a good therapeutic approach; other antibiotics are reserved for complications, and, usually, *Campylobacter*-induced arthritis is self-limiting.

## Shigella

*Shigella*, also Gram-negative, is often linked with Reiter disease which will be discussed later. Important are infections with *Shigella dysenteriae* and *Shigella flexneri*. Within 4 weeks of diarrhoea, oligoarthritis preferring knees and ankles is observed. Already at this initial time, sacroiliac pain may occur. Usually, joint manifestations subside within 3 months but cases lasting more than a year are also seen. Microbiology of faeces taken after the onset of the arthritis usually is not successful, but should be attempted because some patients release *Shigella* intermittently. Testing with agglutinating antibodies may be useful, but it is hampered by cross-reactivity with *Escherichia coli*. The most important diagnostic criteria of reactive arthritis after gastrointestinal infection are summarized in Table 6. Possible courses are shown in Figure 1.

**Table 6**  Important features of reactive arthritis after infection with *Yersinia*, *Salmonella*, *Campylobacter* or *Shigella*

| | |
|---|---|
| Patients with arthritis after gastrointestinal infection (%) | 3(–33*) |
| Mean age at onset (years) | 30 (10–70) |
| Male:female ratio | 1:1–10:1 |
| HLA-B27-positive (%) | 80 |
| Time between onset of enteritis and arthritis (days) | 10–20 |
| Duration of disease (weeks) | 20 |
| Average number of joints involved | 3–4 |
| Patients with monoarthritis (%) | 4–20 |
| Patients with sacroiliitis (%) | 7–10 |

**Yersinia* arthritis
Modified from Keat A, N Engl J Med. 1983;309:1606

## Reiter syndrome

In 1916, Hans Reiter described a patient suffering from arthritis, non-gonococcal urethritis and conjunctivitis following a bout of bloody diarrhoea. These symptoms are the classical clinical triad of Reiter syndrome. An overview of additional clinical features is given in Table 7.

Recently, it was demonstrated that 80% of the patients suffering from Reiter syndrome exhibit the HLA-B27 antigen. It is accepted that Reiter syndrome occurs in genetically susceptible individuals after infection with bacteria like *Chlamydia trachomatis* in the genitourinary tract or *Salmonella*, *Shigella*, *Yersinia* or *Campylobacter* in the gastrointestinal system. Table 8 lists infectious bacteria known to cause Reiter syndrome.

Bacterial fragments have been found in the synovial tissues of patients, yet intact organisms have not been cultured. There are various clinical findings in Reiter syndrome. The arthritis occurs within 3 weeks after dysentery or urethritis. Usually, only few joints are involved. This asymmetrical oligoarthritis predominantly manifests in the joints of the lower extremities. Though most

Acute infection

Persisting inflammation

⇓

Genetic disposition

Yes                 No

⇓               ⇓

No joint involvement       Oligo-(poly) arthritis

⇓     ⇓

Oligoarthritis     Healing

(+sacroiliitis)

⇓  ⇓

Recurring    Recurring, chronic

⇓  ⇓

Complete remission   Ankylosing spondylitis

**Figure 1** Possible manifestations of reactive arthritis after acute enteritis. Genetically susceptible individuals (HLA-B27-positive) develop typical joint affections, which usually recover completely. In some cases, recurring joint involvement is seen which can finally remit or progress to ankylosing spondylitis

joints show only moderate swelling, occasionally the knees can be involved markedly. Even Baker cysts may occur. In contrast to rheumatoid arthritis, local enthesopathy targeting the tendinous insertions into bones is prominent. Therefore 'sausage digits', describing the uniformly swollen fingers or toes, might appear. In severe, recurring or chronic courses, the axial skeleton is involved in a manner similar to ankylosing spondylitis. Urogenital symptoms do not necessarily indicate an infection at that site; individuals developing post-dysenteric Reiter syndrome sometimes also exhibit a sterile urethritis 1–2 weeks after diarrhoea. Two skin lesions are typical for Reiter syndrome: painless ulcers of the glans penis, termed balanitis circinata, and keratoderma blenorrhagica, a hyperkeratotic skin lesion. Unilateral or bilateral conjunctivitis may occur in early disease and is mild and transient. Uveitis, usually unilateral, is clinically

**Table 7**   Clinical symptoms in Reiter disease

| |
|---|
| Main symptoms |

Non-gonococcal urethritis (90)[*]
Conjunctivitis, occasionally iritis, iridocyclitis (63)
Arthritis, typically asymmetrical oligoarthritis of the lower extremities (100)
Dermatosis (total 79)

    Balanitis circinata (46)
    Keratoderma blenorrhagica (22)
    Onychopathy (6)
    Psoriasis (rare)

Aphthous stomatitis (27)

Additional symptoms

Diarrhoea (18)
Enthesopathy (52)
Sacroiliitis, spondylitis
Organ manifestations

    Carditis
    Pleuritis
    Hepatosplenomegaly
    CNS involvement
    Fever

[*] Figures in parentheses show percentage of cases in which these symptoms occur (modified from Calin A et al. J Rheumatol. 1983;10:624–8

**Table 8**   Bacteria pathogenetically important in Reiter disease

Unspecific (non-gonococcal) urethritis
   *Chlamydia trachomatis*
   *Ureaplasma urealyticum*

Gastrointestinal infection
   *Shigella flexneri* 1b and 2a
   *Salmonella typhimurium, S. enteritidis, S. cholerae suis* (?), *S. heidelberg* (?)
   *Yersinia enterocolitica* (type 3 and 9), *Y. pseudotuberculosis* (type 1)
   *Campylobacter jejuni*
   *Brucella abortus* (?)

more important. Anterior iritis may occur and spare choroid and retina. Other manifestations are seen only in long-term chronic courses. In this context, aortic regurgitation, IgA-glomerulonephritis, amyloidosis, neuropathies and pleuritis may occur in rare cases.

Laboratory tests for infectious agents are required, in addition to the investigation of inflammatory parameters. Course and prognosis vary and appear to be related to infectious organism and HLA-B27 expression of the host. Arthritic episodes last several weeks to 6 months. Only few patients have a single self-limiting arthritic period; up to 50% experience recurrent episodes. Undetected infection of the synovium with *Chlamydia* has been proposed to cause recurrent arthritis. Low back pain and sacroiliitis correlate with HLA-B27, but not with recurrent symptoms of the peripheral joints.

NSAIDs are the therapeutic first choice to treat joint symptoms. Sulphasalazine may be successful, if NSAIDs do not suffice in controlling arthritis. Interestingly, in a controlled study, tetracycline-treated patients recovered faster than the placebo group. Still, this observation could only be seen in *Chlamydia*-induced Reiter syndrome, in contrast to *Yersinia*- and *Campylobacter*-induced arthritis.

## Arthritis accompanying chronic inflammatory bowel disease (CIBD)

The inflammatory joint manifestations accompanying Crohn disease and ulcerative colitis are quite similar, though the pathological and clinical features of these CIBD differ markedly. In about 20% of CIBD patients, peripheral arthritis involving the small peripheral joints is seen. Moreover, in about 5–10% of cases of colitis ulcerosa and Crohn disease, arthritis manifests as sacroiliitis or spondylitis of the axial joints and may be indistinguishable from uncomplicated seronegative ankylosing spondylitis. A synopsis of the clinical characteristics is given in Table 9.

### Peripheral arthritis

Peripheral arthritis is characterized by acute asymmetrical joint swellings, especially of the lower extremities, mostly the knees and ankles. However, the small joints of the toes may also be involved. Periarticular inflammation and tendinitis, especially of the Achilles' tendon, are common. Interestingly, even though the extent of bowel inflammation does not correspond to the occurrence of joint inflammation, sufficient treatment of the gastrointestinal disorder also treats peripheral arthritis in CIBD. As in *Yersinia*-induced reactive arthritis, erythema nodosum is a typical feature of this variety of arthritis, besides uveitis and ulcers of the oral mucosa. There is no HLA-B27 association with peripheral arthritis. Therapeutic strategies are directed towards the underlying gastrointestinal disease because this arthritis does not usually damage the joints seriously, nor does it cause functional impairment. Both NSAID and steroids are useful therapeutic instruments; however, steroids are not usually necessary if only the joints are affected.

### Axial involvement

As already mentioned, this type of arthritis accompanying CIBD may be indistinguishable from the typical course of uncomplicated primary ankylosing spondylitis. About 80% of patients exhibit the HLA-B27-positive phenotype. In contrast to the idiopathic form of ankylosing spondylitis, 30% of patients are female.

Unlike peripheral arthritis, there is usually no temporal correlation between arthritis onset and the course of joint manifestations and the activity of the underlying gastrointestinal disease. Frequently, inflammation of the joints attenuates prior to the onset of gastrointestinal symptoms. Treatment follows the same criteria as those in idiopathic ankylosing spondylitis.

**Table 9**  Rheumatological characteristics of chronic inflammatory bowel diseases (CIBD)

| Disease | Frequency of joint lesions | Onset after initial GI symptoms | Duration of symptoms | Involvement of joints | Clinical course of arthritic symptoms | Outcome |
|---|---|---|---|---|---|---|
| Ulcerative colitis (peripheral form) | Up to 20% | 6 months to years | Average 7 weeks | Larger joints, asymmetric, lower extremities preferred, mono-, oligo-arthritis, polyarthritis possible | Corresponding to GI manifestations, especially in extensive bowel involvement | Complete remission if remission of colitis complete, minor residual symptoms possible |
| Crohn disease (peripheral form) | Up to 20% | 10–48 months | | Oligoarthritis mostly of the middle and large joints | Relationship between arthritis and enteritis | Depends on course of Crohn disease |
| Ulcerative colitis (axial form) | 1–25% | 33% before 42% simultaneous 25% after | Years | Ileitis, spondylitis | Arthritic symptoms dominate over GI symptoms without correlating with ulcerative colitis or Crohn disease | Short remissions possible; differential diagnosis to ankylosing spondylitis difficult |
| Crohn disease (axial form) | 3–16% | | | (Mono-), oligo-, poly-arthritis (7%), iliosacral arthritis (4%), ankylosing spondylitis, migrating | No correlation with GI symptoms | After antibiotic therapy, complete remission possible |
| Whipple disease | 65–90% | Acute onset possible several years before first GI symptoms | Palindromic, hours to days or chronic | Mono-, oligo-, poly-arthritis, preferring large joints, sacroiliitis and spondylitis possible | Bone pain, secondary to osteomalacia and osteoporosis possible | Often complete remission |
| Intestinal bypass arthritis | 20–30% | Some weeks up to years | Chronically recurring for days up to weeks | Mono-, oligo-, poly-arthritis, mostly knees and ankles, sometimes joints of the upper extremities | Chronic, recurring | Complete remission possible |

## Intestinal bypass arthritis

Jejunocolic and jejunoiliac bypass surgery, most commonly performed in the United States, may also cause arthritis characterized by recurring inflammation of joints, mostly of the knees, ankles and wrists, but also of the small finger joints. Usually, this form of arthritis does not cause deformities, but lesions of the skin, like erythema nodosum or generalized erythema, are not rare. Circulating immune complexes containing bacterial antigen are found in several patients. After reanastomy of the bypassed loops, arthritis remits completely. Pathogenetically, the mechanism postulated is that certain bacteria spread in the blind loop unphysiologically. Upon reaching the circulation, the antigenic material may initiate the mechanisms already mentioned above.

## Whipple disease

In addition to arthritis and recurring high fever, the triad of steatorrhoea, diarrhoea and weight loss is characteristic for the rare Whipple disease. Furthermore, lymphadenopathy, pneumonia, pleuritis, pericarditis, hyperpigmentation, thyroiditis and even central nervous symptoms may be found. Mostly, males older than 30 years are affected (Table 10).

Therefore, Whipple disease must be considered in all patients suffering from arthritis of unknown origin in combination with high fever and other organ manifestations. Joint symptoms frequently occur years (up to 10 years)

**Table 10**   Clinical findings in Whipple disease

| | |
|---|---|
| Generalized<br>  Fever<br>  Weight loss | Serous membranes<br>  Pericarditis<br>  Pleural effusion<br>  Ascites |
| Locomotor system<br>  Polyarthritis<br>  Sacroiliitis<br>  Ankylosing spondylitis<br>  Myopathy | Skin<br>  Hyperpigmentation<br>  Purpura (non-thrombocytopenic) |
| CNS<br>  Dementia<br>  Myoclonal attacks<br>  Spastic paralysis<br>  Acute encephalopathy<br>  Hypersomnia<br>  Ophthalmoplegia | Haematopoietic system<br>  Lymphadenopathy<br>  Anaemia<br>  Leukocytosis |
| | Cardiovascular system<br>  Arterial hypertension<br>  Myocarditis<br>  Endocarditis<br>  Sudden death |
| Eye<br>  Retrobulbar neuritis<br>  Bilateral central scotoma<br>  Oedema of the papilla<br>  Vitritis | Endocrine glands<br>  Panhypopituitarism<br>  Hypothyreosis<br>  Impotence |
| Ear<br>  Presbyacusis | |

prior to the onset of the intestinal manifestation of Whipple disease. Usually, symptoms start acutely and last for hours to days, but some may persist for years.

Arthritis characteristically presents with oligo- or poly-articular involvement, usually affecting knees, ankles, shoulders, elbows and fingers. Diarrhoea and severity of joint involvement do not correlate; persisting functional impairment or deforming lesions are uncommon.

The correct diagnosis is established by biopsy of the small intestine mucosa showing PAS-positive granules in macrophages. Electron microscopy demonstrates intracellular micro-organisms, recently designated as *Tropheryma whippelii*. As defined by molecular biological methods, these bacteria belong to the group of Gram-positive actinomycetes.

The exact pathogenetic mechanisms leading to this disease are still incompletely understood. Deficient cellular immunity, especially of the T cells, appears to play a major role since the proliferative response upon stimulation is decreased. However, after antibiotic therapy, T-cell function recovers.

Good therapeutic results are achieved with tetracycline which is to be given for at least 12 months. If some symptoms exacerbate, erythromycin is a good alternative. Late exacerbations may occur; therefore life-long care for the patients is required. Complications, especially of the central nervous system, have to be treated with an aggressive antibiotic regimen.

## Arthritis associated with hepatitis B

During the long incubation period of hepatitis B and prior to the onset of clinical symptoms of hepatitis, about 10–30% of patients experience arthritic symptoms. Pathogenetically, an excess of viral antigen compared with small amounts of circulating antibodies result in the formation of immune complexes that enrich in the synovia and cause the arthritis. The mean age of patients is 30 years and there is no sex predominance.

Sudden onset in many joints, symmetrically involving the small finger joints, is one of the typical features of this arthritis. However, asymmetrical migrating joint manifestations are not unusual. With an average duration of several weeks, the arthralgias usually last between several days and 6 months. Interestingly, icterus is absent in most patients. In icteric patients, arthralgias have usually already subsided by the onset of icterus. Arthritis is frequently accompanied by itching dermatitis, usually with urticaria or patchy, sometimes papular or petechial, usually occurring on the legs, but also the arms, trunk or face. Prior to arthritis, malaise, sore throat, nausea, limb pain and subfebrile temperatures are common.

Even though the clinical features of rheumatoid arthritis and hepatitis-B-virus-induced arthritis appear to be similar, the typical laboratory findings in rheumatoid arthritis, increased ESR, $\alpha$2-protein and hypochromic anaemia, are missing in hepatitis-B-induced arthritis. Increased transaminases, antibodies of the IgM subclass against HBs-, or detection of HBc-antigen point towards the correct diagnosis. For the therapeutic approach, NSAIDs, specially aspirin, are helpful. Prognostically, hepatitis-B-induced arthritis subsides after weeks without leaving sequelae.

## Behçet disease

Oral and genital aphthous ulcerations in combination with uveitis are the classical triad of Behçet disease. However, as a systemic vasculitis, Behçet disease may involve other organs like skin, joints, veins, arteries, gastrointestinal tract and meninges. The diagnosis requires the detection of oral ulcerations in combination with two other symptoms, as outlined in Table 11.

The typical oral ulceration is a painful 0.2–2-cm round lesion, and heals within 1–3 weeks, usually without leaving a scar. Frequently, there is an interval of several years after the first oral ulceration and involvement of the eyes. The

**Table 11**    Diagnostic criteria* of Behçet disease

| | |
|---|---|
| Oral ulcers | Recurrent aphthous lesions (at least 3 in 12 months) |
| | And at least two of the following |
| Genital ulcers | Recurrent |
| Eye affliction | Anterior/posterior uveitis<br>Retinal vasculitis |
| Skin affliction | Erythema nodosum<br>Pseudo-folliculitis<br>Papulopustular eruptions<br>Acne-like nodules |
| Pathergy test positive | Erythema (2 mm) 24–48 h after needle pricked to depth of 5 mm |

*Must be confirmed by a physican
Adapted from O'Duffy JD, Primer on the rheumatic diseases; 1993

characteristic hypopyon iritis is rare, possibly due to the now-common early anti-inflammatory therapy. Usually, during exacerbation, more than 50% of patients have arthralgias or mild synovitis of the small and large joints. In HLA-B27-positive patients, sacroiliitis may be seen. The mucosal ulcerations can be found in the entire gastrointestinal tract, preferring the terminal ileum, caecum and the ascending part of the colon, clinically presenting as abdominal pain, bleeding or even perforation. Endoscopic biopsy may be necessary to distinguish from granulomatous colitis. A positive HLA-B51 is an additional support of the correct diagnosis.

Treatment depends on clinical manifestations. Oral or topical steroids alone are used to treat mucosal ulcers and mild systemic manifestations. In addition, dapsone and colchicin and even thalidomide are used for the treatment of mucosal lesions. If the CNS is involved (often presenting as aseptic meningitis with headache, fever, stiff neck and pleocytosis of the cerebrospinal fluid, or vasculitis of the CNS) or for severe ocular involvement, steroids alone are not sufficient and should be combined with an immunosuppressive treatment, such as chlorambucil. Anticoagulation has been discussed controversially for recurrent phlebitis in Behçet disease.

Recently, IFN-$\alpha$ has been used in clinical trials.

## Further reading

Krause A, Baerwald C. Pathogenese rheumatischer Erkrankungen. Rolle von Infektionen. Internist. 1993;34:806–16.

Burmester GR. Enteropathische Arthropathien. In: Kalden JR, ed. Klinische Rheumatologie. 1st Ed. Heidelberg, London, New York: Springer Verlag; 1988.

Imman RD. Reactive arthritis after infectious enteritis. In: Schumacher RD, ed. Primer on the rheumatic diseases. 10th Ed. Atlanta, Georgia, USA: Arthritis Foundation; 1993:166–8.

Fan PT, Yu DTH. Reiter's syndrome. In: Schumacher RD, ed. Primer on the rheumatic diseases. 10th Ed. Atlanta, Georgia, USA: Arthritis Foundation; 1993:158–61.

Hermann E, Meyer zum Bueschenfelde KH. Immunogenetics of the seronegative spondylarthropathies – Pathogenetic role of HLA-B27. Akt Rheumatol. 1994;19:77–83.

Williams KM et al. Demonstration of crossreactivity between bacterial antigens and class I human leukocyte antigens by using monoclonal antibodies to Shigella flexneri. Infect Immun. 1990;58:1774–81.

# 9
# The skin in chronic IBD

## W. CH. MARSCH, J. WOHLRAB and M. CORNELY

Chronic inflammatory bowel diseases (CIBD) of infectious or non-infectious aetiology may produce premonitory or concomitant skin disorders which differ in prevalence and specificity (Table 1).

Ulcerative colitis (UC) is more often associated with indicative dermatological features or definite skin disorders than is Crohn disease (CD), i.e. 10% compared with 5%. Two of the skin diseases most likely to occur in CIBD are erythema nodosum and pyoderma gangrenosum[1-4]. They may precede the clinical appearance of UC and CD by a year or more.

Erythema nodosum is characterized by painful inflammatory nodules, usually limited to the extensor aspects of the lower legs and forearms. The hypersensitivity reaction to microbial and other antigens involves the septal blood vessels of the subcutis (septal panniculitis).

Pyoderma gangrenosum is a non-infective cutaneous ulceration which presents with an early pustular or nodular eruption. The lesions become turgid and

**Table 1**  Skin disorders found in association with CIBD

| Crohn disease | | Ulcerative colitis |
|---|---|---|
| Perianal fissures, fistulae and abscesses in 50% of cases | | |
|     1–7 (16%) | Erythema nodosum | 4–10% |
|     < 1% | Pyoderma gangrenosum | 1–10% |
| | Acquired zinc deficiency (state of malabsorption) | |
| | Epidermolysis bullosa acquisita | |
| | Pyostomatitis vegetans | |
| Cobblestone plaques | | |
| Linear fissures and ulcers | | |
| Extraintestinal (metastatic) lesions with specific histology (lips, genitals, anus, lower legs, trunk, peristomal area) | Oral lesions: aphthous ulcers | Vesiculo-pustular eruption |
| Cutaneous polyarteritis nodosa | | Vasculitis allergica (= necrotizing vasculitis) |

ulcerate rapidly. The edges of the ulcers are dusky, often raised and undermined. Painful nodular erythemas at the extensor parts of the lower extremities, clinically identical to erythema nodosum, may develop multiloculated perforating necroses and present the typical appearance of pyoderma gangrenosum (Figures 1a and b). In about half of pyoderma gangrenosum cases, CIBD is also diagnosed, at that time or a later date, UC being more frequent than CD.

Furthermore, both bowel disorders may cause an acquired zinc deficiency[5,6] with cutaneous symptoms which may present the first clinical signs. These are characterized by pluriorificial erythrosquamous and erosive or pustular lesions which resemble psoriasis (Figure 2a), candidiasis or papulopustular acne (Figure 2b).

States of malabsorption may be combined with exacerbation of psoriasis[7]. Epidermolysis bullosa acquisita is a chronic mechanobullous condition of the skin and mucous membranes. Minor traumas induce subepidermal blisters just below the basal lamina (dermolytic blister with deposits of IgG and complement), particularly over the joints. The lesions heal with atrophic scars and milia formation. Serious scarring of the oesophagus may also occur. Almost 30% of cases are seen in conjunction with either UC or CD[8–10].

Pyostomatitis vegetans[11,12] presents with extensive oral papillary projections with deep fissures and occasional pustules. This very rare disease is seen in both of the CIBD and is nosologically regarded as an oral variant of pyoderma gangrenosum or pyoderma vegetans, the latter mainly affecting intertriginous areas as vegetating plaques.

CD is different from UC in that the patients may have a long-term history of perianal complications, a particular disposition to diverse oral lesions and the potential to develop specific extraintestinal so-called metastatic manifestations at the skin.

Perianal and perirectal fistulae and abcesses as well as anal recurrent fissures are seen in about 50% of CD patients. The extent of these fistulae can be best evaluated by modern magnetic resonance imaging (MRI)[13]. The prevalence rate can rise to 80% if the colon is affected[14]. Remarkably, these perianal complaints may be the initial symptoms in 8–16% of later CD patients[15].

Oral symptoms (Table 1) comprise lesions with specific or, more often, non-specific histology, especially aphthous ulcers which are also seen in UC. Oedema and corrugated thickening of buccal mucosa, and furthermore cobblestone lesions with linear ulcers lying deep in the folds, are specific for CD.

Extraintestinal manifestations of CD at the skin (metastatic cutaneous CD) occur at different topographical regions. The lips[16,17], penis, vulva and anal region, solely or in combination, may develop persistent erythematous swellings ('chronic cellulitis'), predominantly in cases of large-bowel involvement (Figures 3a and b). These swellings exhibit non-caseating epithelioid cell granulomas identical to those of the intestinal primary lesions. The cutaneous manifestations may predate the appearance of bowel lesions by several months. Other locations of metastatic cutaneous CD are the legs[18] and the trunk (sometimes the peristomal area), which may present subcutaneous nodules or plaques and secondary ulceration[19,20]. Clinical knowledge and recognition combined with an

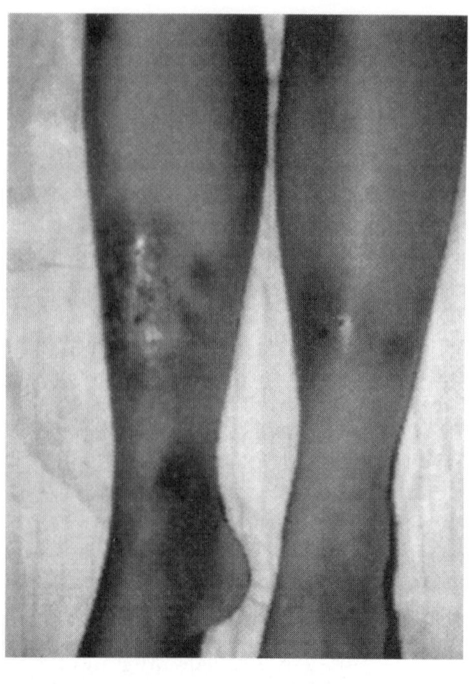

(a)

(b)

**Figure 1**  (a) Erythematous nodules with multiloculated perforating necroses prior to recognition of CD. (b) Detail

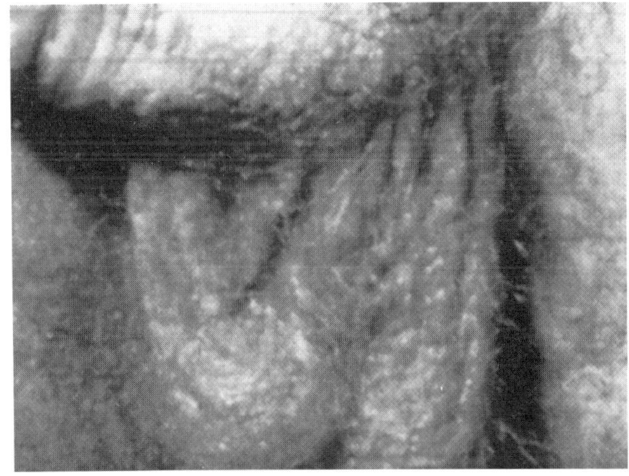

(a)

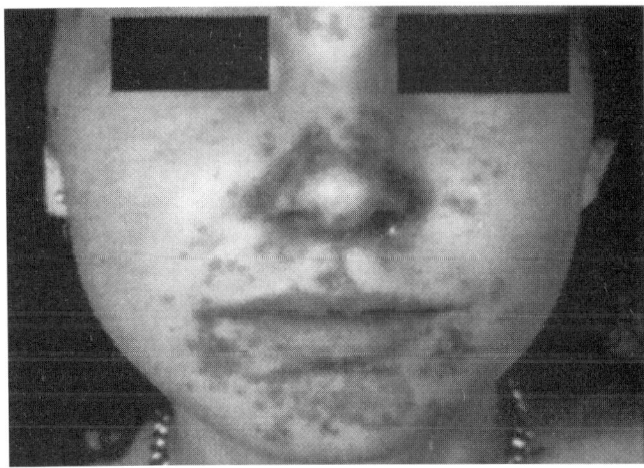

(b)

**Figure 2** Acquired zinc deficiency in CD. (a) 'Eczema' or 'psoriasis' of the scrotum. (b) Lesions simulating papulopustular acne

easily accessible histology are therefore of great diagnostic value for patient therapy.

In summary, pyoderma gangrenosum, cutaneous lesions indicative of zinc deficiency and the mechanobullous disorder, epidermolysis bullosa acquisita, in young and middle-aged persons might suggest that these patients have incipient UC or CD or may develop the complaint later. Erythema nodosum is not uncommon, but relatively rarely seen in conjunction with CIBD as it has a wide range of pathogenetic causes, such as acute sarcoidosis and yersiniosis.

CD is often preceded by a long period of perianal fistulae, fissures and abscesses and is accompanied by a broad spectrum of oral lesions with non-specific histology. However, recurrent aphthous stomatitis and plaques of

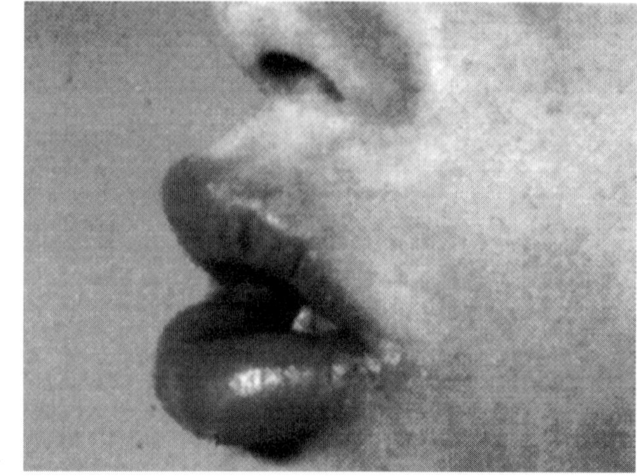

(a)

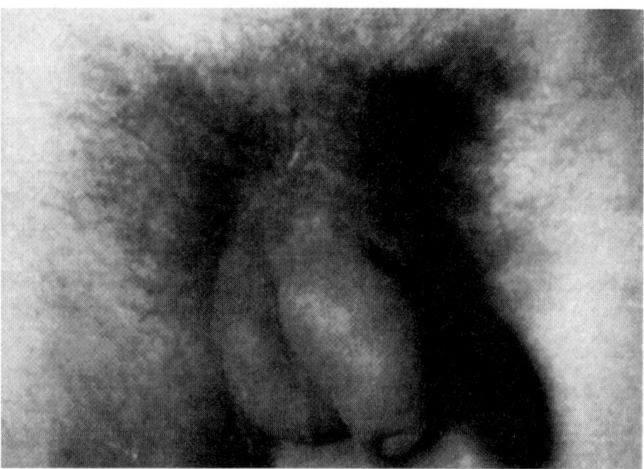

(b)

**Figure 3** Extraintestinal (metastatic) CD. (a) Inflammatory persistent swelling of the lips (cheilitis granulomatosa) with fissuring. (b) Inflammatory persistent swelling of the penile skin ('chronic cellulitis')

cobblestone appearance are most prevalent. Chronic erythematous swellings of the lips (cheilitis granulomatosa; differential diagnoses: Melkersson–Rosenthal syndrome and a localized form of sarcoidosis), the genitals and the anus are typical clinical features of extraintestinal manifestations of CD and display the clear histological features of epithelioid cell granulomas. Again, these clinical signs may be the first symptoms in the course of the disease affecting the large bowel. Dermatology could thus serve as a helpful discipline for the early recognition of CIBD or for co-operative advice concerning treatment of associated skin disorders (Table 2).

**Table 2**  Treatment of associated skin diseases beyond the basic treatment for CIBD

| | |
|---|---|
| Erythema nodosum | Potassium iodide<br>Corticosteroids |
| Pyoderma gangrenosum | Cyclosporin A (new aspect: topical application)<br>Azathioprine<br>Corticosteroids<br>Hyperbaric oxygen |
| Acquired zinc deficiency | Zinc substitution<br>(+ essential fatty acids) |
| Epidermolysis bullosa acquisita | Difficult, but long-term prognosis good:<br>corticosteroids, azathioprine,<br>cyclosporin A, dapsone + minocycline,<br>vitamin E, gold[10] |
| Pyostomatitis vegetans | Corticosteroids |
| Perianal fissures and fistulae of specific histology | Metronidazole[21] |
| Oral aphthous ulcers<br>  Specific<br>  Non-specific | <br>Metronidazole[22]<br>Corticosteroids |
| Extraintestinal manifestations of CD<br>  Cheilitis granulomatosa | Metronidazole[22]<br>Difficult: intralesional corticosteroids[23] |

# References


1. Gregory B, Ho VC. Cutaneous manifestations of gastrointestinal disorders. Part II. J Am Acad Dermatol. 1992;26:371–83.
2. Kirsch B, Gerhardt H, Gladisch R, Heine M, Rohr G, Weiss J. Dermatosen bei chronisch entzündlichen Darmerkrankungen. Akt Dermatol. 1992;18:17–22.
3. MacCallum DI, Kinmont PDC. Dermatological manifestations of Crohn's disease. Br J Dermatol. 1968;80:1–8.
4. Mir-Madjlessi SH, Taylor JS, Farmer RG. Clinical course and evolution of erythema nodosum and pyoderma gangrenosum in chronic ulcerative colitis. Am J Gastroenterol. 1985;8:615–20.
5. Bailly A, Devuyst J, Quarre J et al. Acrodermatitis enteropathica and Crohn's disease. J Am Acad Dermatol. 1984;11:525–6.
6. Hendricks KM, Walker WA. Zinc deficiency in inflammatory bowel disease. Nutr Rev. 1988;46:401–8.
7. Yates VM, Watkinson G, Kelman A. Further evidence for an association between psoriasis, Crohn's disease and ulcerative colitis. Br J Dermatol. 1982;106:323–30.
8. Metz G, Metz J, Horst F. Epidermolysis bullosa acquisita bei Morbus Crohn. Hautarzt. 1975;26:321–6.
9. Ray TL, Levine JB, Weiss W, Ward PA. Epidermolysis bullosa acquisita and inflammatory bowel disease. J Am Acad Dermatol. 1982;6:242–52.
10. Van't Veen AJ, Heule F, Vuzevski VD, den Hengst CW. Epidermolysis bullosa acquisita. Br J Dermatol. 1994;131:724–5.
11. Ballo FS, Camisa C, Allen CM. Pyostomatitis vegetans. J Am Acad Dermatol. 1989;21:381–7.
12. Van Hale HM, Rogers RS, Zone JJ. Pyostomatitis vegetans: a reactive mucosal marker for inflammatory disease of the gut. Arch Dermatol. 1985;121:94–8.
13. Skalej M, Makowiec F, Weinlich M, Jenss H, Laniado M, Starlinger M. Kernspintomographie bei perianalem Morbus Crohn. Dtsch Med Wschr. 1993;118:1791–6.
14. Makowiec F, Starlinger M, Weinlich M, Becker HD. Natural history of perianal fistulas in Crohn's disease. Gastroenterology. 1992;102:A657.
15. Rankin GB, Watts HD, Elnyk CS, Kelley ML. National cooperative Crohn's disease study. Extraintestinal manifestations and perianal complications. Gastroenterology. 1979;77:914–20.

16. Kint A, de Brauwere D, de Weert J, Hendrickx R. Cheilitis granulomatosa und Crohnsche Krankheit. Hautarzt. 1977;28:319–21.
17. Talbot T, Jewell L, Schloss E, Yakimeto W, Thomson ABR. Cheilitis antedating Crohn's disease: case report and literature update of oral lesions. J Clin Gastroenterol. 1984;6:349–54.
18. Shum DT, Guenther L. Metastatic Crohn's disease. Arch Dermatol. 1990;126:645–8.
19. Perret C, Bahmer F. Extensive necrobiosis in metastatic Crohn's disease. Dermatologica. 1987;175:208–12.
20. Rütten A, Wenzel P, Goos M. Kutaner metastatischer Morbus Crohn. Hautarzt. 1989;40:782–4.
21. Brandt LJ, Bernstein LH, Boley SJ et al. Metronidazole therapy for perianal Crohn's disease. A follow-up study. Gastroenterology. 1982;83:383–7.
22. Duhra P, Paul C. Metastatic Crohn's disease responding to metronidazole. Br J Dermatol. 1988;119:87–91.
23. Tatnall FM, Dodd HJ, Sarkany J. Crohn's disease with metastatic cutaneous involvement and granulomatous cheilitis. J R Soc Med. 1987;80:49–51.

# 10
# Pregnancy in CIBD – a non-problem?

## S. BONDESEN

## INTRODUCTION

The interrelationship between chronic inflammatory bowel diseases (CIBD) and pregnancy has been an issue of interest since the recognition of the entities, ulcerative colitis (UC) and Crohn disease (CD). Several reviews on pregnancy in CIBD have analysed data and conclusions from the hitherto published studies[1–7]. The question of whether management of pregnancy in CIBD presents special problems cannot be answered with a further review as categorically as it is posed in the title of this chapter. Thus, our knowledge in this field is still mainly based on retrospective observations of patient populations from different settings and recruited over decades during which medical and surgical treatment has changed. In reports, the description of the patient population is not always adequate with regard to disease activity, drug treatment, earlier surgical treatment and other factors that may have influenced pregnancy and disease. The outcome of pregnancies in UC and CD from reports published before 1980 is shown in Table 1[8–14] and Table 2[15–20], respectively. From these data, the general opinion is that pregnancy is uneventful in patients with CIBD and that disease is unaffected by pregnancy[6,7]. Recently, case-control studies on pregnancy in CIBD have emerged giving more precise data on the outcome of pregnancy in a 'modern' CIBD population.

**Table 1** Outcome of pregnancy in ulcerative colitis reported before 1980

| Reference | No. of pregnancies | Normal birth (%) | Miscarriage (%) | Still-birth (%) | Fetal abnormality (%) |
|---|---|---|---|---|---|
| Abramson et al.[8] | 46 | 78 | 6 | 2 | 0 |
| Crohn et al.[9] | 150 | 89 | 8 | 1 | 0 |
| McDougall[10] | 100 | 80 | 13 | 3 | 0 |
| Banks et al.[11] | 78 | 81 | 3 | 2 | 1 |
| de Dombal et al.[12] | 107 | 84 | 7 | 2 | 3 |
| McEwan[13] | 50 | 88 | 8 | 2 | 0 |
| Webb and Sedlack[14] | 79 | 76 | 16 | 1 | 3 |
| Total | 610 | 83 | 8 | 2 | 1 |

**Table 2**  Outcome of pregnancy in Crohn disease reported before 1980

| Reference | No. of pregnancies | Normal birth (%) | Miscarriage (%) | Still-birth (%) | Fetal abnormality (%) |
|---|---|---|---|---|---|
| Crohn et al.[15] | 84 | 87 | 6 | 1 | 0 |
| Fielding and Cooke[16] | 98 | 84 | 13 | 2 | 0 |
| Schofield et al.[17] | 34 | 71 | 24 | | 6 |
| de Dombal et al.[18] | 60 | 88 | 5 | 5 | 2 |
| Norton and Pattersom[19] | 19 | 84 | 11 | 0 | 0 |
| Homan and Thobjarnasson[20] | 42 | 74 | 17 | 2 | 0 |
| Total | 337 | 81 | 12 | 3 | 1 |

The aim of this presentation is to review more recently published studies and to point out different aspects of the management and counselling of the patient.

## DOES PREGNANCY INFLUENCE THE DISEASE?

### Ulcerative colitis

Current prophylactic treatment regimens have been shown to reduce the frequency of disease attacks in a year from about 70–80% to 20–50% depending on different factors[21]. A patient – pregnant or not – is, thus, exposed to a certain risk of flare-up of symptoms. Whether this risk is lower or higher and whether the symptoms are of a different severity in the pregnant state is the question. Three recent studies have analysed relapse frequencies and severities in UC and CD[22–24]. Table 3 shows the proportion of changes in disease activity in patients that have inactive or active disease at conception in two retrospective studies in patients from referral hospital[23,24]. An equal proportion of patients with inactive disease experienced relapse, whereas twice as many patients with active disease experienced an improvement in one study[23] compared with the other[24]. Further, there was no uniformity in the two studies in the fractions of patients with unchanged symptoms or worsening. In the study of Nielsen et al.[24], the prevalence of active disease during pregnancy and for 6 months postpartum was compared with the period outside the pregnant state. No difference was found since active disease was present

**Table 3**  Ulcerative colitis: clinical activity during pregnancy

| Reference | Initial activity | Activity during pregnancy | | |
|---|---|---|---|---|
| | | Unchanged (%) | Improved (%) | Worse (%) |
| Willoughby and Truelove[23] | Inactive, $n = 129$ | 70 | — | 30 |
| | Active, $n = 55$ | 27 | 40 | 33 |
| Nielsen et al.[24] | Inactive, $n = 133$ | 65 | — | 35 |
| | Active, $n = 19$ | 37% | 21% | 41% |

33%/patient-year in both situations. This was in accordance with other observations[12] and shows that risk of active disease is not influenced by pregnancy. However, in a study by Mogadam et al. based on a questionnaire survey[22] it was found that, in patients with inactive or mild disease at conception, symptoms increased in 28% and, in those with more severe disease, symptoms increased in 44%. These figures, thus, suggest that pregnancy may influence activity if moderately active disease is present at conception. This was also found for the post-partum period, i.e 13% vs 24% exacerbation. In this study, it is not possible specifically to establish the relapse rate of *inactive* UC, but, for CD and UC together, the study reports a 13% relapse in the quiescent patients as opposed to a 51% rate of deterioration in patients who had active disease at conception.

From these studies, it may be concluded that pregnancy does not influence disease course and that patients with inactive disease at conception are at 15–30% risk of renewed symptoms. In patients with active disease, the disease course during pregnancy is variable with a risk of worsening of symptoms that may be more marked in patients with moderate disease activity. Viewing all patients, i.e. active and inactive, an increase in disease activity, possibly necessitating change in medical therapy, may be expected in 25% of cases.

## Crohn disease

In Crohn disease, the patient is at a risk of symptomatic disease of 40–50% per year[21]. These figures are relevant for the time before the introduction of mesalamine prophylaxis. It should also be stressed that no studies exist as to the efficacy and tolerance of this drug or SASP during pregnancy. Table 4 shows the course of CD during pregnancy in two hospital-based studies. Khosla et al.[25] found a relatively low relapse rate of 15%, and noted that patients with low activity at conception generally maintained low activity throughout the pregnancy. The relapse rate was twice as high in the study by Nielsen et al.[26]. This difference may be due to chance or differences in the patient populations and treatment. The proportion of patients experiencing a worsening of disease when active at conception seemed higher in both studies compared with those with inactive disease at conception and an influence of pregnancy on disease severity in these patients is thus suggested. However, Nielsen et al.[26] found that active disease during pregnancy was 44%/patient-year compared with 38% outside this period, a difference that was not significant ($p > 0.05$). This shows that the prevalence of activity of disease in CD is not influenced by the pregnant state. Similarly, Mogadam et al. in a ques-

**Table 4**  Crohn disease: clinical activity during pregnancy

| Reference | Initial activity | Activity during pregnancy | | |
|---|---|---|---|---|
| | | Unchanged (%) | Improved (%) | Worse (%) |
| Khosla et al.[25] | Inactive, $n = 52$ | 85 | — | 15 |
| | Active, $n = 20$ | 30 | 35 | 35 |
| Nielsen et al.[26] | Inactive, $n = 57$ | 61 | — | 39 |
| | Active, $n = 13$ | 28 | 26 | 48 |

tionnaire-based study[27] found the relapse rate in patients with quiescent or mildly active disease to be 22% and a worsening 28% in those with more active disease. Thus, the course of CD is not influenced by pregnancy and a worsening of clinical activity, necessitating a change in treatment policy, may be expected in up to 25% of pregnant women.

## Concluding remarks

The physician may advise the patient that pregnancy will not influence the course of her disease. A risk of worsening of symptoms always exists and a need for change in the medical management may arise. The course of the disease cannot be predicted but it may be more benign if the disease is completely controlled before conception.

## WILL THE PREGNANCY PROGRESS NORMALLY?

### Ulcerative colitis

The more recent studies comprising data on about 700 pregnancies in UC, show that, in general, outcome of pregnancy is similar to that found in the background population with a similar proportion of deliveries at term of a normal child (see Table 5)[23,24,27]. Willoughby and Truelove[23] found no increased incidence of complications, i.e. miscarriages, malformations or stillbirths. Birth weights were also similar to the background population and, comparing treated and non-treated groups, no signs of toxicity of SASP or corticosteroids were found. Mogadam et al.[27] found a markedly low number of fetal complications, 7 of 309 pregnancies (UC and CD), and no significant difference between treated and non-treated patients. In fact, prematurity and low birth weight was significantly less frequent in treated UC patients than the background population, which might be explained by a more effective monitoring of pregnancy in the CIBD patients. Nielsen et al.[24] found no general increase in complications in UC patients compared with the background population. However, in contrast to the other studies, a significantly higher proportion of premature deliveries (< 37 week) and spontaneous abortions was seen in patients with active disease at conception. The main conclusion of this study was that active disease increases the risk of early termination of pregnancy, possibly unrelated to medication. In a study from an obstetric facility, 85% of the UC patients were treated with sulphasalazine and corticosteroids, and significantly lower infant birth weights

**Table 5**  Ulcerative colitis: outcome of pregnancy

| Reference | No. of pregnancies | Normal birth (%) | Miscarriage (%) | Still-birth (%) |
|---|---|---|---|---|
| Willoughby and Truelove[23] | 216 | 79 | 11 | 1 |
| Mogadam et al.[27] | 309 | 97 | 1 | 1 |
| Nielsen et al.[24] | 173 | 76 | 9 | 0 |

were found compared with the normal population, suggesting an influence of disease and medication on pregnancy outcome[28]. Most recently, a case-controlled study from an obstetric unit confirmed that low birth weight is more prevalent in pregnancies of UC patients than controls[29]. Further, in another case-controlled study, premature deliveries were significantly more frequent in the patient group and the risk of miscarriage was slightly increased[30].

**Table 6** Crohn disease: outcome of pregnancy

| Reference | No. of pregnancies | Normal birth (%) | Miscarriage (%) | Still-birth (%) |
|---|---|---|---|---|
| Mogadam et al.[27] | 172 | 96 | 3 | 1 |
| Khosla et al.[25] | 80 | 70 | 27 | 1 |
| Nielsen et al.[26] | 109 | 70 | 9 | 4 |

## Crohn disease

In the study by Mogadam et al.[27], the rate of birth complications was comparable to the background population. However, the complications that occurred (malformations, still-birth, low birth weight, miscarriage) were only found in the CD group receiving SASP and corticosteroids when compared with patients with UC. Khosla et al.[25] studied a group of patients of which the majority had low clinical disease activity and found a 35% rate for miscarriages in the group with active disease. This figure was higher than the background population. Nielsen et al.[26] found a significantly increased risk of premature delivery, i.e. 20%, in the whole patient group, with an over-representation in the group of patients with active disease and in the operated patients. Other complications were not increased, i.e. infant deaths and malformations.

Recent case-controlled studies support the observation that the outcome of pregnancy in CD may not be entirely normal. Thus, Porter and Stirrat, in an obstetric hospital-based study[29], demonstrated a significant increase in the birth of children with low birth weight which was not correlated with disease activity. In a European multicentre case-controlled study, a significantly increased rate of premature delivery, compared with matched controls (16% vs 7%), was shown[31]. Baird et al., in an interview-based case-controlled study, found a significantly increased rate of miscarriages (20% vs 12%) and premature deliveries (25% vs 10%) compared with matched neighbour controls[32]. In a case-controlled study of an obstetric population, the outcome of pregnancy in CD and UC combined demonstrated a significantly lower birth weight in patients versus controls, whereas rate of prematurity, although higher in patients, did not reach statistical significance[30]. In a recent retrospective analysis of 78 pregnancies[33], abnormal outcome was seen in 55% of pregnancies with active CD vs 12% with inactive disease ($p < 0.001$) irrespective of treatment. This again underlines the potential influence of disease activity on the outcome of pregnancy.

## Concluding remarks

Most pregnancies in CIBD are completed uneventfully with a normal child as a result. Recent studies have shown that, in UC and CD, preterm delivery and low birth weight is more prevalent than normal. In the subset of pregnancies in which disease is active or becomes active, a higher risk of spontaneous abortion, preterm delivery and low birth weight seems to be present and is most evident in CD. Preterm birth confers an increased perinatal morbidity and mortality[34]. However, reports on the general outcome of pregnancies in CIBD have not suggested such an increase. This may be due to a greater awareness of possible complications in pregnant women with concomitant bowel disease. The task of the gastroenterologist should be to advise patients who wish to become pregnant to await an inactive stage of the disease. Patients may be informed of an increased risk of preterm delivery, possibly related to disease activity, and that optimal disease control increases the likelihood of a normal delivery. These considerations seem especially relevant for patients with CD.

## CAN IBD BE TREATED WITHOUT RISK DURING PREGNANCY?

### Use of drugs

Although concern about teratogenicity or adverse effects on the pregnancy of drugs used in CIBD may be warranted, no evidence exists to this effect, since no increase in fetal malformations or still-birth has been registered in the published series of pregnancies of about 2000. Mogadam et al. commented on possible toxic effects to the fetus since still-birth and malformations in their series were only seen in the pregnancies of CD patients treated with SASP and corticosteroids[27]. This was also noticed in SASP-treated patients with UC in the study by Willoughby and Truelove[23]. These complications are rare events and, in order to discover a small, significant and important increase related to drug toxicity, carefully controlled observations would be required in groups of at least 1500 pregnancies, according to the statistical power demanded[27].

Only 10–12% of a prednisolone dose reaches the fetus unmetabolized and active and the drug is considered safe in CIBD as well as other corticosteroid-treated conditions[7]. During sulphasalazine treatment, the mother-to-cord plasma concentration ratio of the predrug and sulpha moiety is 1:1, whereas this ratio is between 1:2 and 1:1 for 5-aminosalicylic acid and *N*-acetylated metabolite. The absolute amounts of substance transferred to the fetus are, however, relatively small[35]. Only one report on suspected fetal malformations related to SASP treatment has been published[36].

Mesalamine is now widely used in CIBD and teratogenicity has, as yet, not been noted. An open study on mesalamine administered to 19 pregnant patients (10 UC and 9 CD) at doses from 0.8 to 2.4 g (mean 1.7 g) did not demonstrate side-effects of this new treatment in either mother or child. One miscarriage occurred[37]. A recent report[38] describes a case of fetal renal insufficiency in the kidney after mesalamine. The drug was given in high doses (4 g) from the second trimester for 6 weeks. The case was highly suggestive of nephrotoxicity due to mesalamine, and a renal biopsy from the newborn child showed interstitial and glomerular changes that resembled those found from indomethacin toxicity.

Azathioprine and 6-mercaptopurine reaches the placenta and fetus freely[7] and, in spite of an evident teratogenic potential, this has not been proven in its extensive clinical use. In the survey by Present et al.[39], 13 children were born to patients who had taken 6-mercaptopurine. In three pregnancies, patients were taking the drug at conception and for 3–4 weeks of the first term. No congenital abnormalities were found in any of the children. The results of 16 pregnancies in 14 women treated with azathioprine in combination with corticosteroids or SASP have been reported[40]. The pregnancies were uneventful and the children – observed for a period from 6 to 16 years – developed normally. The positive results of pregnancies in transplanted patients[41] receiving this medication may pave the way for extended use in CIBD. However, in spite of these findings, continuation of azathioprine during the first trimester of pregnancy should be sufficiently motivated by the severity of the case to be treated.

Possible toxicity of other drugs used in CIBD, i.e. metronidazole and cyclosporin, should always be considered in each individual case, especially weighing the benefits of the drug in the given situation (prophylaxis, disease severity) against the, albeit theoretical, risk of toxicity to the fetus. However, disease control does seem to be absolutely necessary for the conclusion of pregnancy with a good result for the baby as well as the mother, as discussed above.

### Concluding remarks

The patient may be advised that medication during pregnancy is or may become necessary according to the activity of her disease for the optimal result of pregnancy. The drugs that are used have not been proven to be toxic to the child, although a theoretical minimal risk cannot be ruled out. It is a matter for the physician to advise her about the medical treatment that is best suited to her disease at the moment.

## Surgery during pregnancy

As shown by recent studies, UC colectomy has been performed without risk to the mother. In the study by Nielsen et al.[24], three colectomies in fulminant UC were followed by uneventful pregnancies and deliveries. In the study by Mogadam et al.[27], seven colectomies in UC and two resections in CD patients were performed, resulting in five abortions. In the study by Nielsen et al.[26], five patients with CD were operated during pregnancy; two ended in spontaneous abortion and two with infants of very low birth weight. Woolfson et al.[33] reported six operations in 78 pregnancies among CD patients. Of these, four were emergencies and resulted in one miscarriage, one premature baby and one small-for-gestational-age. Compared with the group of patients who did not receive surgical treatment, complications were not significantly increased. At any rate, operation should be decided on at an early stage of increasing symptoms, maintaining the patient in a good general condition pre- and post-operatively[6,42]. Weight loss during pregnancy > 5% of prepregnancy weight may, in itself, result in growth retardation of the fetus and a small-for-date child[43] which suggests a place for nutritional monitoring and early dietary intervention. Cases have been reported of severe CIBD during pregnancy treated with complete parenteral nutrition and of a pregnancy supported to full term and delivery of a normal baby[44,45].

## Is delivery influenced by earlier surgery?

The method of delivery in CIBD, in general, is not different from that in the control population[29,30] and special considerations as to the use of Caesarean section are only relevant when there is rectal/vaginal involvement in CD. Deliveries in patients with an ileo-anal pouch anastomosis are, likewise, usually normal with no permanent effects on continence in the mother[46,47]. Special care should be taken in application of episiotomies in this situation because of a potential risk of permanent sphincter damage, and it may be discussed whether this risk should be taken or Caesarean section applied routinely.

## FINAL REMARKS

The recent data published show good results of pregnancies in CIBD, such as had been found in earlier studies. This is possibly due to the specialized treatment of disease and obstetric care. Any CIBD patient may develop a flare-up of disease during pregnancy and experience tells us that improvement in the outcome for the mother and the baby should be sought, probably in the management of disease by close monitoring and an active therapeutic attitude. The optimal results of pregnancy are obtained in patients who have inactive or only mild disease from conception to delivery. From case-controlled studies, it is now clear that pregnancies in CIBD are complicated significantly by premature deliveries and miscarriages and further knowledge of medical and nutritional management in this field is required.

## References


1. Fielding JF. Inflammatory bowel disease and pregnancy. Br J Hosp Med. 1976;April:354–8.
2. Järnerot G. Fertility, sterility and pregnancy in chronic inflammatory bowel disease. Scand J Gastroenterol. 1982;17:1–4.
3. Vender RJ, Spiro M. Inflammatory bowel disease and pregnancy. J Clin Gastroenterol. 1982;4:231–49.
4. Warsof SL. Medical and surgical treatment of inflammatory bowel disease in pregnancy. Clin Obstet Gynecol. 1983;26:822–31.
5. Korelitz BI. Pregnancy, fertility and inflammatory bowel disease. Am J Gastroenterol. 1985;80:365–70.
6. Donaldson RM. Management of medical problems in pregnancy – inflammatory bowel disease. N Engl J Med.1985;312:1616–19.
7. Miller JP. Inflammatory bowel disease in pregnancy: a review. J R Soc Med. 1986;79:221–5.
8. Abramson D, Jankelson IR, Milner LR. Pregnancy in idiopathic ulcerative colitis. Am J Obstet Gynecol. 1951;61:121–9.
9. Crohn BB, Yarnis H, Crohn EB et al. Ulcerative colitis and pregnancy. Gastroenterology. 1956;30:391–403.
10. MacDougall I. Ulcerative colitis and pregnancy. Lancet. 1956;ii:641–3.
11. Banks BM, Korelitz BI, Zetzel L. The course of nonspecific ulcerative colitis: a review of twenty years experience and late results. Gastroenterology. 1957;32:983–1012.

12. de Dombal FT, Watts JM, Watkinson G et al. Ulcerative colitis and pregnancy. Lancet. 1965;ii:599–602.

13. McEwan HP. Ulcerative colitis and pregnancy. Proc R Soc Med. 1972;65:279–81.

14. Webb MJ, Sedlack RE. Ulcerative colitis in pregnancy. Med Clin N Am. 1974;58:823–7.

15. Crohn BB, Yarnis J, Korelitz BL. Regional ileitis complicating pregnancy. Gastroenterology. 1956;31:615–24.

16. Fielding JF, Cooke WT. Pregnancy and Crohn's disease. Br Med J. 1970;iii:550–3.

17. Schofield PF, Turnbull RB, Hawk WA. Crohn's disease and pregnancy. Br Med J. 1970;ii:364.

18. de Dombal FT, Burton IL, Goligher JC. Crohn's disease and pregnancy. Br Med J. 1972;iii:550–3.

19. Norton RA, Pattersom JF. Pregnancy and regional ileitis. Obstet Gynecol. 1972;40:711–12.

20. Homan WP, Thobjarnasson B. Crohn's disease and pregnancy. Arch Surg. 1976;111:545–7.

21. Peppercorn MA. Sulfasalazine, pharmacology, clinical use, toxicity and related new drug-development. Ann Intern Med. 1984;101:377–86.

22. Mogadam M, Korelitz BI, Ahmed SW, Dobbins WO, Baiocco PI. The course of inflammatory bowel disease during pregnancy and postpartum. Am J Gastroenterol. 1981;75:265–9.

23. Willoughby CP, Truelove SC. Ulcerative colitis and pregnancy. Gut. 1980;21:469–74.

24. Nielsen OH, Andreasson B, Bondesen S, Jarnum S. Pregnancy in ulcerative colitis. Scand J Gastroenterol. 1983;18;735–42.

25. Khosla R, Willoughby CP, Jewell DP. Crohn's disease and pregnancy. Gut. 1984;25:522–6.

26. Nielsen OH, Andreasson B, Bondesen S, Jacobson O, Jarnum S. Pregnancy in Crohn's disease. Scand J Gastroenterol. 1984;19:724–32.

27. Mogadam M, Dobbins WO, Korrelitz BI, Ahmed S. Pregnancy in inflammatory bowel disease: effect of sulfasalazine and corticosteroids on fetal outcome. Gastroenterology. 1981;80:72–6.

28. Schade RR, van Tiel DH, Gavaler JS. Chronic idiopathic ulcerative colitis. Pregnancy and fetal outcome. Dig Dis Sci. 1984;29:614–19.

29. Porter RJ, Stirrat GM. The effects of inflammatory bowel disease on pregnancy: a case-controlled retrospective analysis. Br J Obstet Gynaecol. 1986;93:1124–31.

30. Fedorkow DM, Persaud D, Nimrod CA. Inflammatory bowel disease: A controlled study of late pregnancy outcome. Am J Obstet Gynecol. 1989;160:998–1001.

31. Mayberry JF, Waterman IT. European survey of fertility and pregnancy in women with Crohn's disease: a case control study by European collaborative group. Gut. 1986;27:821–5.

32. Baird DD, Narendranathan M, Sandler RS. Increased risk of preterm birth for women with inflammatory bowel disease. Gastroenterology. 1990;99:443–6.

33. Woolfson K, Cohen Z, Mcleod RS. Crohn's disease and pregnancy. Dis Colon Rectum. 1990;33:869–73.

34. Creasy RK. Pre-term birth prevention: where are we? Am J Obstet Gynecol. 1993;168;1223–30.

35. Christensen LA, Rasmussen SN, Hansen SH, Bondesen S, Hvidberg E. Salazosulfapyridine and metabolites in fetal and maternal fluids with special reference to 5-aminosalicylic acid. Acta Obstet Gynaecol Scand. 1987;66:433–5.

36. Hoo JJ, Hadro TA, Von Behren P. Possible teratogenicity of sulfasalazine (letter). N Engl J Med. 1988;318:1128.

37. Habal FM, Hui G, Greenberg GR. Oral 5-aminosalicylic acid for inflammatory bowel disease in pregnancy: safety and clinical course. Gastroenterology. 1993;105:1057–602.

38. Colombel JF, Brabant G, Gubler M-C et al. Renal insufficiency in infant: side-effect of prenatal exposure to mesalazine? Lancet. 1994;344:620–1.

39. Present DH, Meltzer SJ, Krumholz MP et al. 6-Mercaptopurine in the management in inflammatory bowel disease. Am Col Phys. 1989;111:641–9.

40. Alstead EM, Ritchie JK, Lennard-Jones JE et al. Safety of azathioprin in pregnancy in inflammatory bowel disease. Gastroenterology. 1990;97:443–6.

41. Framarino di Malatesta ML, Poli L, Pierucci F et al. Pregnancy and kidney transplantation: clinical problems and experience. Transplant Proc. 1993;25:2188–9.

42. Cookset G, Gunn A, Wotherspoon WC. Surgery for acute ulcerative colitis and toxic mega-colon during pregnancy. Br J Surg. 1985;72:121–4.

43. Gross S, Librach C, Cecutti A. Maternal weight loss associated with hyperemesis gravidarum: a predictor of fetal outcome. Am J Obstet Gynecol. 1989;160:906–9.

44. Rivera-Alsina ME, Saldana LR, Stringer CA. Fetal growth sustained by parenteral nutrition in pregnancy. Obstet Gynecol. 1984;64:138–41.

45. Treadern JC, Falconer GF, Turnberg LA, Irving MH. Maintenance of pregnancy in a home parenteral nutrition patient. J Parent Ent Nutr. 1984;8:199–202.
46. Metcalf A, Dozois RR, Beart RW, Wolff BG. Pregnancy following ileal pouch–anal anastomosis. Dis Colon Rectum. 1985;28:859–61.
47. Santos MC, Thompson JS. Late complications of the ileal pouch–anal anastomosis. Am J Gastroenterol. 1993;88:3–9.

# 11
# The risk of cancer in IBD: a plea for surveillance?

## A. SONNENBERG and P. BANSAL

## INTRODUCTION

A long history of ulcerative colitis is associated with a markedly increased risk of developing colorectal cancer. A similar but considerably weaker risk is also associated with Crohn colitis. Multiple studies have described the epidemiology underlying these associations and how the risk of colorectal cancer becomes modulated by patient characteristics and various clinical parameters. Despite our extensive knowledge about the clinical epidemiology of colorectal cancer in inflammatory bowel disease (IBD), it has proven exceedingly difficult to translate this knowledge into generally accepted guidelines on how to manage the individual patient. Studies testing the protective influence of surveillance colonoscopy have failed to show an unequivocal benefit of such measures. The present chapter starts with a description of the epidemiology and the risk factors for IBD-associated colorectal cancer. In the subsequent two sections, we review the arguments for and against surveillance colonoscopy before we conclude with our own recommendations.

## EPIDEMIOLOGY OF COLORECTAL CANCER IN IBD

All clinical investigations following patients with ulcerative colitis over a prolonged period of time have noted an increase in the occurrence of colorectal cancer[1-4]. The cumulative fraction of patients with ulcerative colitis who develop colorectal cancer depends on the length of time since the onset of the disease and the extent of colonic involvement[4]. The risk starts only 8 years after the onset of ulcerative colitis. During each year of the second decade of pancolitis, about 0.5% of all patients develop colorectal cancer (Figure 1). The rise becomes steeper during the third decade, as 1% per year develop colorectal cancer during the third decade. After 40 years of ulcerative colitis involving most of the colon, about 30% of all patients will have developed colorectal cancer unless they underwent a prophylactic colectomy. In the general popula-

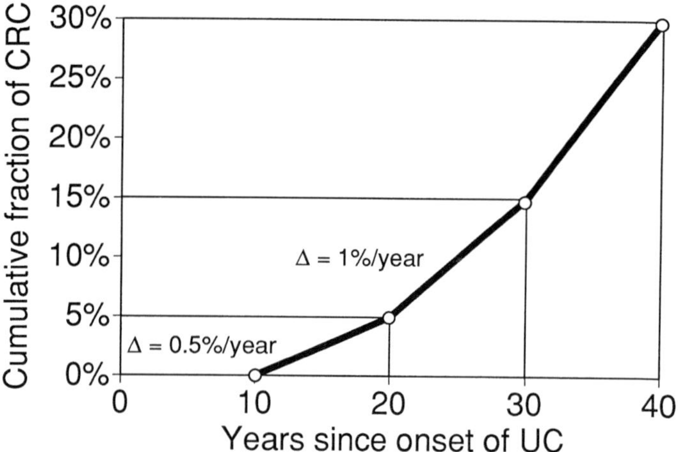


**Figure 1**  Cumulative fraction of patients with ulcerative colitis (UC) who develop colorectal cancer (CRC)

tion, the lifetime risk for developing colorectal cancer is about 6%, i.e. one fifth or less compared with the risk associated with ulcerative colitis[5]. In a population-based study from Sweden, Ekbom and coworkers compared directly the incidence of colorectal cancer in ulcerative colitis with the expected incidence of the general population[6]. Overall, the incidence was 6 times higher in ulcerative colitis than in the general population. The incidence ratio was 1.7 in ulcerative proctitis, 2.8 in left-sided colitis, and 14.8 in pancolitis. In a similar study comparing the incidence of colorectal cancer in Crohn disease and the general population, the same authors found a 2.5-fold increased risk associated with Crohn disease[7].

The risk affects men and women alike, and is similar in patient populations from different countries[4]. Compared with colorectal cancers in the general population, the colonic distribution of IBD-associated cancers is shifted towards the more proximal parts of the large bowel[8,9]. However, this difference is not striking as half of all IBD-associated cancers still occur in the rectosigmoid area. Although the inflamed mucosa may harbour multiple cancers simultaneously and these cancers tend to be less differentiated, overall, IBD-associated cancers do not carry a worse prognosis than regular colorectal cancers, and a 5-year survival rate of 50% is found in patients with or without IBD[9,10].

The most important patient characteristic concerns the extent of colonic involvement. Similar to the work of Ekbom et al.[9] cited above, others have shown a markedly increased risk associated with pancolitis, but only a moderate risk if the disease was confined to the left colon[4,11]. Besides the length of IBD history, onset of ulcerative colitis in childhood was claimed to be associated with a particularly high risk[1,11,12]. Others have suspected that patients aged 50 years and older run a particularly increased risk for colorectal cancer[4]. Obviously, duration of the disease, young age at onset, and old age at time of the colitis are all interrelated, and it has remained difficult to disentangle the separate contribution of each individual factor. Brommé et al. have identified the presence of sclerosing cholangitis as an independent risk factor for the development of colonic dysplasia, the precursor lesion of colon cancer[13]. However, these results need confirmation by other authors. Although multivariate analysis was used to adjust for the joint contribution of sclerosing cholangitis and disease duration, it remains to be shown whether sclerosing cholangitis actually represents an independent risk factor or whether it reflects only the influence of other disease parameters, such as extent, severity and duration of the underlying colitis.

## ARGUMENTS IN FAVOUR OF SURVEILLANCE

In order to be suitable for a screening or surveillance programme, a given disease must fulfil several criteria[14]. For instance, the disease must advance through different stages over an appreciable amount of time that provides enough room for medical intervention. The initial stage and its parameters must be associated with the end stage of the disease in an unambiguous fashion. It must represent itself as a well-defined clinical entity that can be diagnosed unequivocally with the appropriate tools. Diagnosis and treatment of the initial stage should be less harmful than the outcome of the disease itself. All these points seem to apply to colorectal cancer in IBD. The inflamed mucosa progresses from low- to high-grade dysplasia before it turns cancerous. Dysplasia can be diagnosed in random biopsies obtained during colonoscopy. The time lag between mild and severe dysplasia is on the average 3 years[15]. Therefore, colonoscopies at a yearly interval should be able to diagnose the transition from normal colon to dysplasia in a timely fashion and lead to prophylactic colectomy before the cancer develops.

Choi and coworkers[16] analysed 41 patients who developed carcinoma associated with ulcerative colitis. Cancer was detected at a significantly earlier Dukes' stage in 19 patients undergoing surveillance than in 22 patients without surveillance. The 5-year survival rate was 77% in the surveillance group compared with 36% in the non-surveillance group. (It has been pointed out, however, that patients who come to medical attention only after their cancers have developed are more likely to present with more advanced carcinoma than patients enrolled in a surveillance programme and monitored on a regular basis[17]. Thus, the authors could not rule out the possibility that the benefit of their surveillance programme was related to regular physician contacts rather than frequent colonoscopies.) There is ample literature to attest to the seeming benefit of surveillance colonoscopy[18-23]. Most authors interpreted the outcome of their surveillance programmes, lasting anywhere between 9 and 15 years, as supporting the idea of regular colonoscopies. The articles contain a fair list of patients in whom detection of dysplasia led to prophylactic colectomy or in whom cancers were diagnosed that would have gone unnoticed otherwise.

## ARGUMENTS AGAINST SURVEILLANCE

None of the studies cited above compared the success rate of surveillance in cases with prospectively and randomly chosen controls, and the arguments raised in favour of surveillance were based solely on the interpretation of uncontrolled observations. In a study by Lashner et al., 91 cases assigned to the surveillance group were compared with an *historical* cohort of 95 patients chosen from a registry of IBD patients[24]. No benefit of surveillance could be appreciated, as two more colorectal cancers occurred in the case than control population, and cancer-related survival was equal in both groups.

In interpreting the results of previous studies, it is important to differentiate between incidental findings of high-grade dysplasia or cancer and cases that were truly discovered as result of the surveillance programme. Anthony Axon and his group have assembled a rather helpful list of six criteria to exclude incidental cases that do not truly reflect a success of surveillance[25,26].

1. Since surveillance is supposed to result in detection of severe dysplasia or early cancer, advanced cancer of Dukes' stage C must not be counted as success of surveillance.
2. Cancers that are detected during surgery for other reasons than high-grade dysplasia, such a debility or failed medical therapy, cannot be counted as success.
3. One has to disregard cancers found in operative specimens of patients operated for low-grade dysplasia.
4. Cancers detected through other means than regularly scheduled colonoscopy, e.g. air-contrast barium enema or flexible sigmoidoscopy, should be excluded. Similarly, cancers that are found during colonoscopic follow-up of a suspicious finding established by other means should be excluded.
5. The colonoscopic surveillance is restricted to patients with colitis extending beyond the left colon. Moreover, most physicians will not start surveillance before 8–10 years have elapsed since the onset of the disease. Therefore, it unduly inflates the success rate of any surveillance programme if such cancers are considered in favour of surveillance.
6. There is a conceptual difference between a screening colonoscopy, performed only once to assess the severity and the extent of the colitis, and surveillance colonoscopy performed repeatedly to assess progress of the disease. For instance, a screening colonoscopy is performed in patients who are referred to the programme for the first time or who become re-admitted to the programme after a prolonged period of defaulting.

Axon and coworkers have compiled the results of 12 studies dealing with surveillance and applied their criteria to the data (Figure 2)[25,26]. Of the 92 cancers identified in the total population of 1916 patients with ulcerative colitis, only 11 Dukes' A and B cancers could be ascribed to the benefit of surveillance. The number of colonoscopies was available for 11 of the 12 studies. In all, 3807 colonoscopies had been invested to detect eight early cancers, i.e. 476 colonoscopies per cancer. By current American payment standards, this number corresponds to more than $500 000 spent on the detection of one Dukes' A or B cancer.

The limited success of surveillance is, in part, due to ambiguity that lies in the diagnosis of dysplasia. Low-grade dysplasia is a common feature of any prolonged colitis that develops in a time-dependent manner. After 20 years of

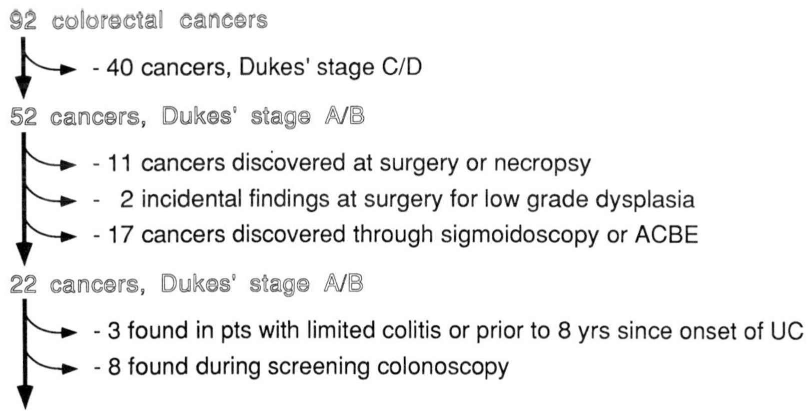



**Figure 2** Compiled data from twelve published studies on cancer surveillance in 1916 patients with ulcerative colitis. Data adapted from Reference 26

ulcerative colitis, 30% of all patients harbour low-grade dysplasia, after 30 years this proportion rises to 50%, and after 40 years to 80%. Although the time lag between low- and high-grade dysplasia is on the average 3 years, this difference has little bearing on the individual patient, in whom dysplasia may even be reversible. Because the distribution of colonic dysplasia is patchy and tissue samples obtained through biopsies represent only a tiny fraction of the overall surface, its occurrence is easily missed. Moreover, colorectal cancer can develop in mucosa devoid of any dysplasia lesions. In the acutely inflamed mucosa, it is frequently difficult to differentiate unequivocally between cell dysplasia and reactive or regenerative cytological abnormalities, i.e. atypia. Although the criteria of low- and high-grade dysplasia are well standardized, their application remains liable to subjective interpretation by the individual pathologist.

In their compilation of previously published data on surveillance, Axon et al. also analysed the association between dysplasia and the occurrence of cancer (Table 1)[26]. The fraction of patients with cancers was increased in patients with low-grade dysplasia, This fraction of patients was even further increased in

**Table 1**  Associations of dysplasia with colorectal cancer

| | | Cancer | | |
|---|---|---|---|---|
| | No. of studies | Yes | No | Total |
| All patients in surveillance | 12 | 93 (4.5%) | 1951 | 2044 |
| Low-grade dysplasia | 11 | 26 (8.3%) | 287 | 313 |
| High grade dysplasia | 12 | 35 (34.7%) | 66 | 101 |

Data from Reference 26

patients with high-grade dysplasia, but many of the cancers occurred in patients without any dysplasia at all.

## CONCLUSIONS AND RECOMMENDATIONS

A Danish cohort of 1161 patients with ulcerative colitis were followed closely over a mean time period of 12 years[27]. The patients were seen on a regular basis at least once per year with radiological or colonoscopic examinations reserved for cases with changes in their symptoms. While all patients were kept on a maintenance therapy with sulphasalazine, acute exacerbations were treated immediately with short glucocorticoid courses. The active approach to therapy included surgery when debilitating symptoms were not manageable with medical treatment. The cumulative colectomy rate 25 years after diagnosis was 32%. Except for the first year after diagnosis when the risk of death was 2.5, no excess mortality was found among the patient population as compared with the general population. Only six patients developed colorectal cancer compared with an expected number of 6.6 calculated from the incidence rates for colorectal cancer in the Danish population. The authors concluded that, under close medical supervision and liberal use of colectomy in cases of failed medical therapy, patients with ulcerative colitis do not run an increased risk of death from colorectal cancer.

The results of a recent case-control study from Sweden seem to support this conclusion[28]. From a population of 3112 patients with ulcerative colitis, the investigators selected 102 cases with colorectal cancer and 196 controls without cancer. Two controls were matched to each case for sex, extent and duration of disease. The results of the study are shown in Figure 3. Physician contacts were more frequent among controls, and barium enemas and endoscopies also tended to be more frequent among controls than cases. Completion of at least one

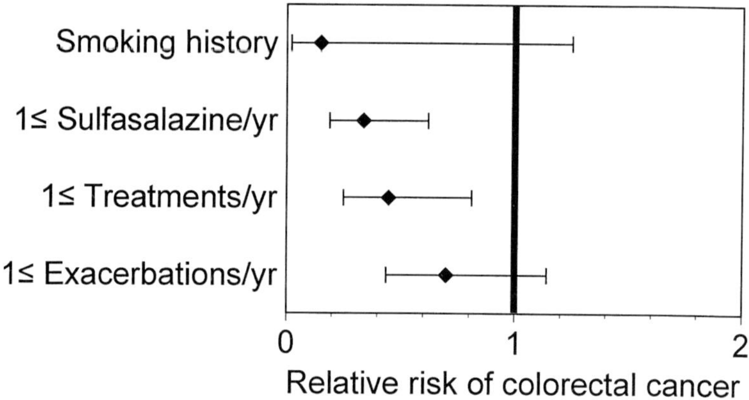


**Figure 3**   Relative risk of colorectal cancer in patients with ulcerative colitis. Risk ratios are shown with their 95% confidence interval; a ratio smaller than 1.0 indicates a reduced risk of cancer. Risks are compared against subjects without smoking history or with less frequent sulphasalazine therapy, pharmacotherapies, and exacerbations. Data adapted from Reference 28

course of therapy per year and therapy with sulphasalazine exerted a protective influence. Patients with history of smoking and with more than one disease exacerbation per year also experienced a reduced risk, although their risk reduction failed to reach statistical significance. In our interpretation of the results from this study, disease exacerbations and frequent courses of pharmacotherapy appear to represent proxy variables for close medical attention paid to patients with long-standing and severe ulcerative colitis. The protective influence of sulphasalazine might be consistent with the protective effect of aspirin against colorectal cancer in the general population.

Currently, there are no data to suggest that surveillance colonoscopy protects against colorectal cancer or extends life expectancy of patients with ulcerative colitis. The results of previously published surveillance studies suggest that frequent physician contacts rather than colonoscopies represented the primary protective influence. This statement is not meant to belittle the contribution of colonoscopy in protecting against death from colorectal cancer. Obviously, patients benefited from screening colonoscopy and colonoscopic pursuit of newly developed symptoms or suspicious findings obtained by other diagnostic means. However, frequent colonoscopies scheduled at annual intervals provide little additional advantage at the expense of recurrent distress, unacceptable to many patients as evidenced by the low rate of compliance and frequent discontinuation. The low yield and the heavy workload have led many European gastroenterologists to advise against surveillance[26,29,30]. Their recommendations also reflect a working environment of socialized medicine, where the individual physician stands to gain little by performing additional colonoscopies. On the other hand, for an American gastroenterologist working in a fee-for-service system and a highly litigious society, these have been at least two extraneous incentives to schedule frequent colonoscopies[17,31].

Based on available data from the literature, the following recommendations can be made:

1.  A screening colonoscopy should be performed 10 years after onset of ulcerative colitis or in any patient who is referred to a gastroenterologist for the first time many years after the onset of his/her disease.
2.  Patients should have regular clinical appointments and should be seen by a physician at least once per year.
3.  A colonoscopy should be performed whenever new symptoms arise.
4.  Patients with high-grade dysplasia should undergo a colectomy. In addition, some physicians may want to concentrate surveillance on high-risk patients, i.e. patients over 50 years old with long-standing disease or with low-grade dysplasia.

## References


1.  Devroede GJ, Taylor WF, Sauer WG, Jackman RJ, Stickler GB. Cancer risk and life expectancy of children with ulcerative colitis. N Engl Med. 1971;285(1):17–21.
2.  Devroede G, Taylor WF. On calculating cancer risk and survival of ulcerative colitis patients with the life table method. Gastroenterology. 1976;71:505–9.
3.  Katzka I, Brody RS, Morris E, Katz S. Assessment of colorectal cancer risk in patients with ulcerative colitis: Experience from a private practice. Gastroenterology. 1983;85:22–9.

4. Gyde SN, Prior P, Allan RN et al. Colorectal cancer in ulcerative colitis: a cohort study of primary referrals from three centres. Gut. 1988;29:206–17.
5. Gloeckler Ries LA, Schatzkin A, Kaplan R. Colon and rectum. In: Miller BA, Gloeckler Ries LA, Hankey BF et al. eds. SEER cancer statistics review: 1973–1990, National Cancer Institute. NIH Publication No. 93-2789, 1993:VI.17.
6. Ekbom A, Helmick C, Zack M, Adami HO. Ulcerative colitis and colorectal cancer. N Engl J Med. 1990;323:1228–33.
7. Ekbom A, Helmick C, Zack M, Adami HO. Increased risk of large-bowel cancer in Crohn's disease with colonic involvement. Lancet. 1990;336:357–9.
8. Ritchie JK, Hawley PR, Lennard-Jones JE. Prognosis of carcinoma in ulcerative colitis. Gut. 1981;22:752–5.
9. Gyde SN, Prior P. Thompson H, Waterhouse JAH, Allan RN. Survival of patients with colorectal cancer complicating ulcerative colitis. Gut. 1984;25:228–31.
10. Choi PM, Zelig MP. Similarity of colorectal cancer in Crohn's disease and ulcerative colitis: implications for carcinogenesis and prevention. Gut. 1994;35:950–4.
11. Sugita A, Sachar DB, Bodian C, Ribeiro MB, Aufses AH Jr, Greenstein AJ. Colorectal cancer in ulcerative colitis. Influence of anatomical extent and age at onset on colitis–cancer interval. Gut. 1991;32:167–9.
12. Edwards FC, Truelove SC. The course and prognosis of ulcerative colitis. Gut. 1964;5:15–22.
13. Broomé U, Lindberg G, Löfberg R. Primary sclerosing cholangitis in ulcerative colitis – A risk factor for the development of dysplasia and DNA aneuploidy? Gastroenterology. 1992;102:1877–80.
14. Morrison AS. Screening in chronic disease, 2nd edn. New York: Oxford University Press; 1992.
15. Lashner BA, Hanauer SB, Silverstein MD. Optimal timing of colonoscopy in ulcerative colitis. Ann Intern Med. 1988;108:274–8.
16. Choi PM, Nugent FW, Schoetz DJ Jr, Silverman ML, Haggitt RC. Colonoscopic surveillance reduces mortality from colorectal cancer in ulcerative colitis. Gastroenterology. 1993;105:418–24.
17. Sachar DB. Clinical and colonoscopic surveillance in ulcerative colitis: Are we saving colons or saving lives? Gastroenterology. 1993;105:588–97.
18. Lennard-Jones JE, Morson BC, Ritchie JK, Williams CB. Cancer surveillance in ulcerative colitis. Lancet. 1983;2:149–52.
19. Rutegård J, Åhsgren L, Stenling R, Janunger KG. Cancer surveillance in an unselected population. Scand J Gastroenterol. 1988;23:139–45.
20. Rosenstock E, Farmer RG, Petras R, Sivak MV Jr, Rankin GB, Sullivan BH. Surveillance for colonic carcinoma in ulcerative colitis. Gastroenterology. 1985;89:1342–6.
21. Löfberg R, Broström O, Karlén P, Tribukait B, Öst Å. Colonoscopic surveillance in long-standing total ulcerative colitis – A 15 year follow-up study. Gastroenterology. 1990;99:1021–31.
22. Nugent FW, Haggitt RC, Gilpin PA. Cancer surveillance in ulcerative colitis. Gastroenterology. 1991;100:1241–8.
23. Woolrich AJ, DaSilva MD, Korelitz BI. Surveillance in the routine management of ulcerative colitis: The predictive value of low-grade dysplasia. Gastroenterology. 1992;103:431–8.
24. Lashner BA, Kane SV, Hanauer SB. Colon cancer surveillance in chronic ulcerative colitis: Historical cohort study. Am J Gastroenterol. 1990;85:1083–7.
25. Lynch DAF, Lobo AJ, Sobala GM, Dixon MF, Axon ATR. Failure of colonoscopic surveillance in ulcerative colitis. Gut. 1993;34:1075–80.
26. Axon ATR. Cancer surveillance in ulcerative colitis – a time for reappraisal. Gut. 1994;35:587–9, 801.
27. Langholz E, Munkholm P, Davidsen M, Binder V. Colorectal cancer risk and mortality in patients with ulcerative colitis. Gastroenterology. 1992;103:1444–51.
28. Pinczowski D, Ekbom A, Baron J, Yuen J, Adami HO. Risk factors for colorectal cancer in patients with ulcerative colitis. A case-control study. Gastroenterology. 1994;107:117–20.
29. Fozard JBJ, Dixon MF. Colonoscopic surveillance in ulcerative colitis – dysplasia through the looking glass. Gut. 1989;30:285–92.
30. Gyde S. Screening for colorectal cancer in ulcerative colitis: dubious benefits and high costs. Gut. 1990;31:1089–92.
31. Pembrook L. Low-grade dysplasia called best criterion for positive CA screen in ulcerative colitis. Gastroenterology Endoscopy News. 1993;May issue:22.

# Section III
# Measures of disease activity, prognosis and quality of life

# 12
# Measuring disease activity: do we need new indices?

H. GOEBELL

## INTRODUCTION

It is a constant wish of physicians and surgeons who treat and observe patients with inflammatory bowel diseases to have reproducible criteria for a quantitative judgment of their patients' disease states. In ulcerative colitis, the large bowel as the area of inflammation is easily accessible. Endoscopic, histological and clinical criteria can be used to define the activity of the process. This is much more difficult in Crohn disease, where endoscopy and histology can rarely give enough information on the patient's problem.

## ULCERATIVE COLITIS

In this disease, the inflammation is located only in the mucosa and submucosa of the large bowel. The disease process is always present in the rectum and spreads to the more proximal parts continuously. The clinical presentation of patients varies from mild to very severe. Truelove and Witts[1] have developed a classification which includes the number of loose stools, the grade of bleeding, the existence of fever, anaemia, elevation of the ESR and the level of albumin in the serum. This classification is still widely used for clinical assessment (Table 1). The investigation of the rectum by rectoscopy allows the inflammatory state to be judged by macroscopic and microscopic evaluation. The histological findings can be graded according to the severity. This grading, together with the clinical assessment, makes it possible to define the patient's state and the response under therapy. An index provided by Rachmilewitz et al. has been developed for this purpose and proven to be suitable[2].

## CROHN DISEASE

There have been many approaches to the definition of parameters for the assessment of Crohn disease. A number of laboratory criteria have been investigated,

**Table 1** Classification of ulcerative colitis

|  | Mild | Moderate | Severe |
| --- | --- | --- | --- |
| Diarrhoea | $\leq 4$ | $\geq 6$ | $\geq 10$ |
| Anal bleeding | Mild | Severe | Continuously |
| Fever | No | $\geq 37.8°$ C | $\geq 38.8°$ C |
| Haemoglobin | Normal or > 11.0 g/dl | < 10 g/dl | < 8.0 g/dl |
| ESR | < 30 mm | > 30 mm | > 50 mm |
| Albumin | Normal | 3–4 g/dl | < 3 g/dl |

From Truelove and Witts[1]

mainly the acute-phase reactants like C-reactive protein, orosomucoid, $\alpha$-antitrypsin or haptoglobin, or other biological markers like the sedimentation rate or elevation of the thrombocyte count. These parameters may reflect the inflammatory activity but they give only a limited view of the problem. Being aware of the great variation in presentation of patients with Crohn disease, indices have been developed to define the state of a patient as objectively as possible. The main purpose of an index is its use in therapeutic studies, especially in multicentre studies. The two major contributions towards a better and safer treatment with drugs in Crohn disease have been made by the National Cooperative Crohn's Disease Study[3] in the USA and the European Cooperative Crohn's Disease Study[4] (ECCDS) with the use of the Crohn disease activity index (CDAI), which was developed by Best et al. for the American study[5]. The CDAI proved to be a very valuable tool for the assessment of the success or non-success of treatment with steroids and/or salazopyrine. Indices are mandatory for studies of this kind.

Another purpose is the use in an individual patient. An index can help the doctor to get a better idea of the actual state of the disease and to make a better decision on the treatment.

When looking at the indices, we come to the question of how we define the activity and severity of Crohn disease. A patient can have very active inflammation but feel quite well, and, on the other hand, he can be physically and socially handicapped without very much inflammatory activity. The definitions of activity and severity therefore are the most difficult problems, inherent in all indices and a matter of discussion. In Table 2, we have defined parameters for

**Table 2** Different parameters which characterize activity, severity or both in Crohn disease

| Activity | Activity–severity overlap | Severity |
| --- | --- | --- |
| Extraintestinal manifestations | Diarrhoea | Abdominal pain |
| Fever | Loss of weight | Stricture |
| ESR | Malnutrition | Palpable mass |
| Active phase reactants | Malabsorption | Fistulae |
| Albumin | Retarded growth | Abscess |
| Thrombocytes | Amenorrhoea |  |
| Iron |  |  |
| Haemoglobin |  |  |

activity, severity and an area of overlap. Extraintestinal manifestations (erythema nodosum, arthritis, iritis) and fever are easy to recognize; the other parameters are alterations of laboratory values. Maybe the most important is the decrease in albumin levels. Signs related to severity are abdominal pain, often related to strictures, a palpable mass, fistulae and abscess formation. An area of overlap is in the field of diarrhoea (caused either by inflammation/exudation or by malabsorption of bile acids in the distal ileum), loss of weight, malnutrition as a secondary consequence and malabsorption.

The most widely used index is the Crohn disease activity index (CDAI) of Best et al.[5]. It contains eight parameters: pain in the abdomen (with a score from 0 to 3), the number of liquid stools, a score for the general well-being (from 0 to 4), extra intestinal lesions and fever, the use of antidiarrhoeic drugs, the presence of an abdominal mass, haematocrit, and the loss of weight. It has been criticized because many of the parameters are open to subjective judgment.

Only the extraintestinal signs and the haematocrit are related to the inflammatory activity. The other parameters reflect either the severity or both. A borderline of 150 is taken, with values below reflecting quiescent disease and above active disease. Moreover, a change in values of more than 60 points has been used as an indicator of evolution or regression of inflammation. An evaluation of the CDAI on the clinical rating of 452 patients of the ECCDS has shown that it reflects the clinical judgment with $r = 0.88$, but not the laboratory rating ($r = 0.573$)[6].

Van Hees et al.[7] have developed the Dutch Index. This index contains, nearly exclusively, data which can be raised objectively: albumin level, ESR, weight, sex, temperature, resection of bowel and extraintestinal lesions. In addition, the more subjective presence or absence of an abdominal mass (score 1–5) and diarrhoea are assessed. The borders of activity are defined as: no disease, below 100; slight disease, between 100 and 150; moderate disease, between 150 and 210; and severe disease, above 210 points. The evaluation of the Dutch Index on the 452 patients of the ECCDS has shown that it is highly correlated with a rating based on laboratory data ($r = 0.742$) and worse with a clinical rating ($r = 0.672$)[6].

Based on the data of the 452 patients of the European Crohn's Disease Study, another European Index of Severity and Activity (SAI) has been developed (Table 3). It contains parameters for the severity (number of loose stools, abdominal pain with a score from 0 to 3, palpable mass, anal lesions or fistulae and loss of weight) and for the activity (extraintestinal lesions, fever, haematocrit, albumin). The influence of objective parameters of the activity is higher in this index than in the CDAI and approaches that of the Dutch Index. The borderlines are: below 120 for quiescent or mild disease; between 120 and 240 for moderate disease; and above 240 for severe and very severe disease. According to the evaluation in the 452 patients of the ECCDS, the CDAI has a preponderance of signals for the severity and the Dutch Index for the activity of the disease[6]. The European SAI tries to evaluate both the severity and the activity in a balanced manner.

The use of indices has been the topic of a recent investigation by the International Organisation for the Study of Inflammatory Bowel Diseases (IOIBD)[8]. Two problems have been studied by a group of physicians and sur-

**Table 3**  Severity–Activity Index (SAI) with an example

| Variable | Example | | Coefficient | | Result |
|---|---|---|---|---|---|
| Number of watery stools per day (weekly total/7) | 5 | × | 10 | = | 50 |
| Abdominal pain (grading 0–3, weekly total/7) | 2 | × | 50 | = | 100 |
| Anal/perianal lesions (yes = 1, no = 0) | 1 | × | 30 | = | 30 |
| Palpable mass (yes = 1, no = 0) | 1 | × | 30 | = | 30 |
| Extraintestinal lesions (yes = 1, no = 0) | 1 | × | 40 | = | 40 |
| Weight[*] (1 – weight/standard weight) | (1 – 0.77) | × | 100 | = | 23 |
| Haematocrit (%) | 33 | × | – 4 | = | – 132 |
| Albumin (g/L) | 27 | × | – 2 | = | – 54 |
| Constant | | | 270 | = | 270 |
| Index | | | | | 357 |

Interpretation: the patient has very active and severe disease. Values below 60 indicate quiescent disease, 60–120 mild disease, 120–240 moderately severe disease, above 240 very severe disease.
[*] In this example, weight = 50 kg, standard weight = 65 kg. Taken from Reference 10.

geons in these studies: the calculation of the indices and the eliciting of data. Ten case histories of patients with Crohn disease were estimated for CDAI by seven clinicians. A considerable observer variation resulted within each single patient and, furthermore, at least two of the observers were far out of the range of the others. Obviously, the CDAI was misunderstood by these observers. A detailed discussion on the handling of the CDAI followed and then the calculation took place again. This time, the results were much better than the first time but still showed variation. The next investigation concerned the handling of the Dutch Index with the same ten case histories and seven observers. The results of five of the observers were very close together, but two were totally out of range and resulted from a false calculation of the index. In a further trial, six patients were interviewed and examined by six experienced physicians. The CDAI and the Dutch Index were calculated. The variation of the individual assessments was wide for the CDAI, e.g. in one patient, it varied between 50 and 500. Again, the variation in the Dutch Index was smaller. These studies show that eliciting data in an individual patient is also open to considerable variation. Therefore, before using an index, the staff should have trained together to guarantee a consensus for raising the data.

Recently, Modigliani and his group have developed an endoscopic index for the assessment of Crohn disease[9]. It turned out that endoscopic criteria do not correlate with the clinical picture of the disease very well. Therefore, as long as the treatment of Crohn disease is made according to the clinical state of activity and severity, the clinical indices should be used.

## CONCLUSIONS

The use of indices is well established both in ulcerative colitis and in Crohn disease. It is obvious that they can only offer an approximation to the real state of the patient. In ulcerative colitis, it is much easier than in Crohn disease to come close to a combined assessment of the inflammatory status and the clinical problems. So, we need new investigations, mainly for Crohn disease, to integrate histological, endoscopic and clinical data. Eventually, they might lead to new indices in this field.

## References


1. Truelove SC, Witts LJ. Cortisone in ulcerative colitis: final report on a therapeutic trial. Br Med J. 1955;2:1041–8.
2. Rachmilewitz D and an international study group. Coated mesalazine (5-aminosalicylic acid) versus sulphasalazine in the treatment of active ulcerative colitis: a randomised trial. Br Med J. 1989;298:82–6.
3. Summers RW, Switz DM, Sessions JT et al. National Cooperative Crohn's Disease Study: Results of drug treatment. Gastroenterology. 1979;77:847–69.
4. Malchow H, Ewe K, Brandes JW et al. European Cooperative Crohn's Disease Study (ECCDS): Results of drug treatment. Gastroenterology. 1984;86:249–66.
5. Best WR, Becktel JM, Singleton JW, Kern F. Development of a Crohn's disease activity index (National Cooperative Crohn's Disease Study). Gastroenterology. 1976;70:439–44.
6. Goebell H, Wienbeck M, Schomerus H, Malchow H. Evaluation of the Crohn's Disease Activity Index (CDAI) and the Dutch Index for severity and activity of Crohn's disease. Med Klin. 1990;85:573–6.
7. Van Hees PAM, van Lier HJJ, van Elteren PH et al. Effect of sulphasalazine in patients with active Crohn's disease: a controlled double-blind study. Gut. 1981;22:404–9.
8. de Dombal FT, Softley A. IOIBD-report No 1: observer variation in calculating indices of severity and activity in Crohn's disease. Gut 1978;28:474–81.
9. Mary JY, Modigliani R. Development and validation of a Crohn's disease endoscopic index of severity: a prospective multicentre study. Gut. 1989;30:983–9.
10. Goebell H, Malchow H, Wienbeck W. Evaluation of an index for severity and activity of Crohn's disease (Severity-Activity Index). Eur J Gastroenterol Hepatol. [In preparation].

# 13
# Prognostic indicators for remission, relapse and postoperative recurrence in IBD

## G. R. D'HAENS and P. J. RUTGEERTS

## INTRODUCTION

Crohn disease and ulcerative colitis are chronic inflammatory diseases of the gastrointestinal tract of unknown aetiology. They are both characterized by alternating episodes of disease activity, or 'relapses', and episodes of mild symptoms or even absence of symptoms, called 'remission'. For many years, clinicians have studied clinical and biochemical 'indicators' which could predict disease reactivation. They would permit a timely intensification of medical therapy, i.e. before full-blown systemic disease has developed. Although *induction* of remission can successfully be accomplished in most cases, the optimal strategy for *maintenance* of remission in both Crohn disease and ulcerative colitis is often debatable. We will discuss a number of parameters and their reliability to guide the clinician.

**Crohn disease** can present with a large number of different clinical 'patterns', each of which has its own characteristic symptoms, complications and response to therapeutic actions. Knowledge of the disease pattern is not only important in the approach of every individual patient, but it should be taken into account in clinical trials too.

In about half the Crohn disease patients, surgical intervention becomes unavoidable at a certain point in the evolution. Even if all grossly involved tissue can be resected, the likelihood of disease recurrence in the future is high. Several risk factors have been identified with regard to frequency and severity of recurrent Crohn disease. A number of trials which study the therapeutic benefit of certain drugs in recurrence prevention are currently being conducted.

**Ulcerative colitis** is an inflammatory mucosal disease limited to the colon. Although the disease course can be fulminant and require urgent colectomy, the condition is usually less debilitating than Crohn disease. A number of useful parameters have been identified for the prediction of relapses and the need for urgent colectomy. We will discuss relapse-provoking factors, a few well-known risk factors for the development of dysplasia and cancer in long-standing ulcerative colitis, and risk factors for the development of pouchitis after colectomy and construction of an ileal pouch–anal anastomosis.

## PROGNOSTIC INDICATORS FOR RELAPSE AND REMISSION IN CROHN DISEASE

### Disease patterns

The clinical presentations of Crohn disease can be classified by:

1. Initial location of the inflammation
2. Extent of disease
3. Behaviour of the disease
4. Operative history (i.e. primary vs recurrent disease)[1–3].

The three major subgroups with regard to initial location are ileocolonic Crohn disease (40–55%), purely colonic (15–25%) and small intestinal disease (30–35%). There can be accompanying upper gastrointestinal or anorectal inflammation, but these seem less useful as prognostic indicators. Ileocolonic Crohn disease is characterized by the highest operation and reoperation rates (73% and 44%, respectively). Intestinal obstruction, fistulae, abscess and uncontrollable anal disease are the most common indications for intervention. Surgical intervention in *small bowel* disease is necessary in cases of intestinal obstruction, i.e. eventually in about half the patients. Surgical indications in *colonic* disease include toxic megacolon, strictures, poor response to medical therapy with severe rectal bleeding and perianal disease.

Healing of inflammatory lesions with medical treatment differs significantly throughout the GI tract. Whereas oesophageal lesions heal quickly and completely, gastroduodenal and small intestinal ulcers show little change on follow-up visualization. Colonic and anal ulcerations do heal, though slowly and often incompletely[4,5].

It is also prognostically important to distinguish localized from diffuse ileal or colonic inflammation, the latter of which has a poorer outcome and response to therapy. The Mount Sinai classification of disease 'behaviour' is based on the clinical observation that many patients, throughout their disease course, either develop mainly 'obstructive' symptoms, due to a *fibrostenotic* type of inflammation, or fistulae and abscesses due to a *penetrating* type of inflammation. A third group of patients can be classified into the category of mainly '*inflammatory*' disease, including those with severe systemic symptoms. Of course, one type may progress to one of the others with time and overlapping features can occur. Fibrostenotic disease will often lead to surgical therapy, whereas inflammatory disease requires intensive medical treatment. Fistulizing Crohn disease can be managed either way depending on the individual case[1].

### Clinical indices

Several clinical indices have been developed for assessment of disease activity, and to reach a consensus in patient evaluation in multicentre trials. The oldest index is the Crohn Disease Activity Index (CDAI), which is mainly based on frequency of stools, abdominal pain and, importantly, 'general well-being'. Although this index is strongly influenced by subjective criteria, it appears to be the most sensitive in the prediction of clinical relapse. The Van Hees Index and other indices have also been shown to be useful but appear to be somewhat less reliable. Strangely enough, the correlation between the different indices is rather poor[6,7].

## Laboratory parameters

The correlation of a large number of serum proteins with disease activity and their predictive value have been studied extensively. C-reactive protein (CRP) is the most widely used parameter which corresponds closely with clinical indices, response to therapy and remission. The likelihood of relapse appears to be higher if CRP levels remain persistently elevated[8,9]. Serum concentrations of other acute-phase reactants such as orosomucoid, $\alpha_2$-globulin and $\alpha_1$-antitrypsin also reflect the grade of activity of the disease, and pronounced elevation of haptoglobin levels would even be suggestive of fistulae or abscesses. It should be emphasized, however, that in some cases acute-phase reactants are normal with clinically active disease and vice versa.

The erythrocyte sedimentation rate (ESR) is a cheap and rapid test but its correlation with disease activity is markedly weaker[10–12]. Brignola and his colleagues in Bologna developed a biochemical 'prognostic index': $- 3.5 + (ESR \times 0.03) + (acid\ \alpha_1\text{-glycoprotein} \times 0.013) + (\alpha_2\text{-globulin} \times 2)$. Indices of the patients who suffered relapse in the 18-month follow-up period were significantly higher (cut-off value $+ 0.35$, $p < 0.0001$) than the indices of those who stayed in remission[13].

Circulating levels of a large number of immunological markers and cytokines are increased in active Crohn disease (e.g. IL-6), but with the exception of soluble interleukin-2 receptor (sIL2-r), correlations with disease activity have not been established. In addition, Crabtree et al. demonstrated that the sIL2-r level is also a reliable marker of relapse[14]. Tumour necrosis factor-$\alpha$ (TNF-$\alpha$) concentrations in stool correlate with clinical disease activity in children with IBD[15]; its prognostic value is still unknown. The level of fibrinopeptide A, an indicator of subclinical activation of coagulation, appears to be another valuable parameter of disease activity; failure to return to normal predicts early relapse[16]. Neopterin is a product of human macrophages when stimulated by $\gamma$-interferon. Urinary concentrations provide useful information about the activation state of the cellular immune system, but the predictive value remains to be determined[17].

## Permeability tests

Increased intestinal permeability is a well-documented feature of active Crohn disease. Permeability tests with both Cr-EDTA and lactulose/mannitol are sensitive markers of gut integrity and Crohn disease activity during remission. Moreover, Wyatt et al. demonstrated that the dual sugar lactulose/mannitol test could predict relapses in 75% of patients[18].

## Endoscopic markers

The French GETAID (Groupe d'Etudes Therapeutiques des Affections Inflammatoires Digestives) demonstrated the absence of any correlation between endoscopic observations and clinical disease activity in Crohn colitis and came to the conclusion that adjustment of steroid therapy based on endoscopic findings is of no benefit. The endoscopic picture has no prognostic value with regard to disease relapse[19]. This thesis does not apply to postoperative recurrent Crohn disease in the neoterminal ileum, where the endoscopic features were found to be predictive of the future clinical evolution[20].

## Disease modifiers in Crohn disease

A number of disease- and patient-related parameters should be taken into account in the prognosis of the clinical course. An increased frequency of relapses is associated with:

1. Younger age (< 25 y)
2. Younger age at diagnosis (< 20 y)
3. Shorter interval between relapses (≤ 2 y)
4. Presence of colonic disease.

In addition, lifestyle issues modify the course of the disease. Patients with Crohn disease are more likely to be smokers than are matched controls. Not only do heavily smoking (>10 cigarettes/day) Crohn patients have an increased risk of operation and reoperation, but their risk of postoperative recurrence is markedly increased as well. Fistulae and abscesses develop more frequently in heavy smokers than in non-smokers, and relapses appear to be more severe[21,22].

It remains unclear whether the use of oral contraceptive medication increases the risk of Crohn disease. Epidemiological data are controversial, but the most recent reports have not demonstrated any association[23,24].

## THE PROBLEM OF POSTOPERATIVE RECURRENCE OF CROHN DISEASE

Follow-up studies have shown that clinical symptoms recur in about 10% of patients per year following resection. Risk factors for early recurrence include failure of medical therapy preoperatively, diffuse ileocolitis, young age and smoking[25]. Endoscopic signs of recurrence can often be observed shortly after the operation. We reported recurrent ileal inflammation in 73% of patients at 1 year, and in 85% of patients at 3 years after ileo(colonic) resection of all grossly diseased tissue. The severity of the lesions (number and size of aphthous or larger ulcerations) correlated well with the clinical course of the patients over the following years[20].

The virulence of the inflammatory activity is often comparable before surgery and at the time of clinical recurrence; in addition, the type (fibrostenotic versus perforating) and the length of ileal inflammation were found to be similar before and after surgery[26–28]. The presence of granulomas and 'free resection margins' (i.e. absence of microscopic inflammatory activity) does not seem to influence recurrence rates or severity[29].

However, if a permanent ileostomy is performed rather than a classical ileocolonic anastomosis, the recurrence rate appears to be significantly lower, probably due to the absence of bacterial colonization.


## ULCERATIVE COLITIS: CLINICAL COURSE

### Ulcerative colitis and the need for urgent colectomy

Chakravarty and colleagues in New Zealand compared clinical and biochemical parameters in patients with acute ulcerative colitis for whom medical therapy had failed and who required urgent colectomy with those in whom colectomy could be avoided[30]. There were no significant differences between the groups in age or sex, age at onset of disease, duration of disease, haemoglobin level or white cell count. There was a tendency towards higher ESR and greater extent of colitis (proximal to the splenic flexure) in the colectomy group. The most significant predictors of colectomy, however, were serum albumin levels ($p = 0.0001$) and severity of diarrhoea ($p = 0.0001$)[30]. Another study demonstrated a higher success rate of medical therapy with milder disease, limited extent, shorter duration, lower ESR and higher haemoglobin levels[31].

The importance of body temperature and the number of stools passed was reported somewhat later: maximum body temperature below 38°C and a stool frequency of less than 8 per day were predictive for response to medical therapy[32]. The Truelove and Witts criteria, although initially believed to predict the prognosis, were later found to correlate poorly with outcome. In other studies, CRP-levels, state of nutrition and endoscopic observations were the best predictive factors[33].


### Relapse-provoking factors in ulcerative colitis

In many relapses of ulcerative colitis a precipitating factor can be identified. Intestinal, respiratory or systemic infections can all acutely exacerbate colitis symptoms. *Clostridium difficile* is a very common pathogen which, even in the absence of earlier antibiotic therapy, is responsible for an important number of colitis relapses. Other infectious agents such as *Salmonella, Campylobacter, Entamoeba histolytica* and enteroviruses also need to be searched for if symptoms worsen. CMV-infection can provoke severe relapses, especially during immunosuppressive therapy, such as corticosteroids or azathioprine treatment.

Idiosyncratic reactions to sulphasalazine or 5-ASA preparations can cause exacerbation of symptoms when these drugs are initiated or increased; symptoms may be masked by concomitant administration of steroids. Ischaemic colitis, though more frequent in the older population, has been reported in young patients with inflammatory diseases and secondary mesenteric vein thrombosis or thromboembolism. Adenocarcinoma of the colon should always be considered in patients with long-standing extensive ulcerative colitis[34].

## Prediction of relapse

The same laboratory parameters as used in Crohn disease have been studied in ulcerative colitis and have been shown to be of some benefit in the prediction of relapses. In addition, elevated $PGE_2$ levels in rectal dialysate from asymptomatic patients who had discontinued maintenance therapy with sulphasalazine were predictive of relapse[35].

## Prediction of long-term clinical course in ulcerative colitis

A careful study from the university of Copenhagen including more than 1000 patients clarified a number of important issues regarding the long-term prognosis of ulcerative colitis. After 10 years of follow-up, their colectomy rate amounted to 24%. At any point in time, 90% of the patients were fully capable of work. The only significant factor with regard to relapses was disease activity in the foregoing years, which was predictive of continuing disease activity with a 70–80% probability. In each year, about 50% of patients remained in clinical remission. The cumulative rate of a relapsing course was 90% after 25 years of follow-up[36].

## Prediction of the development of malignancy

It is now generally accepted that the risk of colon cancer is considerably increased in long-standing ulcerative colitis. The risk increases steadily from 2% after 10 years of colitis to more than 25% after more than 30 years. Additional risk factors besides duration include increasing extent of disease, and possibly older age at disease onset and the presence of cholestatic liver function abnormalities[37,38]. The benefit of routine screening programmes remains, nevertheless, a controversial issue.

## Prediction of the development of pouchitis after ileal pouch–anal anastomosis

Inflammation of the ileal pouch after colectomy with ileo-anal anastomosis occurs in 5–20% of patients. The incidence of pouchitis is, curiously enough, twice as high in patients who exhibited extraintestinal manifestations prior to their colectomy (40% vs 20%)[39]. Pouchitis was not influenced by pouch design, sepsis, age or sex. Patients with indeterminate colitis have a higher incidence and more severe disease. The presence of daytime or night-time incontinence also has an association with pouchitis[39,40].

## References

1. Sachar DB, Andrews HA, Farmer RG et al. Proposed classification of patient subgroups in Crohn's disease. Gastroenterol Int. 1992;5:141–54.
2. Farmer RG. Factors in the long-term prognosis of patients with inflammatory bowel disease. Am J Gastroenterol. 1981;75:97–103.
3. Farmer RG, Whelan G, Fazio VW. Long-term follow-up of patients with Crohn's disease; relationship between the clinical pattern and prognosis. Gastroenterology. 1985;88:1818–25.
4. Olaison B, Sjodahl R, Tagesson C. Glucocorticoid treatment in ileal Crohn's disease; relief of symptoms but not of endoscopically viewed inflammation. Gut. 1990;31:325–8.

5. Modigliani R, Mary JY, Simon JF et al. Clinical, biological and endoscopic picture of attacks of Crohn's disease. Evolution on prednisolone. Gastroenterology. 1990;98:811–18.
6. Wright JP, Alp MN, Young GO, Tigler-Wybrandi N. Predictors of acute relapse of Crohn's disease; a laboratory and clinical study. Dig Dis Sci. 1987;32:164–70.
7. Kjeldsen J, Schaffalitzky de Muckadell OB. Assessment of disease severity and activity in inflammatory bowel disease. Scand J Gastroenterol. 1993;28:1–9.
8. Fagan EA, Dyck RF, Maton PN et al. Serum levels of C-reactive protein in Crohn's disease and ulcerative colitis. Eur J Clin Invest. 1982;12:351–9.
9. Boirivant M, Leoni M, Taricotti D, Fais S, Squarcia O, Pallone P. The clinical significance of serum C reactive protein levels in Crohn's disease. J Clin Gastroenterol. 1988;10:401–5.
10. Cellier C, Sahmoud T, Froguel E et al. Correlations between clinical activity, endoscopic severity and biological parameters in colonic or ileocolonic Crohn's disease. A prospective multicentre study of 121 cases. Gut. 1994;35:231–5.
11. Brignola C, Lanfranchi GA, Campieri M et al. Importance of laboratory parameters in the evaluation of Crohn's disease activity. J Clin Gastroenterol. 1986;8:245–8.
12. Weeke B, Jarnum S. Serum concentration of 19 serum proteins in Crohn's disease and ulcerative colitis. Gut. 1971;12:297–302.
13. Brignola C, Campieri M, Bazzocchi G, Farruggia P, Tragnone A, Lanfranchi GA. A laboratory index for predicting relapse in asymptomatic patients with Crohn's disease. Gastroenterology. 1986;91:1490–4.
14. Crabtree JE, Juby LD, Heatley RV, Lobo AJ, Bullimore DW, Axon ATR. Soluble interleukin 2-receptor in Crohn's disease: relation of serum concentration to disease activity. Gut. 1990;31:1033–6.
15. Braegger CP, Nicholls S, Murch SH, Stephens S, McDonald TT. Tumor necrosis factor-$\alpha$ in stool as a marker of intestinal inflammation. Lancet. 1992;339:89–91.
16. Edwards RL, Levine JB, Green R et al. Activation of blood coagulation in Crohn's disease: increased plasma fibrinopeptide A levels and enhanced generation of monocytes tissue factor activity. Gastroenterology. 1987;92:329–37.
17. Prior C, Bollbach R, Fuchs D et al. Urinary neopterine, a marker of clinical activity in patients with Crohn's disease. Clin Chim Acta. 1986;155:11–22.
18. Wyatt J, Vogelsang H, Hubl W, Waldhoer T, Lochs H. Intestinal permeability and the prediction of relapse in Crohn's disease. Lancet. 1993;341:1437–9.
19. Landi B, N'Guyen Anh T et al. Endoscopic monitoring of Crohn's disease treatment: a prospective, randomized clinical trial. Gastroenterology. 1992;102:1647–53.
20. Rutgeerts P, Geboes K, Vantrappen G, Beyls J, Kerremans R, Hiele M. Predictability of the postoperative course of Crohn's disease. Gastroenterology. 1990;99:956–63.
21. Tobin MV, Logan RFA, Langman MJS, McConnell RB, Gilmore IT. Cigarette smoking and inflammatory bowel disease. Gastroenterology. 1987;93:316–21.
22. Sutherland LR, Ramcharan S, Bryant H, Fick G. Effect of cigarette smoking on recurrence of Crohn's disease. Gastroenterology. 1990;98:1123–8.
23. Lesko SM, Kaufman DW, Rosenberg L et al. Evidence for an increased risk of Crohn's disease in oral contraceptive users. Gastroenterology. 1985;89:1046–9.
24. Lashner BA, Kane SV, Hanauer SB. Lack of association between oral contraceptive use and Crohn's disease: a community-based matched case-control study. Gastroenterology. 1989;97:1442–7.
25. Sachar DB, Wolfson DM, Greenstein AJ, Goldberg J, Styczynski R, Janowitz HD. Risk factors for postoperative recurrence of Crohn's disease. Gastroenterology. 1983;85:917–21.
26. Heimann TM, Greenstein AJ, Lewis B, Kaufman D, Heimann DM, Aufses AH. Prediction of early symptomatic recurrence after intestinal resection in Crohn's disease. Ann Surg. 1993;218:294–9.
27. Cameron JL, Hamilton SR, Coleman J, Sitzmann JV, Bayless TM. Patterns of ileal recurrence in Crohn's disease. Ann Surg. 1992;215:546–51.
28. Greenstein AJ, Lachman P, Sachar DB et al. Perforating and non-perforating indications for repeated operations in Crohn's disease: evidence for two clinical forms. Gut. 1988;29:588–92.
29. Wolfson DM, Sachar DB, Cohen A et al. Granulomas do not affect postoperative recurrence rates in Crohn's disease. Gastroenterology. 1982;83:405–9.
30. Chakravarty BJ. Predictors and the rate of medical treatment failure in ulcerative colitis. Am J Gastroenterol. 1993;88:852–5.

31. Meyers S, Lerer PK, Feuer EJ, Johnson JW, Janowitz HD. Predicting the outcome of corticoid therapy for acute ulcerative colitis. J Clin Gastroenterol. 1987;9:50–4.
32. Lennard-Jones JE, Ritchie JK, Hilder W, Spicer CC. Assessment of severity in colitis: a preliminary study. Gut. 1975;16:579–4.
33. Oshitani N, Kitano A, Fukushima R et al. Predictive factors for the response of ulcerative colitis during the acute phase treatment. Digestion. 1990;46:107–13.
34. Hermens DJ, Miner PB. Exacerbations of ulcerative colitis. Gastroenterology. 1991;101:254–62.
35. Lauritsen K, Laursen LS, Bukhave K, Rask-Madsen J. Use of colonic eicosanoid concentration as predictors of relapse in ulcerative colitis: double-blind placebo-controlled study in sulphasalazin maintenance treatment. Gut. 1988;29:1316–21.
36. Langholz E, Munkholm P, Davidson M, Binder V. Course of ulcerative colitis: analysis of changes in disease activity over years. Gastroenterology. 1994;107:3–11.
37. Lashner BA, Siverstein MD, Hanauer SB. Hazard rates for dysplasia and cancer in ulcerative colitis. Results from a surveillance program. Dig Dis Sci. 1989;34:1536–41.
38. D'Haens GR, Lashner BA, Hanauer SB. Pericholangitis and sclerosing cholangitis are risk factors for dysplasia and cancer in ulcerative colitis. Am J Gastroenterol. 1993;88:1174–8.
39. Becker JM, Dunnegan D. Ileal pouch function and dysfunction following ileal pouch anal anastomosis. In: MacDermott RP, ed. Inflammatory bowel disease, current state and future approach. Amsterdam: Elsevier; 1988:689–93.
40. Santos MC, Thompson JS. Late complications of the ileal pouch–anal anastomosis. Am J Gastroenterol. 1993;88:3–10.

# 14
# Quality of life in IBD: does it reflect activity of disease?

R. W. SUMMERS

## INTRODUCTION

The traditional inflammatory bowel diseases (IBD) qualify as chronic diseases, i.e. the cause(s) is/are unknown, the course is capricious, and the therapy is empiric and largely palliative. The major objectives of therapy are to modify the course of the disease, and, currently, patients and physicians alike must learn to cope with the disease rather than to cure it.

Physicians have always recognized that health is more than the absence of disease. Similarly, illness has an effect on the patient greater than the symptoms which it causes. Patients feel ill and the illness interferes with their daily lives. Even the word 'dis-ease' implies that the afflicted experience uneasiness or lack of true satisfaction with life. While the goal of therapy has always been to alleviate the symptoms and signs of disease, it is also recognized that the cure or a solution to all problems is not possible. The responsibility remains to help the sufferer to cope with those problems which cannot be dealt with medically. The goal is to aid the patient in minimizing the dysfunction and in feeling as well as possible within the confines of the illness. Because all aspects of IBD cannot be defined in terms of physical problems, interest in 'quality-of-life' assessment in chronic diseases has grown progressively over the past 20 years. Assessment of quality-of-life issues is an important measure in outcomes research, but it can also be useful in the day-to-day management of patients.

## DEFINING TERMS AND IMPROVING DESCRIPTIONS

What then are quality-of-life issues which stem from inflammatory bowel disease and how should they be defined? Humans have attempted to describe, define and achieve quality of life from the beginnings of recorded time. Happiness and satisfaction are the objectives of all humankind, yet there is no agreement on the definition of the good life.

Quantification of the disease impact on life
A measure of care beyond physical problems
Life satisfaction or happiness
A state of physical, mental and social well-being
The perceived discrepancy between aspirations and achievement

There is a growing recognition that biological processes and malfunction alone are insufficient to describe a patient's health status. A variety of dimensions or domains are used to describe well-being and satisfaction.

1. Physical factors always come to mind first, including disease and organ-specific factors as well as systemic factors
2. Psychological or emotional factors
3. Social factors, such as interpersonal relationships, leisure or recreational activities, and participation in organized social activities
4. Sexual factors, such as desire, interest, activity and body image
5. Economic factors, such as employment and insurance

## RECOGNITION OF THE ISSUES IN THE 70s

Early studies recognized the importance of assessing quality of life in clinical studies. Measurement of these factors was quite crude and imprecise in its application. As an example, Bergman and Krause[1] measured quality of life using only three categories in their evaluation of patients with Crohn disease 10 years postresection:

I. Good general health, able to work full time, unrestricted leisure
II. Reduced ability to work, restriction in leisure less than 50%
III. Unable to work, leisure severely restricted

In a group of patients undergoing a 'radical resection', 87% had a category I, 9% a category II and less than 4% a category III. Radical resection was judged to be superior to a more limited resection in surgical management.

Gazzard et al.[2] studied 85 outpatients with Crohn disease using two general indices, the morbid anxiety index (MAI) and the Eysenck personality questionnaire (EPQ). Women were similar to a control group, but men were more neurotic and introverted. They felt that patients lived optimistic useful lives and that successful adaptation to the disease was more closely related to their personality than to the activity or extent of the disease. Mallet et al.[3], however, studied 40 patients and asked them to assess the impact of their disease on their lives. They described their worst problem and then a derived questionnaire was given to another 95 patients. Urgency, incontinence, abdominal or rectal pain and lassitude were major problems limiting work, social life and leisure. Symptoms often reduced their earning capacity and interfered with their lives, but did not always correlate with disease activity or extent. Meyers et al.[4] assessed the quality of life following surgical resection in comparison with retrospective recall of the same factors before operation. They utilized a questionnaire to evaluate physical symptoms, relationships, school or work performance, recreation, sexuality and body image. Quality of life was perceived to improve long-term after resection, even with evidence of recurrent disease.

These early studies were descriptive and the measurements were limited in scope, general and unvalidated. Furthermore, most of the tests were applied retrospectively, i.e. they were not part of a prospective study design. However, they were most important in calling attention to the assessment of a broad array of life's qualities beyond the ordinary symptoms usually noted in IBD, such as diarrhoea, bleeding and abdominal pain.

## DEVELOPMENT OF INSTRUMENTS TO MEASURE QUALITY OF LIFE IN THE 80s

In 1988, a group of investigators from McMasters launched a series of studies to develop instruments to measure quality of life in inflammatory bowel disease. Guyatt et al.[6] started with the premise that they would stress the patient's subjective experience by developing qualitative and semiquantitative descriptions of how IBD patients' lives were limited in work and social activities, home and married life and emotional function. Detailed interviews were held with 43 patients with ulcerative colitis and 54 patients with Crohn disease. They encouraged spontaneous responses in these areas and also elicited responses from lists generated from experienced clinicians and the literature. A number of important variables were identified:

Primary bowel symptoms
  Frequent bowel movements
  Loose bowel movements
  Abdominal cramps
  Pain in the abdomen
Systemic symptoms
  Fatigue
  Feeling unwell
  Worn out
Emotional impairment
  Frustrated
  Depressed
  Worried about surgery
Social impairment
  Avoiding events without bathrooms
  Cancelling social events
  Functional impairment
  Cannot attend school/work

From a somewhat longer list, a disease-specific IBD questionnaire (IBDQ) was then developed as a measure of health status by selecting 32 of the most frequent and important items identified by these patients. The questionnaire was then subjected to testing by administration to another 97 patients, using a personal interview, repeated a second time and given to a group of controls. The results were compared with a clinical assessment of disease activity[5–7].

The following quantitative tests assessed the quality of the instrument:

**Reproducibility**  Repeat tests gave similar results in subjects without a change in disease activity.

**Responsiveness**  IBDQ scores changed directly with change in disease activity.

**Validity**  The components of the instruments correlated with changes in global assessment of disease activity and with other components internally.

A similar approach to quality-of-life assessment in IBD has been reported by Farmer et al. using interview techniques[8]. It should be pointed out that Love et al. have shown that self-administered forms can yield data as reliable as those obtained by personal interview[7].

Other investigators have collected quality-of-life data using so-called generic instruments. These standardized instruments have been used extensively and are well accepted and widely validated. They have the advantage of being able to make comparisons between diseases which are clinically very dissimilar, e.g. rheumatoid arthritis and ulcerative colitis. They may not be as responsive or as reproducible because many of the questions may not apply to the disease being evaluated. Drossman et al.[9] have applied the Sickness Impact Profile (SIP) in IBD, and also combined it with the disease-specific Rating Form of IBD Patient Concerns (RFIPC). Clearly, useful information was elicited about the worries and concerns of patients beyond their bowel symptoms. Patients with Crohn disease reported greater impairment of function and perceived themselves to be more ill than patients with ulcerative colitis[9]. These authors state that measures to assess the broad range of patient concerns must be added to the usual biological measures of disease activity in order to obtain an accurate evaluation of the patient's health status[10]. In a larger study, 997 members of the Crohn's and Colitis Foundation of America were mailed the SIP, SCL-90 symptom checklist (for assessment of psychological distress) and Ways of Coping-Revised questionnaire[11]. Coping profiles of ulcerative colitis patients were similar to those of patients with Crohn disease. Patients' self-perceived health status was generally good despite significant symptoms and complications, possibly related to effective coping styles. Patients with Crohn disease had more psychosocial difficulties than those with ulcerative colitis, probably due to more severe bowel symptoms. These studies appear to provide some useful information about large population groups but may not be of as much use when dealing with individuals. A more recent study from the same group developed brief and easy-to-use health status scales for both UC and CD[12]. Items were identified which discriminated active from inactive disease in a large survey of patients. Such scales would be useful in research and clinical care of patients if they are confirmed by other studies to be accurate predictors of prognosis or utilization of health resources. During this decade, every group devised their own quality-of-life questionnaire. This prevented independent validation of the instrument and any comparison between studies.

## REFINEMENTS AND APPLICATIONS OF THE INSTRUMENTS IN THE 90s

At this point, most would agree that IBD has an impact on lives which goes beyond disturbed bowel function. This impact can be described and quantified accurately using a variety of measuring instruments. The next question is of what use are these results? Most of the early investigators were satisfied to describe the alterations in health status in various groups of patients. However, in the past few years, interest has grown in the comparative aspects of quality-of-life parameters before and after medical and surgical interventions or of one medical or surgical therapy against another. Increasing numbers of comparative quality-of-life studies are being performed in both surgical and medical therapy, and examples of each are described below. In addition, specific quality-of-life issues, such as sexual dysfunction, and the cost of illness in financial terms have been explored in greater depth.

### Medical therapy – an example

Both disease-specific and general quality-of-life parameters were evaluated in a placebo-controlled dose–response study of mesalamine in the treatment of pan- or left-sided ulcerative colitis[13]. Three hundred and seventy-four patients with active disease were treated with either placebo, 1 g/d, 2 g/d or 4 g/d mesalazine for a total of 8 weeks.

Response parameters included:

Bowel symptoms:
  Number of trips to the toilet
  Stool consistency
  Rectal bleeding
  Abdominal/rectal pain
  Rectal urgency

General or systemic problems:
  Ability to sleep
  Sexual relations
  Indoor activities
  Outdoor activities
  Work/occupation
  Social activities
  Hobbies/recreation

Mesalamine at 2 g/d and 4 g/d was found to be significantly superior to placebo in improving each of the above parameters. This was yet another independently derived measuring device. However, a number of studies of medical therapies have utilized the McMaster's IBDQ which allows comparison between studies.

## Surgical therapy – an example

Among 971 patients undergoing colectomy and ileal pouch–anal anastomosis (IPAA) in a 9-year period, 30 patients from each year (a total of 240 patients) were compared with 20 cholecystectomy patients each year (a total of 160 patients) using a quality-of-life questionnaire[14]. IPAA patients experienced a greater median stool frequency (6 stools/24 h) in comparison with the cholecystectomy patients (1 stool/24 h) and, similarly, faecal spotting was much more common in IPAA patients. However, overall quality-of-life assessments including evaluation of interpersonal relationships, social and recreational activities, sex life, and fulfilment, were all equal in IPAA and cholecystectomy patients.

A number of medical and surgical studies have compared quality-of-life parameters between medical therapies and between surgical therapies, before and after surgical therapy and between medical and surgical therapies. This trend is encouraging and yet it is important to be certain that the groups are comparable at the beginning of the study and this means that the tests are applied prospectively rather than choosing the patients after the intervention.

A number of studies have utilized quality-of-life testing in very specific domains to emphasize the importance of assessing these dimensions in the management of patients. For example, Moody et al. investigated the importance of sexual dysfunction in two papers[15,16]. Of 50 women with Crohn disease, 45 were in a stable relationship and 24% of patients reported infrequent or no intercourse in comparison with only 4% of controls. The presumed reasons for infrequent relations included the existence of abdominal pain, diarrhoea and fear of faecal incontinence. Dyspareunia is common, and perianal disease, fistulae and vaginal candidiasis all may contribute to the problem in women. A similar study was performed in a larger group of 188 patients with IBD. The frequency of sexual intercourse in women with ulcerative colitis was also reduced for similar reasons. Fear of incontinence, urgency and abdominal pain again were felt to be responsible for the reduction in intercourse, although this remains to be proven. The frequency of intercourse was not decreased in men with IBD in comparison with matched controls. Thus, women were found to experience sexual dysfunction more than matched healthy controls and they need support, sympathetic investigation and supportive management. Even though sexual dysfunction has been assessed in other quality-of-life studies, it tends to be lost and buried in myriads of other details or condensed as a numerical index and the reader does not recognize its importance.

Finally, the question might be asked, do life events or depression exacerbate inflammatory bowel disease? North et al.[17] looked at this issue in a prospective study of 32 patients who had had a flare within the two previous years. The Social Readjustment Rating Scale (measuring life events), the Beck Depression Inventory (a visual analogue scale for depressed mood) and a series of questions to evaluate intestinal symptoms were completed monthly by each subject. A mean of 2.2 exacerbations was seen by each subject. Life events were not temporally associated with changes in intestinal symptoms. Significant associations between changes in intestinal symptoms and mood changes were seen, but there was no directionality in symptom occurrence in a time-lagged analysis. Therefore, even though changes in mood were associated with exacerbations of

IBD, the findings did not indicate that stressful life events or depression precipitated exacerbations in these patients. Even though the issue was not directly addressed, one would need to ask whether the disease activity was a major factor in determining the changes in quality-of-life parameters.

## COMPARATIVE QUALITY-OF-LIFE STUDY OF IBD IN IOWA CONSIDERING DIAGNOSIS, GENDER, AGE AND SEVERITY OF ILLNESS

### Introduction

Our purpose in this study was to compare quality-of-life issues in a number of patient subgroups. It seemed that a number of variables would probably influence the impact of the various domains which have traditionally been a part of quality-of-life assessments. The comparisons which were made were based on divisions of the groups into a number of subgroups:

Crohn disease vs ulcerative colitis
Men vs women patients
Older (> 40 y) vs younger ($\leq$ 40 y)
Inactive or mildly active vs moderately or very active disease

### Patients

We studied 300 patients with inflammatory bowel disease who were members of the Iowa chapter of the Crohn's and Colitis Foundation of America. Questionnaires were mailed to 550 members. Of those 400/550 who returned the questionnaire, 78/400 stated that they did not have IBD. Of those who stated that they had IBD, 22 preferred not to fill out the questionnaire and the study was based on the first 300 consecutive patients who returned the questionnaire.

### Questionnaires

The questionnaires were in various formats and addressed several different issues:

Demographics
Open-ended questions about IBD
List of 82 common individual current problems and concerns.
 The requested responses were ranked as:
 1. Major problem
 2. Minor problem } within the last 2 weeks
 3. No problem
McMaster's IBD questionnaire – 33 questions which have been frequently considered important. The questions address bowel symptoms, systemic symptoms, emotional and social problems. The answers were rated using a Likert scale. Healthy patients have the highest scores.

Comparisons were made using the $\chi$-square test.

## Results

Characteristics of the patients were as follows:

Diagnosis: 100 ulcerative colitis and 200 Crohn disease
Duration of disease: 88 < 5 y and 212 > 5 y
History of surgery: 145 yes and 155 no
Gender: 110 men and 190 women
Education: 7 < high school, 293 high school, 85 college or university, 47 some graduate education
Marital status: 48 single, 214 married, 17 widowed, 24 divorced
Disease activity: 108 in remission, 128 mildly active, 50 moderately active, 10 very active

Therefore, the typical patient was a well-educated married woman with Crohn disease which was of long duration and exhibited little or no activity.

## Comparisons between various subgroups

### Crohn disease vs ulcerative colitis

Patients with Crohn disease had more problems with frequent and loose bowel movements, but fewer complained of bloody bowel movements than patients with ulcerative colitis. While ulcerative colitis patients complained of more weakness and medication side-effects, Crohn disease patients were bothered more by fatigue. In Crohn disease, patients worried more about never feeling better while, in ulcerative colitis, concern was greater about developing cancer.

### Men vs women

There were no significant differences between men and women in bowel function or systemic symptoms, except that women had more problems with fatigue and loss of energy and they tired more easily. There were also no differences in emotional or social function except that women were more often concerned about feeling alone.

### Older (> 40 y) vs younger (< 40 y)

The older group of patients were bothered more by waking at night and had more problems falling asleep. Joint pains were more frequently a problem in the older group and they were more troubled by medication side-effects than younger patients. They expressed less interest in sex and complained about a loss of sexual drive. They were more often concerned about finding a toilet and more frequently avoided events where a toilet was not readily available. Somewhat surprisingly, the older group was more concerned about decrease in potential than the younger group, although they had also had their disease for a longer period of time.

## *Ill vs well patients*

The largest differences between subgroups were in those patients who were moderately and very ill in comparison with those who were well or mildly ill. The more ill patients obviously had more gastrointestinal and systemic problems than the well patients, except that gas and bloating were no more frequently problems in the ill patient than they were in those who were well. However, the differences were just as great in nearly all of the emotional and social categories. This comparison indicates that quality-of-life issues are indicators of disease activity. Although there was overlap among groups, the self-rating of disease activity correlated well with a survey activity index and with the IBDQ numerical index.

In a separate comparison, patients rated their needs in the various domains and their physician's response to those needs. They perceived that physicians almost always addressed their physical needs, but often noted that their needs in the emotional, sexual and social domains were not addressed. This perception points out the importance of recognizing needs of patients beyond their digestive and systemic problems in order to provide comprehensive care. This may be especially important when the disease-specific inflammatory process cannot be completely controlled.

## Conclusions

The results of this study indicated that nearly all of the quality-of-life domains were affected by the activity of the disease. However, even when the disease activity was mild or inactive, psychological, social and sexual concerns continued to be significant for many of the patients. The patients frequently had needs beyond the disease-specific and systemic indicators and these needs were frequently not recognized or addressed by the physician. Therefore, in the comprehensive care of the patient with IBD, it is important to be aware of and address the non-physical as well as the physical needs of the patient.

## SUMMARY OF HOW QUALITY-OF-LIFE STUDIES ARE USEFUL IN IBD

1.  Some quality-of-life studies are descriptive and useful for increasing awareness and understanding of the many ways in which inflammatory bowel disease affects the lives of patients.

2.  Quality-of-life studies can be used to assess disease activity. The psychological, social and sexual dimensions which contribute to the description of quality of life change in parallel to the physical dimensions of the disease.

3.  Quality-of-life studies have been used to assess and compare medical, surgical and some other interventions in the management of inflammatory bowel disease. They add to the understanding of the effect of the intervention and should be included prospectively in clinical research protocols.

4.  Quality-of-life studies can be used in the clinical sphere to plan interventions other than the typical medical or surgical therapies. If the physician

is aware of specific problems, he or she can often address and manage these individual problems. These strategies can help patients cope with their disease even when it is not possible to treat the symptoms of the disease effectively or the inflammatory process itself.

## References


1. Bergman L, Krause U. Crohn's disease: a long-term study of the clinical course in 186 patients. Scand J Gastroenterol. 1977;12:937–44.
2. Gazzard BG, Price HL, Libby GW, Dawson AM. The social toll of Crohn's disease. Br Med J. 1978;2:1117–19.
3. Mallett SJ, Lennard-Jones JE, Bingley J, Gilon E. Colitis. Lancet. 1978;2:619.
4. Meyers S, Walfish JS, Sachar DB, Greenstein AJ, Hill AG, Janowitz HD Quality of life after surgery for Crohn's disease: A psychosocial survey. Gastroenterology. 1980;78:1–6.
5. Mitchell A, Guyatt G, Singer J et al. Quality of life in patients with inflammatory bowel disease. J Clin Gastroenterol. 1988;10:306–10.
6. Guyatt G, Mitchell A, Irvine EJ et al. A new measure of health status for clinical trials in inflammatory bowel disease. Gastroenterology. 1989;96:804–10.
7. Love JR, Irvine EJ, Fedorak RN. Quality of life in inflammatory bowel disease. J Clin Gastroenterol. 1992;14:15–19.
8. Farmer RG, Easley KA, Farmer JM. Quality of life assessment of patients with inflammatory bowel disease. Cleve Clin J Med. 1992;59:35–42.
9. Drossman DA, Patrick DL, Mitchell CM, Zagami EA, Applebaum MI. Health-related quality of life in inflammatory bowel disease: Functional status and patient worries and concerns. Dig Dis Sci. 1989;34:1379–86.
10. Garrett JW, Drossman DA. Health status in inflammatory bowel disease: Biological and behavioral considerations. Gastroenterology. 1990;99:90–6.
11. Drossman DA, Leserman J, Mitchell CM, Li Z, Zagame DA, Patrich DL. Health status and health care use in persons with inflammatory bowel disease: A national sample. Dig Dis Sci. 1991;12:1746–55.
12. Drossman DA, Li Z, Leserman J, Patrick DL. Ulcerative colitis and Crohn's disease health status scales for research and clinical practice. J Clin Gastroenterol. 1992;15:104–12.
13. Robinson M, Hanauer S, Hoop R, Zbrozek A, Wilkinson C. Mesalamine capsules enhance the quality of life for patients with ulcerative colitis. Aliment Pharmacol Ther. 1994;8:27–34
14. Kohler LW, Pemberton JH, Hodge DO, Zinsmeister AR, Kelly KA. Long-term functional results and quality of life after ileal pouch–anal anastomosis and cholecystectomy. World J Surg. 1992;16:1126–32.
15. Moody GA, Probert CSJ, Srivastava EM, Rhodes J, Mayberry JF. Sexual dysfunction amongst women with Crohn's disease: a hidden problem. Digestion. 1992;52:179–83.
16. Moody GA, Mayberry JF. Perceived sexual dysfunction amongst patients with inflammatory bowel disease. Digestion. 1993;54:256–60.
17. North CS, Alpers DH, Helzer JE, Spitznagel EL, Clouse RE. Do life events or depression exacerbate inflammatory bowel disease? A prospective study. Ann Intern Med. 1991;114:381–6.

# Section IV
# Standards and new developments in diagnosis

# 15
# How much endoscopy and when – points to be considered in diagnosis and follow-up

C. ELL

Endoscopic examinations play an essential role in the diagnosis of chronic inflammatory bowel disease. The standards established years ago have remained virtually unchanged up to the present day. Nevertheless, a number of specific aspects need to be modified due to new developments and recently presented research results. Moreover, the spectrum of endoscopic procedures has been expanded by endosonography. New concepts in the field of therapy, in the management of strictures and in the treatment of primary sclerosing cholangitis have been introduced as well (Table 1).

**Table 1**  Diagnostic and therapeutic spectrum of endoscopy in inflammatory bowel disease

Initial diagnosis
Differential diagnosis
Fistula
Follow-up
Pre-operative
Postoperative
Cancer surveillance

Cholestasis and IBD

Strictures

## INITIAL DIAGNOSIS

There is no doubt that colonoscopy represents the leading imaging technique for diagnosing chronic inflammatory bowel disease. This technique serves to provide an initial diagnosis of colitis and to determine the clinical activity of the disease on the mucosal level. Furthermore, colonoscopy allows the extent of the lesion to be assessed and offers first insights upon which a differential diagnosis can be based. There is no doubt that colonoscopy is superior to a double-contrast barium enema X-ray examination of the colon[1]. The latter should be avoided entirely, except in a select number of indications (e.g. endoscopically impassable stenosis). An initial diagnostic examination based on colonoscopy should be carried out at the earliest possible time. A toxic megacolon continues to remain the only contraindication. In the latter case, attempts to apply endoscopic decompression procedures are hazardous and their efficacy doubtful – in contrast to their application in the case of intestinal pseudo-obstruction. Whenever possible, a complete colonoscopy combined with an inspection of the ileum must be performed. Sequential biopsies comprising all representative sections of the colon and the ileum are imperative. The previously held view that an acute colitis marks a contraindication should be seen in a more relative perspective. Colonoscopy is acceptable, even under active disease conditions, if the endoscopist possesses sufficient expertise and proceeds very cautiously[2]. However, if difficulties, such as loop formation or deep ulcerations bearing the risk of perforation, are encountered, the procedure should be restricted to a partial inspection only. If appropriate medical therapy is performed, complete colonoscopy can be carried out at an active-disease-free interval. The application of further diagnostic imaging techniques can be dispensed with if a limited form of ulcerative colitis (e.g. proctosigmoiditis) is endoscopically diagnosed and if the patient is not suffering from additional abdominal complaints, especially in the upper abdominal area. In contrast, oesophago–gastro–duodenoscopy is compulsory in patients presenting with Crohn disease, as up to 15% macroscopic and microscopic Crohn lesions may be identifiable in the upper gastrointestinal tract. The availability of modern enteroscopes with a working length of 2.30 to 2.50 m which offer the same range of treatment as standard gastroscopes has, for the first time, made a reliable inspection of the deeper sections of the duodenum and the upper jejunum technically possible. This method – provided it is available and the endoscopist is sufficiently experienced – should be extensively implemented to assess Crohn lesions in this area because these domains cannot be reliably diagnosed either with the conventional barium meal or by double-contrast X-ray examinations.

There is no doubt that biopsies in combination with endoscopy are an essential part of basic endoscopic diagnosis. The pathohistological evaluation of the extracted tissue samples frequently allows an additional diagnostic distinction to be achieved (e.g. in the case of ischaemic colitis). Moreover, histological examination can provide conclusive evidence of microscopically identifiable colitis (e.g. collagenous colitis), even if mucosal changes are macroscopically inconspicuous. And further, a biopsy is the only method able to reveal dysplasias and early carcinomas. On the other hand, it should be pointed out that, frequently, a clear distinction between ulcerative colitis and Crohn disease cannot be established on the basis of the histology. Therefore, in the attempt to provide a differential diagnosis between ulcerative colitis and Crohn disease, the endoscopic findings, in combination with the results of the other applied imaging methods and the clinical evidence, including the patient's history, should have precedence over the pathohistological findings. In this case, pathology must remain the assistant of endoscopy and clinical examination.

## DIFFERENTIAL DIAGNOSIS

Endoscopy and biopsy allow a conclusive differential–diagnostic identification of microscopic colitis, pseudomembranous colitis and also ischaemic colitis. Differential diagnosis is difficult to achieve in the case of infectious colitis, however, as the latter can simulate the complete range of morphological criteria indicative of Crohn disease and ulcerative disease. Quite often, the combination of a precisely established patient history (chronic–recurrent symptomatic complaints) with the findings of other clinical and diagnostic imaging methods and the microbiological results of stool and biopsy examinations can ultimately serve to distinguish infectious colitis from chronic inflammatory bowel disease. It is only in certain exceptions that the patient's response to therapeutic measures or the course of the disease have to be taken into account when performing differential diagnosis. Whereas the disease can be expected to subside completely within a short period of time if it has an infectious cause, this is not (or rarely) the case with Crohn disease or ulcerative colitis.

## FOLLOW-UP COLONOSCOPY AS A HELP FOR TREATMENT

On the basis of present knowledge, follow-up endoscopy is strictly not to be recommended as a help for treatment decisions. This applies especially to Crohn disease. A carefully conducted extensive multicentre study confirmed that the endoscopically determined conditions had no influence on the recurrence rate after clinical remission. Recurrence rates for both the group with endoscopically established remission and the group exhibiting continued florid inflammatory symptoms were equally high during an 18-month follow-up period[3]. In comparative terms, the body of available data on ulcerative colitis is less clearly outlined as no directly related study exists at present. In smaller test groups, however, there are definite indications that microscopic and endoscopic signs of disease activity may point towards an early recurrence[4]. This set of considerations does not bear the same degree of importance in the case of colitis ulcerosa, on the other hand, because all patients presenting with ulcerative colitis are given 5-ASA medication continuously, so that the question of discontinuing treatment does not arise at all.

Of course, there are certain situations which form exceptions to the general rule of not implementing endoscopy as a help for treatment. This occurs when a patient shows a persistently high degree of disease activity or if his status deteriorates despite adequate drug therapy. In such instances, endoscopy has to be repeated, firstly in order to confirm the diagnosis and secondly to rule out the presence of a further disease (superinfection or pseudomembranous colitis, for example).

## ENDOSCOPY AND SURGICAL MEASURES

It goes without saying that a complete staging procedure, based on diagnostic imaging, has to be carried out when planning an operation on patients afflicted by Crohn disease in order to provide the surgeon with exact data on the pattern and extent of inflammation, thus ensuring the utmost degree of bowel-conservative surgery.

As far as the question of postoperative endoscopic follow-up is concerned, endoscopic control examinations should be avoided after surgical intervention has taken place. This, of course, also holds for proctocolectomy in treating ulcerative colitis. Furthermore, control endoscopy does not appear justified in bowel resection and Crohn disease, particularly if the patient feels comfortable. It is a well-known fact that Crohn lesions in the anastomotic area can be post-surgically detected in 50–70% of all patients within a period of 6–12 months[5].

At present, the value of postoperative remission-maintaining drug therapy has not been conclusively established. In consequence, the endoscopic findings do not require a therapeutic consequence if the patient is asymptomatic.

An endoscopic follow-up examination is compulsory only in cases where the patient complains of persisting symptoms of discomfort, where a continued inflammatory disease activity is detected clinically, or where complaints recur after a temporary improvement of the patient's condition.

## CANCER SURVEILLANCE

The cancer risk rate affecting patients with ulcerative colitis is no doubt distinctly higher than that of the general population[6]. The data pertaining to Crohn disease are not quite as conclusive, although an increased relative risk can be assumed to exist here as well[7]. Carcinoma prevalence increases markedly – by a multiple factor – particularly in cases presenting with pancolitis and those with early onset of the disease (before the age of 20) and a correspondingly long-standing duration of the disease (see also Chapter 11). From these considerations, there follows the recommendation that patients with pancolitis and recurrent attacks of the disease, as well as those patients afflicted over a longer period of time or before the age of 20 should be enrolled in a follow-up therapy programme. A left-sided colitis, Crohn disease, or an outbreak of the disease after the age of 50 are relative indications for admitting patients to such a programme. However, patients suffering from ulcerative proctosigmoiditis are subject to a marginally increased risk requiring no compulsory follow-up treatment programme. Compulsory complete colonoscopy, including biopsy, is recommended for the first-mentioned patient group every 1–2 years. All macroscopically conspicuous lesions (with the exception of pseudopolyps) should be biopsied. In addition, 1–4 biopsies should be taken from inconspicuous mucosa domains every 5–10 cm. Since only a small number of patients will be eligible to participate in such a preventive programme, the physician performing endoscopy should be sufficiently willing and prepared to conduct a relatively extensive investigation.

In view of the fact that colonoscopy is generally simple and straightforward to implement in managing cases of long-standing colitis, the endoscopic inspection should not be limited solely to proctosigmoidoscopy. The prevention programme should begin approximately 10 years after the onset of the disease. If the biopsies do not reveal any dysplasias, follow-up endoscopy is performed periodically every 1–2 years. If, however, microscopic findings are undefined or a low extent of dysplasia formation is detected, a fairly short-term control endoscopy within a period of 3–6 months is justified. In cases of severe dysplasias, proctocolectomy is recommended.

## ENDOSONOGRAPHY

Endosonography allows periproctitic abscesses and fistulae to be detected. This method is superior to the customary proctoscopic examination and also to fistulography, and can lay claim to a success rate comparable to that of magnetic resonance imaging. However, the investigation is often painful for patients with Crohn disease and with extensive perianal lesions, and it cannot be carried out if stenoses are present. Comparative studies on endosonography and MRI have not been presented to date.

## CHOLESTASIS AND CHRONIC INFLAMMATORY BOWEL DISEASE

If laboratory tests (alkaline phosphatase, $\gamma$-GT) yield evidence for a cholestatic involvement in inflammatory bowel disease, endoscopic retrograde cholangiography (ERCP) is imperative. In most cases, the cause of the pathological cholestase parameters is a primary sclerosing cholangitis which can only be detected by ERCP. Mostly, intrahepatic inflammatory cholangitis and discrete or pronounced extrahepatic constrictions of the biliary ducts are usually detected. The routine procedure adopted by our institute involves, besides the extensive extraction of cytological or bioptic samples of material from the bile ducts, the insertion of a nasobiliary probe. If a distinct reduction in the elevated cholestase levels is achieved within a period of several days, a sphincterotomy is carried out and a 10-French plastic end prosthesis is inserted. The prosthesis is replaced every 4–6 months. Therapy as such is continued over a period of 2 years with the aim of establishing a permanent expansion to overcome drainage obstruction. Of course, if a primary sclerosing cholangitis is present, antibiotic coverage has to be ensured before ERCP treatment is initiated in order to prevent an otherwise imminent outbreak of cholangitis. Endoscopic stenting is a therapy technique that has not yet been adequately proven in practice. However, retrospective analyses indicate that long-term improvement can be achieved – at least insofar as stable laboratory parameters can be maintained. It still remains to be seen, though, if this therapy option will, in any way, be able to positively influence the course and the prognosis of the disease.

## ENDOSCOPY AND STENOSES

Blomberg et al. and Breysem et al. were the first to point out the possibility of managing Crohn disease by a dilation treatment. In case studies involving 27 and 18 patients, respectively, long-term treatment success was achieved in two thirds and one half, respectively, of the patient groups[8,9]. In view of the fact that many patients had already undergone previous operations, this treatment option can be recommended under certain preconditions: the stenosis must be easily accessible to endoscopy and it should be a solitary stenosis with a short extension. Anastomotic stenoses are best suited for dilation treatment. Such treatment is contraindicated, however, if the anastomotic area exhibits florid inflammation. Dilation treatment is performed under direct endoscopic supervision by implementing an inflatable high-pressure balloon catheter.

The diameter of the balloon is increased from 10 mm to a maximum of 25 mm. As a rule, 1–5 treatment sessions are required. There have been only anecdotal reports to date on possible complications, such as perforations, caused by the balloon catheter. In general, the treatment is tolerated quite well by patients, if sedatives/analgesics are administered, and can also be conducted on an out-patient basis. Nevertheless, carefully controlled investigations serving to verify the actual efficiency of the technique would be desirable for this indication as well.

## References


1.  Modigliani R, Mary JY. Reproducibility of colonoscopic findings in Crohn's disease: A prospective multicenter study of interobserver variation. Dig Dis Sci. 1987;32:1370–9.
2.  Modigliani R. Endoscopic management of inflammatory bowel disease. Am J Gastroenterol. 1994;89:53–65.
3.  Landi B, N'gugen A, Cortot A et al. Endoscopic monitoring of Crohn's disease: A prospective, randomized clinical trial. Gastroenterology. 1992;102:1647–53.
4.  Riley SA, Mani V, Goodman MJ et al. Microscopic activity in ulcerative colitis: what does it mean? Gut. 1991;32:174–8.
5.  Rutgeerts P, Geboes K, Vantrappen G et al. Natural history of recurrent Crohn's disease at the ileocolonic anastomosis after curative surgery. Gut. 1984;25:665–72.
6.  Ekbom A, Helmick C, Zack M et al. Ulcerative colitis and colorectal cancer. A population based study. N Engl J Med. 1990;323:1228–33.
7.  Ekbom A, Helmick C, Zack M et al. Increased risk of large-bowel cancer in Crohn's disease with colonic involvement. Lancet. 1990;336:357–9.
8.  Blomberg B, Rolny P, Järnerot G. Endoscopic treatment of anastomotic stricture in Crohn's disease. Endoscopy. 1991;23:195–8.

# 16
# IBD: diagnostic relevance of abdominal sonography

W. B. SCHWERK

Recent studies have emphasized the growing use of ultrasonography in the diagnosis of acute and chronic inflammatory bowel disease (IBD), such as appendicitis, acute ileitis, colonic diverticulitis, Crohn disease and ulcerative colitis[1-7]. Endoscopy and contrast radiology are widely accepted as the imaging methods of choice for the evaluation of IBD. These diagnostic modalities basically provide information about mucosal integrity and the luminal aspect of IBD.

In contradistinction to endoscopy and contrast radiology, ultrasound scanning provides cross-sectional imaging of the gut wall itself and displays the transmural aspect of inflammation as well as interloop pathology.

By means of high-resolution sonography or endoscopic ultrasound, five individual wall layers of the normal gastrointestinal tract can be visualized, which are distinguished by different echogenicity and thickness. In-vitro correlations of ultrasound images and histological sections have revealed that ultrasonic gut layers partially correspond to histological tissue layers but also to echoes produced by acoustic interfaces between.

Inflammatory and neoplastic diseases which affect the entire bowel wall or individual layers only, can alter the echoarchitecture of the wall and thus may be recognized by ultrasound scanning.

## ULTRASONIC FINDINGS

Inflammatory bowel disease is associated with a spectrum of echomorphological findings of the bowel and its mesentery, which corresponds to the variability of transmural and interloop pathology (Table 1, Figures 1–6). The ultrasonic patterns of intestinal inflammation are very similar in different inflammatory diseases and are basically non-pathognonomic. On the other hand, sonographic findings in patients with IBD may vary greatly from one patient to another for various reasons (e.g. activity and duration of disease) and may vary even within the same individual when considering different areas of affected bowel loops.

**Table 1**  Correlation of prominent histological features, echographic patterns of the bowel wall, and peristalsis in different states of inflammatory bowel disease[7]

|  | Acute inflammation (mucosal) | Prolonged inflammation (transmural) | Chronic inflammation (transmural) |
|---|---|---|---|
| Prominent histological features | Oedema of mucosa, submucosa, serosa | Cellular infiltration ↑; mural spread of inflammation | Fibrosis, scarring, neovascularization; destruction of anatomic layers; transmural spread of inflammation |
| Echographic patterns of the wall | Slight thickening; visualization of individual ultrasonic layers; luminal narrowing ± | Prominent thickening; accentuated ultrasonic layers; overall echogenicity ↓; luminal narrowing | Prominent thickening; accentuated or poorly defined individual ultrasonic layers; echogenicity ↓; luminal narrowing; hyperechoic halo |
| Motility of segments involved | Normal or hypermotile peristalsis | Decreased or absent peristalsis | Immobile stiff-walled loop |

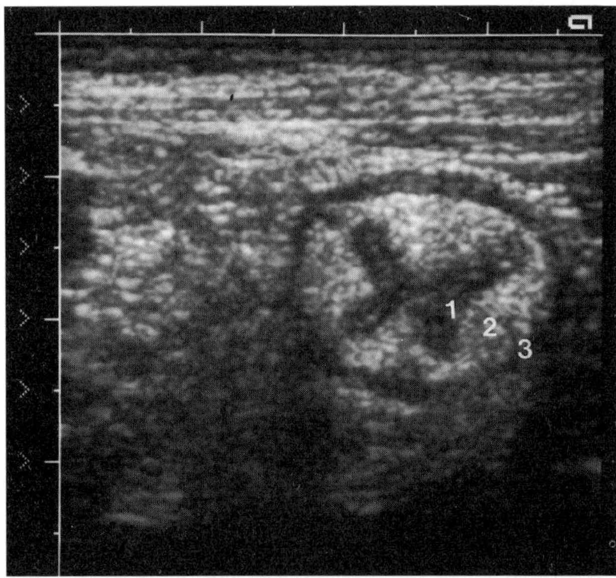

**Figure 1**  Transverse scan of the descending colon showing early manifestation of IBD due to oedematous swelling of the wall and accentuated visualization of layers: hypoechoic mucosa (1), hyperechoic submucosa (2), and hypoechoic muscularis (3)

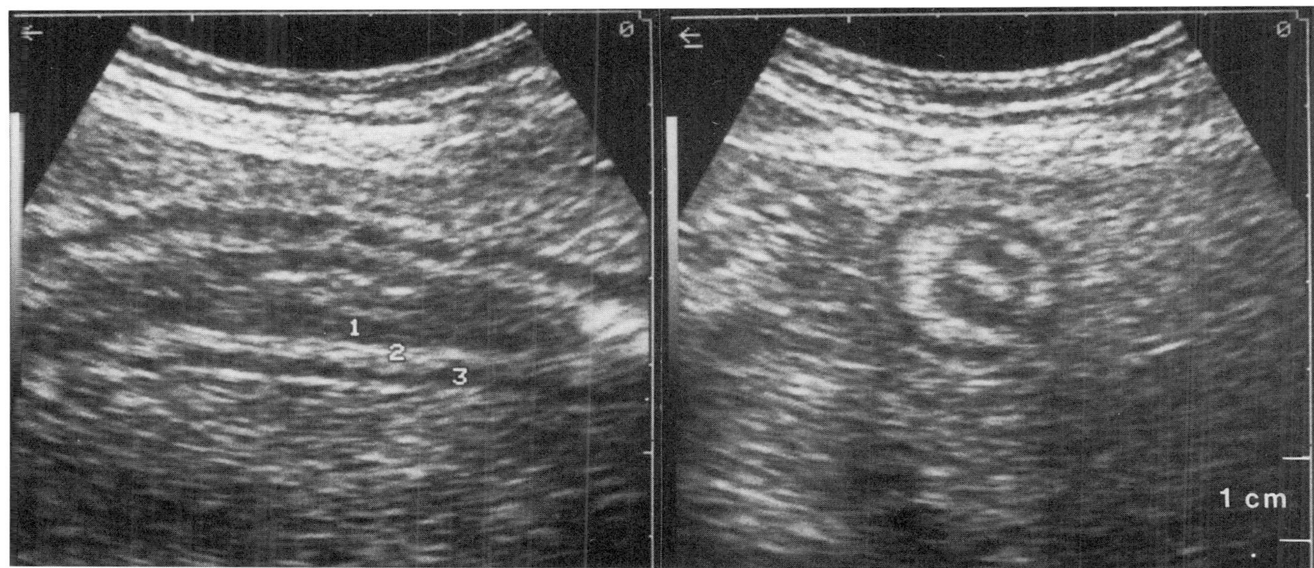


**Figure 2** Longitudinal (left) and transverse (right) scans of the ileum in Crohn disease showing ultrasonic features of transmural inflammation: 'target appearance' in transverse view. For 1–3, see Figure 1. Normal peristalsis along the involved segment

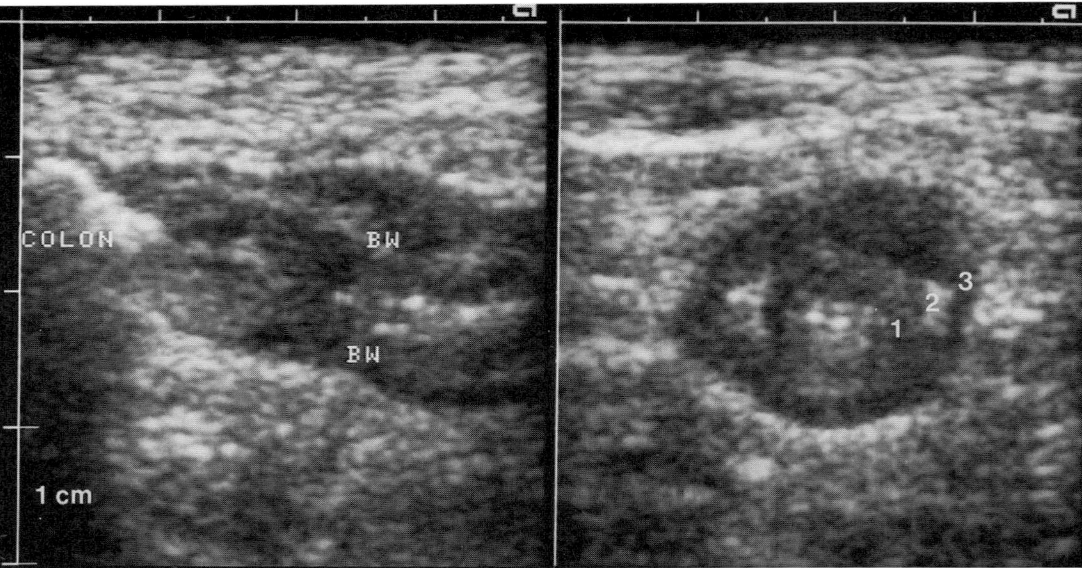


**Figure 3** Longitudinal (left) and transverse (right) scans of the aperistaltic stenotic neoterminal ileum in Crohn disease showing prominent thickening of the bowel wall (BW) with decreased echogenicity of poorly defined wall layers and luminal narrowing. 1–3: see figure 1

The ultrasonic features of IBD mainly concern the thickness and echogenicity of the gut wall or individual layers, integrity of echographic layering, and the appearance of surrounding tissue. As bowel motility and compressibility can be easily assessed during real-time ultrasound observation, these dynamic phenomena should also enter diagnostic evaluation.

Induced by inflammatory mediators, which increase vascular permeability, oedema is a prominent feature of acute intestinal inflammation and accumulates in spaces where loose connective tissue predominates. The resulting mucosal and submucosal oedema leads to thickening of the wall and presents with well-defined ultrasonic layers. On the transverse section of a loop, the alternate hypoechogenic and hyperechogenic concentric layers give rise to the so-called 'target-appearance'. Thickening of both the hypoechogenic mucosa and the hyperechogenic submucosa without substantially reduced motility are the very early sonographic findings in bowel inflammation.

These ultrasonic patterns can be demonstrated almost always in patients with Crohn disease. However, findings are non-specific and may be visualized in other aetiologically identified acute inflammatory bowel diseases (e.g. bacterial, viral, parasitic, eosinophilic, ischaemic and irradiation-induced IBD).

With prolonged intestinal inflammation, increasing cellular infiltration occurs and mural spread of inflammation may develop. The echographic patterns include prominent thickening of the bowel wall showing accentuated ultrasonic layers (target-sign) with an overall decrease in echogenicity, luminal narrowing and reduced peristalsis along the segment involved.

With chronic intestinal inflammation, metaplasia, proliferation, fibrosis, scarring, fissuring ulceration, neovascularization and destruction of anatomic layers additionally contributes to the variety of histopathological patterns, particularly in Crohn disease.

Depending on intensity, histopathological components and mural spread of bowel inflammation, the chronic inflammatory process may be associated with wall thickening, a decrease in echogenicity, poorly defined ultrasonic layers of stiff-walled immobile loops, and stenosis (Figures 3 and 4).

Transmural spread of inflammation in prolonged and chronic intestinal inflammation in Crohn disease leads to omental covering and an increase in mesenteric fat wrapped around the bowel involved. These peri-intestinal changes are responsible for a rigid zone of increased echogenicity ('hyperechoic halo') surrounding the affected loop, particularly when fissuring ulceration and fistulae extend into the mesentery (Figure 4).

With colour Doppler sonography, both the ultrasound features of intestinal inflammation and haemodynamic alterations can be visualized simultaneously. Particularly in the fulminating state of IBD, the associated hypervascularity of the bowel wall can be demonstrated by colour Doppler flow imaging. In our experience, the degree of hypervascularity seen at 'Doppler angiography' seems to parallel the degree of inflammatory activity of disease.

We prospectively investigated the diagnostic accuracy and limitations of high-resolution abdominal sonography in the detection of inflammatory bowel disease[7]. By means of this imaging technique, sensitivity and specificity of the above-mentioned ultrasonic features of IBD were 90.3% and 88.4%, respectively. In 95.7% of patients with Crohn disease and in 86.2% of individuals with

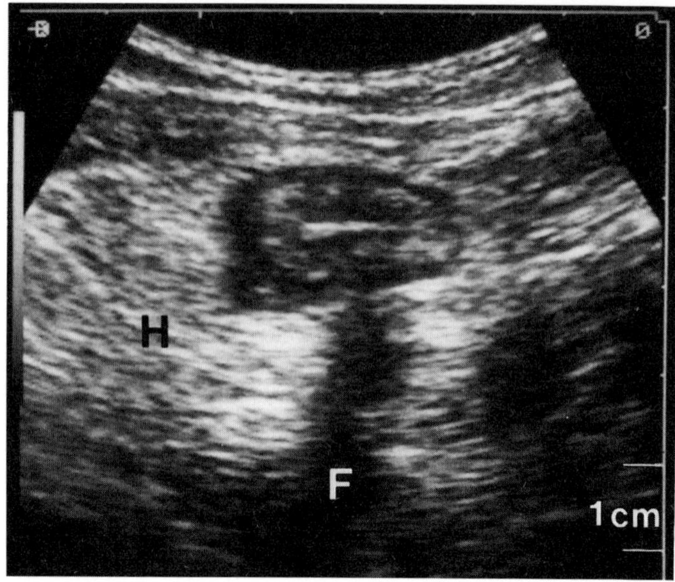

**Figure 4**  Transverse scan of a bowel loop in Crohn disease showing ultrasonic signs of transmural spread of inflammation: echogenic halo (H) and fistulation (F).

ulcerative colitis, sonographic manifestations of inflammatory bowel thickening were identified. Considering separately the detection of small bowel and/or colonic involvement in Crohn disease, we found a high degree of diagnostic accuracy of intestinal sonography, ranging between 89.5% and 100% (Tables 2–4). In ulcerative colitis, target lesions were detected in 94% and 100% of patients with pancolitis or left-sided colitis, respectively, but in only 50% of cases with the disease restricted to the rectosigmoid.

A summary of prospective studies concerning the diagnostic value of ultrasonography in IBD is listed in Table 5.

**Table 2**  Prospective evaluation of abdominal sonography in the detection of inflammatory thickened bowel segments in a study population of 232 patients[7]

| | | Ultrasonography | | | |
| --- | --- | --- | --- | --- | --- |
| Diagnosis | Patients (*n*) | True positive | True negative | False positive | False negative |
| Crohn disease | 128 | 110 | 11 | 2 | 5 |
| Ulcerative colitis | 33 | 25 | 4 | – | 4 |
| Enterocolitis and undetermined colitis | 21 | 14 | – | – | 7 |
| Controls | 50 | – | 45 | 5 | – |

Data indicate number of patients

**Table 3**  Diagnostic value of abdominal sonography in the detection of inflammatory bowel wall thickening[7]

| | |
|---|---|
| Sensitivity | 90.3% |
| Specificity | 88.4% |
| Predictive value positive | 95.5% |
| Predictive value negative | 79.2% |
| Overall accuracy | 90.5% |
| Number of patients | 232 |

**Table 4**  Ultrasound detection of inflammatory thickened bowel segments in correlation to anatomic distribution of Crohn disease in 115 patients[7]

| Site of Crohn disease | Patients (n) | Small bowel | | | | Colon | | | |
|---|---|---|---|---|---|---|---|---|---|
| | | TP | FN | TN | FP | TP | FN | TN | FP |
| Ileum | 40 | 37 | 3 | – | – | – | – | 40 | 0 |
| Ileum and colon | 56 | 56 | 0 | – | – | 51 | 5 | – | – |
| Colon | 19 | – | – | 17 | 2 | 17 | 2 | – | – |
| Total | 115 | | | | | | | | |

Data indicate number of patients. TP/TN, true-positive/negative; FP/FN, false-positive/negative

**Table 5**  Diagnostic value of abdominal sonography in the detection of inflammatory bowel disease (prospective studies)

| Authors | Patients (n) | Sensitivity (%) | Specificity (%) | Predictive value positive (%) | Predictive value negative (%) |
|---|---|---|---|---|---|
| Sonnenberg et al.[3] | 175 | 84 | 91 | | |
| Worlicek et al.[4] | 241 | 72 CD<br>53 UC | | | |
| Pera et al.[6] | 181 | 81 | 79 | | |
| Schwerk et al.[7] | 232 | 90<br>96 CD<br>86 UC | 88 | 96 | 79 |

CD, Crohn disease; UC, ulcerative colitis

## COMPLICATIONS

The transmural inflammatory process in Crohn disease, involving the serosa and mesentery, accounts for common complications of the disease, i.e. stenosis, ileus, fistula and abscess formation, which can be visualized on abdominal sonography.

The ultrasound appearance of enteroenteric, blind ending enteromesenteric, enterocutaneous or enterovesical fistulae depends on whether fistulous tracts are filled with gas, fluid material, or both. Thus, they may be highly echogenic, associated with distal sound shadow, or may present with an hypoechogenic liquid appearance (Figure 4).

There is a wide range of ultrasound patterns of abscesses, particularly associated with Crohn disease, ranging from liquid to solid-like space-occupying lesions, occasionally containing highly reflective gas from bacterial metabolism (Figure 5). In our experience, fistulae and abscesses constituted a more difficult diagnostic problem for transabdominal sonography when they were located in the small pelvis or in the anorectal area in comparison with reliably detected abscesses in other abdominal and retroperitoneal regions (Table 6).

## CONCLUSIONS

Abdominal sonography, using high-resolution technique, is a valuable method for both the imaging diagnosis and follow up of IBD and associated com-

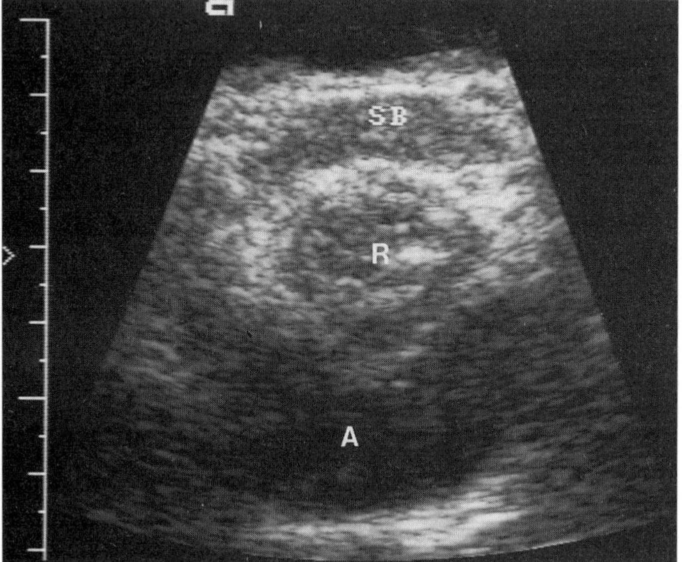


**Figure 5**  Transverse scan of the rectum (R): perirectal abscess (A) complicating Crohn disease

**Table 6**  Ultrasound detection rate of abscesses ($n = 21$) confirmed by surgery or needle aspiration in 20 patients with Crohn disease[7]

| Site of abscesses | $n$ | US true positive | US false negative |
|---|---|---|---|
| Abdominal wall | 3 | 3 | – |
| Intra-abdominal | 9 | 8 | 1 |
| Retroperitoneal/perianal | 9 | 6 | 3 |
| Total | 21 | 17 (81%) | 4 (19%) |

Data indicate number of abscesses

plications. This non-invasive diagnostic modality provides important findings which are complementary to endoscopic and radiographic imaging and may aid for grading disease activity (Table 7).

**Table 7**   Sonographic signs of high-grade disease activity in chronic IBD

- Advanced inflammatory wall thickening
- Tenderness and aperistalsis of involved segments
- Decreased echogenicity of wall layers
- Rigid echogenic halo ($\rightarrow$ transmural spread of inflammation)
- Fistula/abscesses/free peritoneal exudate
- Inflammatory hypervascularity (colour Doppler)

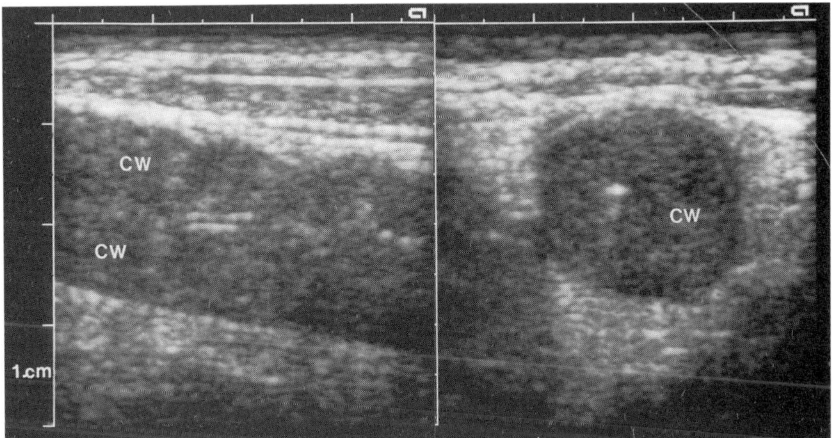


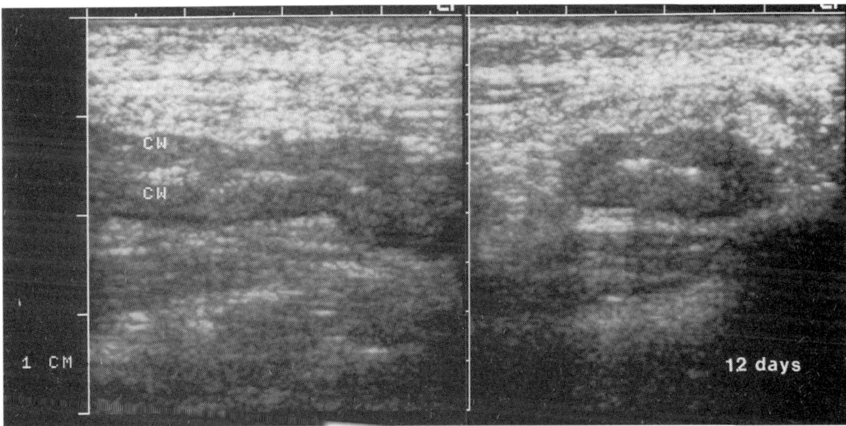


**Figure 6**   Longitudinal (left) and transverse (right) scans of the descending colon in the acute phase of fulminating colitis (top) and 12 days later (bottom) demonstrating regression of hypoechoic inflammatory thickening of colonic wall (CW) after appropriate therapy

Furthermore, intestinal sonography is particularly useful in all patients in whom endoscopy or contrast radiology are not desired or even contraindicated, e.g. patients in the fulminating phase of disease, patients with intestinal obstruction, pregnant women, children and all those who need short-term follow-up examination (Figure 6).

## References


1. Schwerk WB, Wichtrup B, Rothmund M et al. Ultrasonography in the diagnosis of acute appendicitis. Gastroenterology. 1989;97:630–9.
2. Schwerk WB, Schwartz S, Rothmund M. Sonography in acute colonic diverticulitis. A prospective study. Dis Colon Rectum. 1992;35:1077–84.
3. Sonnenberg A, Erckenbrecht J, Peter P, Niederau C. Detection of Crohn's disease by ultrasound. Gastroenterology. 1982;83:430–4.
4. Worlicek H, Lutz H, Thoma B. Sonography of inflammatory intestinal diseases – a prospective study. Ultraschall. 1986;7:275–80.
5. Hoijlund-Pederson B, Gronvall S et al. The value of dynamic US scanning in Crohn's disease. Scand J Gastroenterol. 1986;21:969–72.
6. Pera A, Cammarota T et al. Ultrasonography in the detection of Crohn's disease and in the differential diagnosis of inflammatory bowel disease. Digestion. 1988;41:180–4.
7. Schwerk WB, Beckh K, Raith M. A prospective evaluation of high resolution US in the diagnosis of inflammatory bowel disease. Eur J Gastroenterol Hepatol. 1992;4:173–82.

# 17
# Conventional radiology, CT and MRI in IBD

R. P. SPIELMANN

Conventional X-ray examination of the colon has been largely replaced by endoscopy as pathological findings can be immediately subjected to biopsy and therapeutic intervention. For the small bowel, however, only the proximal and distal segments are accessible to endoscopy. The best overall evaluation of the small bowel is still achieved by using the conventional double-contrast entero-clysis with barium sulphate. This technique, which was introduced by Sellink in the early 70s[1], allows detailed assessment of the intestinal mucosa. It involves placing a tube at the duodenojejunal junction and infusing a dilute barium sulphate suspension which is followed by water or methyl cellulose for distension of the intestinal loops.

The main indication for small bowel enteroclysis is Crohn disease[2–4]. It can occur anywhere in the gastrointestinal tract, but the terminal ileum is affected in most cases. An early radiological sign of Crohn disease is the presence of 'aphthoid ulcers', small elevations of the mucous membrane with a central depot of contrast material. Later, deep longitudinal fissures develop leading to the typical 'cobblestone' appearance. In the early stages of the disease, narrowing of the lumen is caused by spastic contraction of the diseased bowel segment which eventually opens again ('string sign'). Characteristic are 'skip lesions', which are separated by unaffected bowel segments and may demonstrate different stages of the disease. In the advanced stage of the disease, fixed strictures cause hindrance of passage of bowel contents and prestenotic dilation. Deep ulcerations progress into fistulae which may connect with neighbouring structures or open at the skin surface. Because of the large volume of contrast applied, even very delicate fistulae can be identified by small bowel enteroclysis.

Thickening of the intestinal wall can be directly demonstrated with tomographic techniques (ultrasound, CT and MRI). Reduced scanning time and improved resolution has made CT an instrument not only to identify space-occupying lesions such as abscesses and inflammatory tumours, but also to assess the intestinal wall, if the lumen is filled with contrast medium[5]. Furthermore, CT can be used to guide interventional procedures, e.g. percutaneous drainage of abscesses[6].

Inflammatory thickening of intestinal loops can also be demonstrated by MRI if oral contrast agents are applied[7,8]. In general, however, MRI images of the intestines are heavily degraded by motion artifacts due to respiration and peristalsis. Recently, imaging times of the order of one second have become feasible, so that, in future, the inherent high soft-tissue contrast of this technique may contribute to the diagnostic evaluation of inflammatory bowel disease. MRI has already been proved valuable in specific diagnostic problems, e.g. the demonstration of perirectal fistulae, for which imaging in longitudinal planes is an advantage.

The radiological technique of choice to study the mucosal contour of the large bowel is the double-contrast enema with barium sulphate[9]. Colonic lesions in Crohn disease follow a pattern similar to that in the small bowel with early presence of aphthoid ulcers, cobblestone appearance of the mucosa, and segmental distribution of the lesions, which begin on the mesenteric side resulting in asymmetric involvement of the colon wall.

Contrary to Crohn disease, ulcerative colitis generally begins in the rectum and progresses proximally in a continuous fashion. It is restricted to the colon; only in cases with involvement of the entire colon can the terminal ileum also be minimally affected ('backwash ileitis'). The first radiological sign of ulcerative colitis is granularity of the mucosal surface due to oedema and hyperaemia. With progression of the disease, superficial ulcers become visible, which then increase in depth and lead to the destruction of the mucosal membrane. At this stage of the disease, the so-called 'toxic megacolon' can develop, in which case a barium enema should be avoided because of the risk of perforation. Hyperplastic remnants of intact mucosa result in 'pseudopolyposis' of the colon. In the chronic stage of the disease, the colon has an ahaustral rigid appearance. Despite the widespread use of endoscopy, the barium enema has the advantage of less patient discomfort and may be particularly useful for the follow-up of patients.

CT, which is rarely performed in patients with ulcerative colitis, shows less wall thickening than Crohn disease but may demonstrate hypodense submucosal oedema surrounded by hypervascular muscular tissue with contrast enhancement ('target sign') as an unspecific sign of acute inflammation of the bowel wall[10].

In some cases, differential diagnosis between Crohn disease and ulcerative colitis can be a problem, but often the different radiological pattern of bowel involvement allows distinction between the entities. Also radiological differentiation from other inflammatory bowel diseases, e.g. between Crohn disease and *Yersinia* enterocolitis or tuberculous ileitis, may be occasionally difficult.

The use of barium sulphate for contrast material has some well-known drawbacks. The leakage of barium into the peritoneal cavity may lead to severe peritonitis. Therefore, barium may not be applied in cases with suspected perforation, and surgery usually is postponed until all barium-containing contrast material has been removed. Alternatively, water-soluble iodinated contrast material can be used. However, although conventional X-ray investigations with water-soluble contrast material are helpful in identifying disturbances of intestinal motility and strictures, the outline of the mucosa surface is not sufficient for detailed diagnostic assessment. Also using water-soluble contrast material to mark the intestinal lumen, CT offers a potential alternative which has the advantage of imaging the intestinal wall directly.

## References

1. Sellink JL. Organdiagnostik durch künstliche Absorptionsänderungen – Verdauungstrakt. In: Rosenbusch G, Oudkerk M, Ammann E, eds. Radiologie in der medizinischen Diagnostik. Evolution der Röntgenstrahlwendung 1895–1995. Blackwell; Berlin: 1994.
2. Sellink JL. Radiological atlas of common disease of the small bowel. Leiden: Stenfert Kroese; 1976.
3. Antes G. Dünndarmradiologie. Berlin-Heidelberg: Springer, 1986.
4. Maglinte DDT, Chernish SM, Keloin FM, O'Connor KW, Hage JP. Crohn disease of the small intestine: accuracy and relevance of enteroclysis. Radiology. 1992;184:541.
5. Goldberg HT, Gore RM, Margulis AR, et al. Computed tomography in the evaluation of Crohn disease. AJR. 1983;140:227.
6. Casola G, van Sonnenberg E, Neff C, Saba RM, Withers C, Emarine CW. Abscesses in Crohn's disease: percutaneous drainage. Radiology. 1987;163:19.
7. Kaminsky S, Laniado M, Coogoll M, et al. Gadopentetate dimeglumine as a contrast agent: safety and efficacy. Radiology. 1991;178:503.
8. Anderson CM, Brown JJ, Balfe DM, Heiken JP, Borrello JA, Clouse RE, Pilgram TK. MR imaging of Crohn disease: use of perflubron as a gastrointestinal contrast agent. JMRI. 1994;4:491.
9. Margulis AR, Thoeni RF. The present status of the radiologic examination of the colon. Radiology. 1988;167:1.
10. Philpotts LE, Heiken JP, Westcott MA, Gore RM. Colitis: use of CT findings in differential diagnosis. Radiology. 1994;190:445.

# 18
# Diagnosis of perianal fistula and abscess

H.-J. BRAMBS

Perianal fistulae and abscesses are common conditions, easily recognized and readily treated. A small portion of anorectal fistulae and abscesses can be very difficult to manage because of their high level and their complexity with secondary tracks and extensions. In these cases, success of surgical treatment depends on accurate assessment of the disease. If the full extent of the perianal or perirectal sepsis is not recognized clinically or at operation and the fistulae or abscesses are inadequately treated, they will recur and necessitate further surgery. Repeated surgical interventions increase the risk of sphincter damage with subsequent incontinence.

## AETIOLOGY

Fistula in ano is most frequently the result of an infection of the anal glands which ramify in the internal sphincter and in the intersphincteric space discharging into the anal crypts at the linea dentata (Table 1).

Fistulous disease in the perirectal and perianal region may be a complication of chronic inflammation, infiltrating malignancy, radiation therapy, surgical treatment or trauma.

Specific inflammatory processes, such as Crohn disease, lymphogranuloma venereum, tuberculosis and actinomyces, may involve the anal glands that arise

**Table 1**  Aetiology of perianal fistulae and abscesses

Inflammation of the anal glands
Crohn disease
Rare causes:
    Malignant tumours
    Irradiation therapy
    Trauma
    Postoperative effects
    Venereal diseases
    Specific inflammatory diseases (actinomyces, tuberculosis)

at the level of the crypts of Morgagni. In Crohn disease, fistulae begin in deep rectal fissures or in the anal glands and extend through the rectal wall or external sphincter muscle. Acute leukaemia with neutropenia may predispose patients to anal gland infections.

Establishment of the anatomical relationship of fistulae and abscesses to the anal sphincter complex is essential to planning of the therapeutic approach. However, the extent and ramification of fistulae often present a considerable diagnostic problem.


## CLASSIFICATION

Anorectal fistulae and abscesses are classified by their location in relation to the sphincteric muscles and to the muscles of the pelvic floor[1].

Intersphincteric fistulae are the most common type, penetrating the internal sphincter and passing between the internal and external anal sphincters (Table 2).

Trans-sphincteric fistulae are less frequent, passing through both sphincters into the ischiorectal fossa. The majority of these fistulae then track downwards to exit through the skin at variable distances from the anal margin. There may be an upward extension to the roof of the ischiorectal fossa lying under the levator hammock. Occasionally, the upward extension will perforate the levator resulting in a supralevator fistula or abscess lying adjacent to the rectal wall.

Anorectal fistulae are very rare and have an internal opening into the rectum. Sometimes this type of high fistula occurs when there is a high supralevator extension of an intersphincteric fistula which opens into the rectum or forms a supralevator abscess which then tracks down through the levator plate to exit through the ischiorectal fossa.

Small low fistulae are not always associated with anal gland infection. These subcutaneous fistulae are associated with fissures or occasionally occur in a haemorrhoidectomy wound.

Supralevator fistulae may be associated with pelvic or abdominal disease. Such fistulae are usually associated with diverticular disease or Crohn disease and are termed extrasphincteric fistulae. They track downwards lateral to the puborectalis through the levator plane to enter the ischiorectal fossa.


**Table 2**   Classification of perianal fistulae

| | |
|---|---|
| Intersphincteric | |
|    External | |
|    Internal   → | infra- and supralevatoric |
| Trans-sphincteric | |
|    External   → | supralevatoric |
|    Internal   → | infra- and |
| Anorectal | |
| Subcutaneous | |
| Extrasphincteric | |

## DIAGNOSIS

Careful digital examination under anaesthesia by an experienced physician is very accurate in determining fistula geography. However, this examination is limited to palpable lesions and macroscopic alterations of the perianal skin and the crypts of Morgagni. Deep fistulae and abscesses within the ischiorectal fossa and beyond the levator plate may escape detection (Table 3).

**Table 3**  Main objectives to peroperative examination

| |
| --- |
| To define the anatomy of the fistula and abscess in relation to: |
|   The sphincter muscles |
|   The levator plate |
| To determine the activity of the inflammatory lesions |

## Barium enema

Conventional radiographic studies will demonstrate local abscess formation and perianal fistulae in some cases, but have the disadvantage that they do not reveal soft-tissue disease surrounding a fistula. If multiple tracks are seen during barium enema examination, a diagnosis of Crohn disease or an infection complicating leukaemia is suggested.

## Fistulography

Contrast fistulography is often difficult to perform and interpret when the fistulous tracts are multiple and complex[2]. In fistulae and abscesses developing from the anal glands, contrast fistulography has proved disappointing. Only in high fistulae which track to the pelvic space can sinography be an informative technique[3].

## Computed tomography (CT)

CT is being performed increasingly to evaluate extraintestinal complications in patients with chronic inflammatory bowel disease and diverticulitis. The extra-luminal manifestations of these conditions, including abscesses, fistulae, mesenteric inflammation and lymphadenopathia, can be assessed precisely. In patients with Crohn disease, a detailed retrospective study dedicated to the perianal and perirectal region has shown that more than 80% of patients had abnormalities of these regions[4].

The full extent of fistulous tracts and perianal and perirectal abscesses can be clearly defined by CT. However, transverse sections may not depict the relationship of a fistula or an abscess to the course of the levator muscle. Additional problems in interpretation of CT scans are caused by partial-volume effects in this region. Additionally, CT has poor-quality imaging of the anorectal wall structures compared with endoscopic ultrasound[5].

## Endoscopic ultrasound

Currently, endoscopic ultrasound (EUS) is mostly used in the detection and staging of anorectal cancer. EUS is an increasingly used method for exploration of the rectum for the diagnosis of fistulae and abscesses. Good correlation between the preoperative EUS findings and those at surgery in evaluating perianal sepsis and fistulae has been reported[6]. EUS seems to be superior to clinical examination and can detect lesions missed with the routine proctological examination. Transrectal ultrasound delineates the rectal wall layers, the anal sphincter, and the perianal and perirectal tissues[3,7]. However, penetration of the ischiorectal fossa is poor, so that delineation of inflammatory lesions in these areas is limited and high tracks or abscesses may be difficult to see. Additionally, it may be difficult to precisely evaluate recurrent fistulae and lesions after multiple operations. Another drawback of this method is that, in some cases with painful perianal lesions, the procedure has to be performed

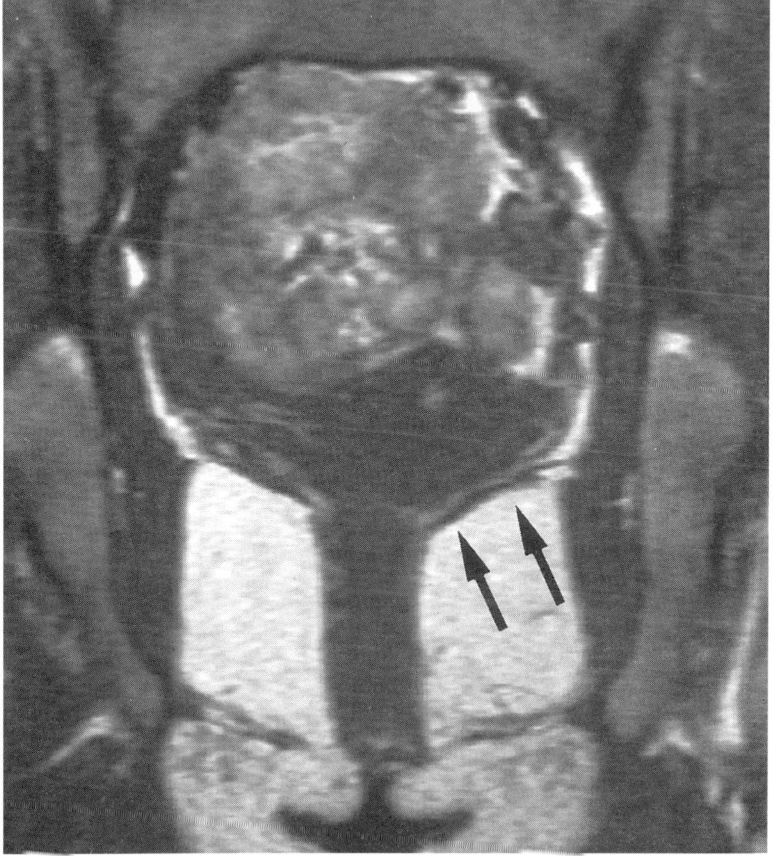

**Figure 1** T1-weighted image. The coronal plane outlines the anatomy of the levator ani (arrows) and delineates the ischiorectal fossa with the signal-intensive fat tissue

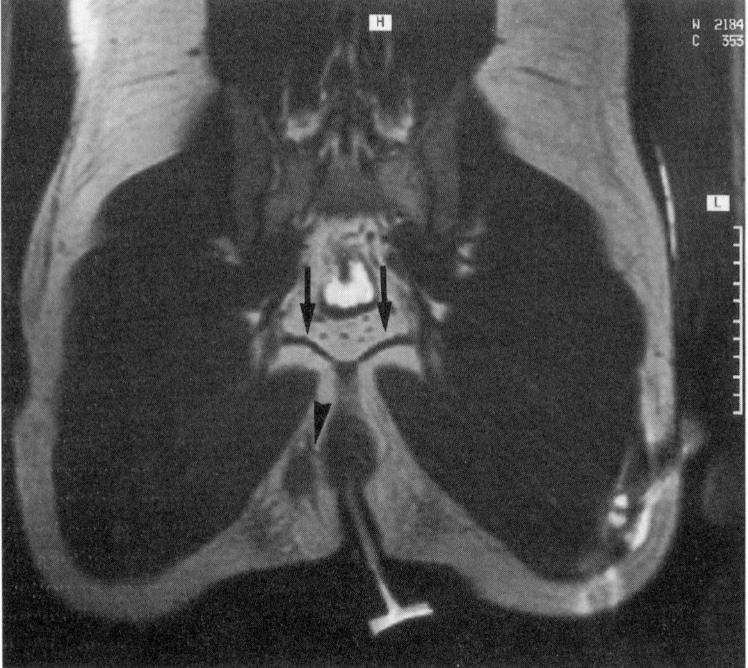

**Figure 2** T1-weighted image, coronal plane. Hypointense fistulous track (arrow head) running from the anal canal to an ischiorectal abscess. Clear delineation of the levator plane

under general anaesthesia. In patients with Crohn disease, EUS is usually easy to perform and not painful. However, narrowing of the anal canal may render the examination impossible.

## Magnetic resonance imaging

Soft-tissue anatomy is superbly displayed with MR imaging (MRI) in multiplanar sections. In the coronal plane, the supralevator and infralevator compartments are well delineated (Figure 1). Sagittal images may provide additional information about the extent of the disease along the coccygeal portion of the levator ani muscle (Figure 2, Figure 3).

MRI has been shown to be very useful in patients with anorectal anomalies because it directly demonstrates the rectal pouch and sphincter muscles in multiple planes. Exact location and development of the sphincter muscles can be estimated and associated anomalies involving the kidney and the spine can be evaluated[8].

In two prospective studies, the great value of MRI in imaging of perianal fistulae and abscesses has been documented[9,10]. The accuracy of MRI is high and, in future, this method could be the investigation of first choice for patients with difficult and recurrent fistulae. MRI was appreciated to be also a useful technique for assessing non-operative treatment methods[9]. Additionally, it could

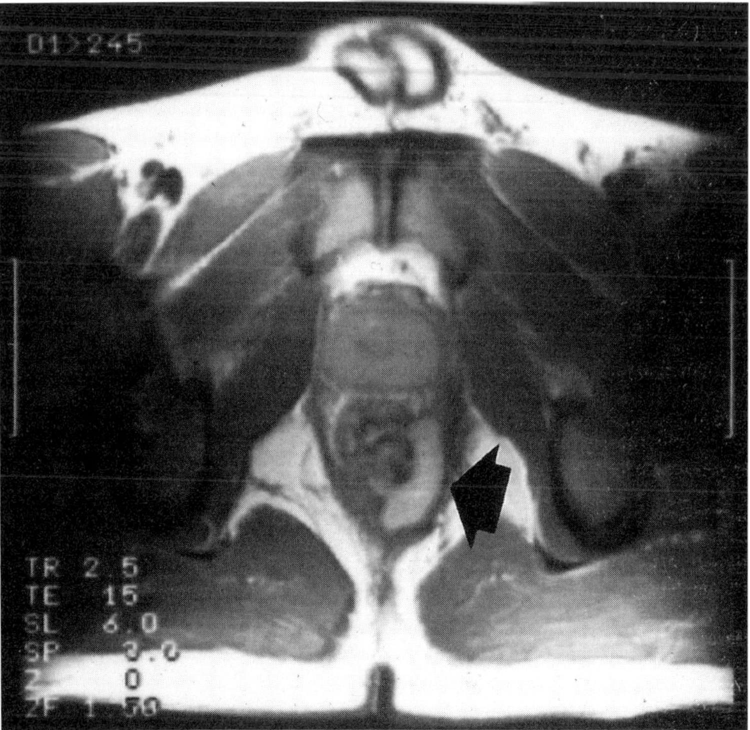

**Figure 3**  Proton density image, axial plane. Hyperintense horseshoe-like intersphincteric abscess (arrow) within the anal canal

be shown that, in T2-weighted sequences, acute inflammatory lesions, such as abscesses and active fistulae, can be differentiated from inactive alterations, such as scars[10].

Technical refinements such as high-resolution endorectal MRI demonstrate the layers of the rectal wall and the interface between the rectum and the perirectal fat. T1-weighted images have high contrast between the rectal wall and the perirectal fat and will improve the diagnostic work-up in patients with perianal and perirectal disease.

## References


1. Parks AG, Gordon PH, Hardcastle JD. A classification of fistula in ano. Br J Surg. 1976;63:1–12.
2. Van Dongen LM, Lubbers EJ. Perianal fistulas in patients with Crohn's disease. Arch Surg. 1986;121:1187–90.
3. Van Outryve MJ, Pelckmans PA, Michielsen PP, van Maercke YM. Value of transrectal ultrasonography in Crohn's disease. Gastroenterology. 1991,191.1171 7.
4. Yousem DM, Fishman EK, Johnes B. Crohn disease: Perirectal and perianal findings at CT. Radiology. 1988;167:331–4.

5. Shank B, Dershaw DD, Caravelli J, Barth J, Enker W. A prospective study of the accuracy of preoperative computed tomographic staging of patients with biopsy-proven rectal carcinoma. Dis Rectum. 1990;33:285–91.
6. Law PL. Talbot RW, Bartram CI et al. Anal endosonography in the evaluation of perianal sepsis and fistula in ano. Br J Surg. 1989;76:752–5.
7. Choen S, Burnett S, Bartram CI, Nicholls RJ. Comparison between anal endosonography and digital examination in the evaluation of anal fistulae. Br J Surg. 1991;78:445–7.
8. Sato Y, Pringle KC, Bergmann RA. Congenital anorectal anomalies: MR imaging. Radiology. 1988;186:157–62.
9. Lunniss PJ, Armstrong P, Barker PG, Reznek RH, Phillips RKS. Magnetic resonance imaging of anal fistulae. Lancet. 1992;340:394–6.
10. Skalej M, Makowiec F, Weinlich M, Jenss H, Laniado M, Starlinger M. Kernspintomographie bei perianalem Morbus Crohn. Dtsch Med Wschr. 1993;118:1791–6.

# 19
# Laboratory tests in IBD – which and when?

J. EMMRICH

Laboratory tests are widely used in inflammatory bowel diseases (IBD) even though estimation of disease activity is rarely superior to an experienced clinician's judgement. The laboratory parameters can be useful for the precise evaluation of the extent, activity and complications of the inflammatory process; they can be helpful in defining situations where symptoms may not be related to active inflammation and can also be useful in predicting the course of the disease and evaluating or comparing drug efficacy in therapeutic trials. Therefore, it is necessary to define precisely the aim of their application. Mainly, there are three reasons for using laboratory tests:

1. They can help in the differential diagnosis of IBD.
2. They can reflect and localize the activity of IBD.
3. They can help to define intestinal and extra-intestinal complications.

It is also necessary to define the limitations of laboratory parameters. They cannot make the diagnosis of IBD and they cannot clearly differentiate between ulcerative colitis (UC) and Crohn disease (CD).

## DIAGNOSIS AND DIFFERENTIAL DIAGNOSIS OF IBD

When patients complain of abdominal pain and long-lasting diarrhoea, first it is necessary to differentiate between inflammatory or non-inflammatory diseases. For this purpose, discriminatory laboratory tests are necessary. Many different tests are available. For clinical practice the most important tests are erythrocyte sedimentation rate (ESR), blood test (haematocrit, leukocytes, differentiation of leukocytes, thrombocytes) and C-reactive protein (CRP). These routine blood tests are simple, easily performed and cheap. With the help of these tests, it is possible to identify an inflammatory disease. The definitive diagnosis is made according to clinical findings, endoscopy, histological examination of biopsies, radiographic examinations and bacteriological investigations.

The differentiation between UC and CD can constitute a diagnostic problem. Therefore, results obtained by different methods should be considered. For example, an additional indication of IBD is the detection of autoantibodies. Many autoantibodies (e.g. antibody binding basolateral membrane of colonic epithelial cells, antibody against pancreatic acinar cells, antibody against mucin of goblet cells, lymphocytotoxic antibody, and antineutrophil cytoplasmic autoantibody) have been reported in the sera of patients with UC and CD[1]. Two major subclasses of antineutrophil cytoplasmic autoantibodies (ANCA) were initially defined by their pattern of indirect immunofluorescence. One is a diffuse granular cytoplasmic pattern (c-ANCA) and the other is a more restricted cytoplasmic distribution with perinuclear highlighting (p-ANCA). The p-ANCA subclass has been recognized in patients with IBD, particularly UC and sclerosing cholangitis[2–4]. In Table 1, the data from the literature[1–8] regarding autoantibodies are summarized. However, the presence of circulating anticolon antibodies and ANCA in patients with UC does not correlate with the severity, duration, course or extent of the disease[2].

**Table 1**  Autoantibodies in IBD (%)

| Autoantibodies | UC | CD | Controls |
|---|---|---|---|
| p-ANCA | 67 | 12 | 3 |
| Antibodies against intestinal goblet cells | 29 | – | – |
| Antibodies against pancreatic acinar cells | 4 | 31 | – |

An increased frequency of IBD in families may implicate genetic factors in the aetiology of these diseases. An association was suspected, especially between UC and HLA-DR2, but there are controversies about these data[1,6,7]. For clinical diagnosis, these factors are not meaningful. Further studies are needed to elucidate this problem.

## INFLAMMATORY ACTIVITY OF IBD

There are many tests which are useful to assess the inflammatory activity at the beginning, or during the course, of the disease. Some of these are ESR, CRP, orosomucoid, leukocyte count, differentiation of leukocytes, haemoglobin, haematocrit, thrombocyte count, serum albumin, $\alpha_2$-globulin and serum iron. But the correlation of these values with the general state of the patient may be interpretable. Clinical activity indices which reflect well-being, pain, diarrhoea, body weight as well as inflammation were used to detect these correlations.

For example, a multiple regression analysis of laboratory values to the Crohn's Disease Activity Index (CDAI)[9] was made by Andre et al.[10] in the case of CD. The authors showed that orosomucoid has the best correlation with CDAI and ESR has the lower correlation but better than CRP. In a study by Goebell[11], the correlation of ESR with CDAI in a group of 300 patients with CD was not good.

Weeke and Jarnum[12] reported that, by analysis of serum concentration of 19 proteins in CD and UC, a good correlation between the laboratory data and the activity of the diseases was observed. They found a large increase in orosomucoid, $\alpha_1$-antitrypsin, antichymotrypsin and haptoglobin. Albumin and transferrin was decreased. Albumin was reduced due to the catabolic process. Various reports have shown that the albumin concentration is inversely proportional to the activity of IBD[13,14]. Other authors[15] correlated CRP with faecal excretion of labelled granulocytes. This method should reveal the inflammation in the gut. They made the point that CRP reflected the activity of CD better than that of UC.

Another investigation made by Fischbach and Becker[16] studied the correlation between 11 laboratory parameters and the detection of faecal granulocytes in a group of 75 patients with CD. The results are presented in Table 2. A significant correlation was found between most parameters and the faecal granulocyte excretion.

**Table 2** Comparison of laboratory findings and clinical indices with the percentage faecal excretion of [111]indium-labelled autologous granulocytes in patients with CD[16]

| | $n$ | $r$ | $p$ |
|---|---|---|---|
| Orosomucoid | 75 | 0.40 | 0.001 |
| $\alpha_1$-Antitrypsin | 75 | 0.43 | 0.001 |
| CRP | 75 | 0.49 | 0.001 |
| ESR | 78 | 0.44 | 0.001 |
| Leukocytes | 78 | 0.26 | 0.01 |
| Thrombocytes | 78 | 0.41 | 0.001 |
| Serum albumin | 78 | − 0.37 | 0.005 |
| Serum Fe | 78 | − 0.45 | 0.001 |
| $\alpha_1$-Globulin | 70 | 0.43 | 0.001 |
| $\alpha_2$-Globulin | 70 | 0.43 | 0.001 |
| Elastase | 35 | No correlation | No correlation |
| CDAI | 59 | No correlation | No correlation |
| van Hees index | 60 | 0.62 | 0.001 |

$n$ = Number of studies; $r$ = Spearman's rank correlation coefficient

Orosomucoid and CRP appear to be the most sensitive acute-phase proteins[10,15–19]. CRP is more suitable because it is easy and quick to measure in all laboratories. CRP is synthesized in the liver preferentially after stimulation by interleukin-6[20]. During the inflammatory process in the gut lymphocytes, monocytes and endothelial cells are activated and produce interleukin-6 and other cytokines. The concentration of CRP is increased rapidly due to inflammation but decreases soon after this process is finished. Patients with CD seem to have higher values of CRP than those with UC[21]. However, normal values could also be found in patients who were obviously ill[13].

These statistical data do not mean that, in individual cases of disease, laboratory parameters are helpful. In our own study, we could confirm the usefulness of thrombocytes as an activity parameter (Table 3). In this study, thrombocytes of 142 patients suffering from UC in the acute phases were counted using a haemocytometer, not a cell counter. We considered that values

**Table 3**  Thrombocytes in UC. Classification of UC into three groups according Truelove and Witts[22]

| Classification of UC | Patients (n) | Thrombocytes (Gpt/µl) | s |
| --- | --- | --- | --- |
| 1 | 79 | 214 | 91 |
| 2 | 44 | 239 | 118 |
| 3 | 19 | 278 | 54 |

greater than 300 Gpt/$\mu$l were pathological. There was a significant difference between to group 1 and group 3, according to the classification of Truelove and Witts[22]. However, the mean values of thrombocytes were normal due to variability of this parameter.

This is confirmed by comparing the individual values of several patients. Patients with severity grade 3 were hospitalized in the acute phases of the disease several times and we found very different values, some of them in the pathological range (Table 4). These data supported the idea that, especially in cases of UC, we must not consider the laboratory data alone.

For the characterization of clinical severity and inflammatory activity of IBD, some activity indices were developed. For CD, the CDAI[9], van Hees index (VHI)[14] and Severity–Activity Index (SAI)[23] were used. In UC, the Disease Activity Index (DAI) according to Rachmilewitz[24] is mostly used. In these indices, laboratory values are represented as parameters for inflammatory activity. Haematocrit is necessary for CDAI; ESR and albumin for VHI; and haematocrit and albumin for SAI. In UC, the DAI includes ESR and haemoglobin.

Laboratory parameters have also been included in prognostic indices. An index was developed for CD by Brignola et al.[25] using ESR, orosomucoid and $\alpha_2$-globulin. This index should predict a relapse. Another prognostic index for CD was published by Wienbeck et al.[26]. For this index, the main laboratory parameter was albumin level. An index higher than 180 points was highly significant for a severe course of CD in the next 2 years.

The conclusion provided by these data is that many parameters could be used to characterize the activity of IBD. Because the laboratory methods should be easy, quick and cheap, we recommend assessing inflammatory activity in the course of IBD by ESR, haemoglobin, haematocrit, thrombocytes, leukocytes and CRP tests.

## LOCALIZATION OF INFLAMMATORY ACTIVITY IN THE GUT

In clinical practice, the localization of inflammation should be made by endoscopy and X-ray examination. In addition, for clinical studies and individual cases, other methods of determination of inflammatory activity in the gut have been developed. Mainly [111]indium-labelled leukocytes, as well as faecal excretion and scintigraphic localization, have been used for this purpose[16,17,27]. Another method for localization of inflammation uses [99]technetium-labelled antibodies against granulocytes. The faecal excretion of radioactivity-bound

**Table 4** Heterogeneity of thrombocyte counts in the acute phases of UC in patients with disease grade 3 according to Truelove and Witts[22]. Cells were counted by haemocytometer. Values set in bold type were increased

| Patient | Thrombocyte counts (Gpt/µl) at different times in the acute phase of the disease | | | | |
|---|---|---|---|---|---|
| DK | **352** | 181 | 211 | **384** | – |
| HK | **368** | **352** | 232 | 210 | 98 |
| FK | 85 | **302** | 209 | 242 | **532** |
| HB | **344** | 234 | 254 | **333** | – |
| NH | **354** | 197 | 242 | 239 | **421** |
| DS | **328** | 232 | 240 | – | – |
| CN | 208 | 281 | 168 | **364** | – |

leukocytes is a good parameter of inflammatory activity[17,27]. In UC, the excretion rate of leukocytes is higher than in CD[15]. However, these tests are expensive, time-consuming and require facilities to work with radioactive substances. In clinical routine, these methods are not helpful.

## LABORATORY PARAMETERS IN INTESTINAL AND EXTRA-INTESTINAL COMPLICATIONS

In CD and UC, many complications and extra-intestinal manifestations are known. In these cases, some laboratory tests may be helpful for diagnosis and to control the course of complications (Table 5). However, other methods, besides laboratory tests such as sonography, endoscopy and biopsy, are necessary.

Extended lesions in the bowel cause increased exudation of protein leading to enteral protein loss. Faecal excretion of $\alpha_1$-antitrypsin and faecal excretion of $^{51}$chromium-tagged serum proteins are markers for this exudative enteropathy[28,31].

The [$^{14}$C]glycocholate breath test demonstrates an impaired physiological reabsorption of conjugated bile acids in the terminal ileum resulting from an inflammatory process. In the short-bowel syndrome after surgery, diarrhoea may be due to non-absorbed bile acids. Using the $H_2$-breath test, pathological bacterial overgrowth in the small bowel can be detected. Impaired vitamin $B_{12}$ resorption in the terminal ileum can be demonstrated with the Schilling test with the addition of intrinsic factor.

Gastrointestinal bleeding is an important clinical sign of disease, especially in UC. Following the loss of blood, a disturbance in the blood coagulation system appears. Fibrinogen increases as an acute-phase protein, and Factor XIII and antithrombin III may be diminished. There is no direct correlation of these values with clinical activity indices, but, in the acute phase of the disease, it is helpful to supplement Factor XIII and antithrombin III, if these are diminished, as support for standard therapy. Table 6 shows the heterogeneity of coagulation parameters in individual patients.

Increased concentrations of alkaline phosphatase and other cholestasis enzymes ($\gamma$-GT, GLDH) suggest the development of a complication of IBD, primary sclerosing cholangitis.

**Table 5**   Laboratory tests for cases with complications

| Complications | Tests |
| --- | --- |
| Malabsorption | Faecal excretion of $\alpha_1$-antitrypsin<br>$H_2$-breath test<br>$^{14}C$-glycocholate breath test<br>Schilling test<br>Vitamin serum levels |
| Disturbed blood coagulation | Factor XIII, AT III |
| Primary sclerosing cholangitis | Alkaline phosphatase, $\gamma$-GT, GLDH |
| Nephrolithiasis | Urinary oxalate, red blood cells |
| Amyloidosis (renal insufficiency) | Electrophoresis, creatinine |

**Table 6**   Parameters of blood coagulation in patients with UC

| Patient | DAI | Fibrinogen (g/L) | TAT (%) | Factor XIII (%) |
| --- | --- | --- | --- | --- |
| AB | 13 | **4.96** | 5.4 | **32** |
| IR | 12 | **4.89** | 3.6 | **58** |
| DS | 12 | **4.53** | 2.6 | 97 |
| SL | 10 | 3.97 | 3.6 | 96 |
| CN | 9 | 2.93 | **7.0** | 87 |
| HR | 7 | **8.16** | 3.9 | **54** |
| RB | 7 | 2.77 | 3.5 | 103 |
| TF | 6 | 2.36 | 3.5 | 52 |

DAI = Disease activity index[24]; TAT = thrombin–antithrombin complex; values set in bold type are pathological

An increased $\gamma$-globulin fraction in electrophoresis can demonstrate the development of amyloidosis. Serum creatinine indicates manifest injury of the glomeruli.

## SUMMARY

Laboratory parameters are part of the range of useful methods in IBD. They are helpful to recognize inflammatory disease, to assess inflammatory activity and to control the course of IBD. However, they cannot differentiate exactly between UC and CD. Essentially, for clinical routine, ESR, haematocrit, leukocytes, differentiation of leukocytes, thrombocytes and CRP should be used. Laboratory parameters are among the main indices of activity in UC and CD and in the prognostic indices. They can support diagnosis of intestinal and extra-intestinal complications.

## References

1. Asakura H, Sugimura K. HLA, antineutrophil cytoplasmic autoantibody, and heterogeneity in ulcerative colitis. Gastroenterology. 1995;108:597–9.

2. Oudkerk Pool M, Ellerbroek PM, Ridwan BU et al. Serum antineutrophil cytoplasmic auto-antibodies in inflammatory bowel disease are mainly associated with ulcerative colitis. A correlation study between perinuclear antineutrophil cytoplasmic autoantibodies and clinical parameters, medical and surgical treatment. Gut. 1993;34:46–50.

3. Rump JA, Schoelmerich J, Gross V et al. A new type of perinuclear anti-neutrophil cytoplasmic antibody (p-ANCA) in active ulcerative colitis but not in Crohn's disease. Immunobiology. 1990;181:406–13.

4. Seibold F, Weber P, Klein R, Berg PA, Wiedmann KH. Clinical significance of antibodies against neutrophils in patients with inflammatory bowel disease and primary sclerosing cholangitis. Gut. 1992;33:657–62.

5. Colombel JF, Reumaux D, Duthilleul P et al. Antineutrophil cytoplasmic autoantibodies in inflammatory bowel disease. Gastroenterol Clin Biol. 1992;16:656–60.

6. Duerr RH, Neigut DA. Molecularly defined HLA-DR2 alleles in ulcerative colitis and an antineutrophil cytoplasmic antibody–positive subgroup. Gastroenterology. 1995;108:423–7.

7. Lee JCW, Lennard-Jones JE, Cambridge G. Antineutrophil antibodies in familial inflammatory bowel disease. Gastroenterology. 1995;108:428–33.

8. Seibold F, Slametschka D, Gregor M, Weber P. Neutrophil autoantibodies: A genetic marker in primary sclerosing cholangitis and ulcerative colitis. Gastroenterology. 1994;107:532–6.

9. Best WR, Becktel JM, Singleton JW, Kern F. Development of a Crohn's disease activity index. National Cooperative Crohn's Disease Study. Gastroenterology. 1977;70:439–44.

10. Andre C, Descos L, Andre F, Vignal J, Landais P, Fermanian J. Biological measurements of Crohn's disease activity – a reassessment. Hepato-gastroenterology. 1985;32:135–7.

11. Goebell H. Different activity indices in Crohn's disease and their possible role. In: Goebell H, Peskar BM, Malchow H, eds. Inflammatory bowel disease – basic research and clinical implications. Lancaster, UK: MTP Press; 1988:253–8.

12. Weeke B, Jarnum S. Serum concentration of 19 serum proteins in Crohn's disease and ulcerative colitis. Gut. 1971;12:297–302.

13. Cooke WT, Prior P. Determining disease activity in inflammatory bowel disease. J Clin Gastroenterol. 1984;6:17–25.

14. van Hees PAM, van Elteren PH, van Lier HJJ, van Tongeren JHM. An index of inflammatory activity in patients with Crohn's disease. Gut. 1980;21:279–86.

15. Saverymuttu SH, Hodgson HJF, Chadwick VS, Pepys MB. Differing acute phase responses in Crohn's disease and ulcerative colitis. Gut. 1986;27:809–13.

16. Beck IT. Laboratory assessment of inflammatory bowel disease. Dig Dis Sci. 1987;32:26–41.

17. Fischbach W, Becker W. Clinical relevance of activity parameters in Crohn's disease estimated by the faecal excretion of 111Indium labeled granulocytes. Digestion. 1991;50:149–52.

18. Buckell NA, Lennard-Jones JE, Hernandez MA, Kohn J, Riches PG, Wadsworth I. Measurement of serum proteins during attacks of ulcerative colitis as a guide to patient management. Gut. 1979;20:22–7.

19. Descos L, Andre F, Andre C, Gillon J, Landais P, Fermanian J. Assessment of appropriate laboratory measurements to reflect the degree of activity of ulcerative colitis. Digestion. 1983;28:148–52.

20. Heinrich PC, Castell JV, Andus T. Interleukin-6 and the acute phase response. Biochem J. 1990;265:621–36.

21. Shine B, Berghouse L, Lennard-Jones JE, Landon J. C-reactive protein as an aid in the differentiation of functional and inflammatory bowel disorders. Clin Chim Acta. 1985;148:105–9.

22. Truelove SC, Witts LJ. Cortisone in ulcerative colitis. Final report on a therapeutic trial. Br Med J. 1955;2:1041–8.

23. Goebell H, Wienbeck M. Schomerus H, Malchow H. Evaluation of the Crohn's disease activity index (CDAI) and the Dutch index for severity and activity of Crohn's disease. Med Klin. 1990;10:573–6.

24. Rachmilewitz D. Coated mesalazine (5-amino-salicylic acid) versus sulphasalazine in the treatment of active ulcerative colitis: a randomized trial. Br Med J. 1989;298:82–6.

25. Brignola C, Campieri M, Bazzocchi G, Farruggia P, Tragnone A, Lanfranchi GA. A laboratory index for predicting relapse in asymptomatic patients with Crohn's disease. Gastroenterology. 1986;91:1490–4.

26. Wienbeck M, Goebell H, Schomerus H, Jesdinsky HJ. Entwicklung eines prognostischen Indexes bei Morbus Crohn. Med Klin. 1987;82:87–91.

27. Fischbach W, Becker W, Mössner J, Koch W, Reiners C. Faecal alpha-1-antitrypsin and excretion of [111]Indium granulocytes in assessment of disease activity in chronic inflammatory bowel diseases. Gut. 1987;28:386–93.

28. Karbach U, Ewe K, Dehos H. Antiinflammatory treatment and intestinal alpha-1-antitrypsin clearance in active Crohn's disease. Dig Dis Sci. 1985;30:229–35.

29. Karbach U, Singe CC, Ewe K. Simplified determination of intestinal protein excretion based on alpha-1-antitrypsin clearance. Z Gastroenterol. 1988;26:169–73.

30. Meyers S, Wolke A, Field StP, Feuer EJ, Johnson JW, Janowitz HD. Fecal alpha-1-antitrypsin measurement: an indicator of Crohn's disease activity. Gastroenterology. 1985;89:13–18.

31. Thomas DW, Sinatra FR, Merritt RJ. Fecal alpha-1-antitrypsin excretion in young people with Crohn's disease. J Pediatr Gastroenterol Nutr. 1983;2:491–6.

# Section V
# Standards and new developments in medical treatment

# 20
# Sulphasalazine, mesalazine and other 5-ASA derivatives

A. DIGNASS and P. LAYER

## INTRODUCTION

Although the aetiologies of ulcerative colitis and Crohn disease still remain elusive, considerable progress has been made in the therapeutic management of these diseases. One of the main principles in the treatment of inflammatory bowel diseases focuses on inhibition of the effects of inflammatory mediators which are involved in the inflammatory process. In this respect, treatment with aminosalicylic acid and its derivatives has become one of the main principles in the treatment of IBD. Since the introduction of sulphasalazine into the treatment of IBD by Nana Swartz in the 1930s, it has been demonstrated that the therapeutic activity of sulphasalazine is attributable to the local action of its 5-ASA moiety[1], whereas most of the sulphasalazine-related side-effects are caused by the sulphapyridine residue, to which 5-ASA is linked in order to prevent absorption of 5-ASA in the proximal gastrointestinal tract. Absorption of 5-ASA in the proximal gastrointestinal tract would make it unavailable to the colonic mucosa where it exerts its desired effects. New formulations of 5-ASA have been developed over the past several years in order to achieve liberation in the distal small intestine and the colon. This chapter will review different 5-ASA preparations, their pharmacokinetic properties and their efficacy in the treatment of inflammatory bowel diseases.

## PHARMACOKINETIC PROPERTIES OF 5-ASA PREPARATIONS

### Sulphasalazine (SASP)

Sulphasalazine is composed of two components: an aspirin analogue, 5-aminosalicylic acid (5-ASA), and a sulphonamide, sulphapyridine, which are covalently linked by a diazo bond. Only small quantities (< 10%) of intact SASP are absorbed by the human small intestinal mucosa and most of the compound is delivered into the distal ileum and colon. In the colon and (to a lesser extent) the distal ileum, sulphasalazine is cleaved into 5-ASA and sulphapyridine by the enzyme, azoreductase, which is produced by the luminal bacterial flora[2]. Sulphasalazine is able to deliver large quantities of sulphapyridine and 5-ASA into the proximal colonic lumen. Sulphapyridine is absorbed quantitatively by the colonic mucosa and undergoes hepatic metabolism (acetylation, glucuronidation, hydroxylation) and subsequent renal excretion. Luminal 5-ASA is acetylated by colonic bacteria and by the colonic epithelium with presumed resecretion back into the lumen. Acetylated 5-ASA does not appear to cross back into the epithelium[3]. The pioneering studies by Azad Khan and colleagues[1] have revealed that the anti-inflammatory activity of suphasalazine is attributable to the 5-ASA moiety, while the sulphapyridine residue has no significant therapeutic effect in inflammatory bowel disease. Indeed, it became obvious that most of the side-effects of sulphasalazine are caused by the sulphapyridine moiety. However, the sulphapyridine residue is necessary for therapeutic efficacy because it prevents the absorption and/or metabolism of 5-ASA in the proximal gastrointestinal tract which would make 5-ASA unavailable to the ileal or colonic mucosa.

## 5-Aminosalicylic acid

Uncoated 5-ASA is rapidly and completely absorbed in the upper gastrointestinal tract after oral administration and acetylated by the gastrointestinal mucosa with formation of the inactive metabolite, acetyl-5-ASA (ac-5-ASA)[4–6]. Consequently, the major portion (> 80%) of the absorbed amount is present in the plasma as ac-5-ASA[6]. 5-ASA is also acetylated in the liver. Systemic elimination of 5-ASA occurs almost exclusively in the acetylated form by renal excretion[5]. The half-lives of 5-ASA and ac-5-ASA vary depending on the dose administered. For 5-ASA, the half-life varies between 40 and 90 min; the half-life of ac-5-ASA is 6–10 h[7]. Approximately half of the absorbed 5-ASA is bound to plasma proteins. The absorption rate of 5-ASA is lower in the colon than in the small intestine.

After direct administration of 5-ASA into the colon by enema or oral slow-release preparations (see below), about 20–30% of the total dose is absorbed and systemically available, whereas the majority is excreted in the faeces[7,8].

## Modern oral slow-release 5-ASA preparations

The pharmacokinetic properties of uncoupled 5-ASA (rapid absorption and inactivation in the proximal gastrointestinal tract) prompted the formulation of new 5-ASA preparations in order to provide delivery of therapeutic amounts of 5-ASA into the distal small intestine and the colon. A well-characterized system to provide delivery of 5-ASA in sufficient amounts into the colon has been described above for sulphasalazine. However, the use of sulphapyridine as a carrier molecule in order to prevent absorption of 5-ASA in the proximal intestine is disadvantageous because the sulphapyridine residue is responsible for most of the side-effects of SASP (rash, arthritis, pericarditis, pancreatitis, pleuritis, reversible infertility in men, pancytopenia because of folate deficiency and other reactions) which are seen in a dose-dependent fashion in 13–60% of patients[9]. Basically, two principal approaches have been used to deliver oral 5-ASA to the small and large bowel:

1. A pharmacological approach with coupling of 5-ASA to a carrier molecule, and
2. A pharmaceutical approach with encapsulation of 5-ASA in a slow-release matrix.

Using these two different approaches, several oral 5-ASA derivatives have been developed.

## Coupling of 5-ASA to carrier molecules

The prototype compound of this group is sulphasalazine which has been described above. SASP still serves as the gold standard to compare the effectiveness of other 5-ASA preparations. Because of the disturbing side-effects mentioned above, other carrier molecules have been developed. One of the most interesting pharmacological approaches is the coupling of two molecules of 5-ASA and synthesis of a 5-ASA dimer (olsalazine; Dipentum®). This 5-ASA dimer is stable within the proximal gastrointestinal tract. In the colon, olsalazine is cleaved by bacterial azoreductase and two molecules of free 5-ASA are released[10]. Other carrier molecules for 5-ASA include inert carriers such as 4-amino-benzoyl-alanin (Balsalazide), 4-amino-benzoyl-glycin (Ipsalazide) and para-amino-benzoic acid (Benzalazine). These new preparations are not currently available in most European countries and the United States.

## Encapsulation of 5-ASA in a slow-release matrix

Release of 5-ASA into the small intestine and the colon can also be achieved by encapsulation of 5-ASA with acrylic resins or ethylcellulose. These preparations also prevent the release and absorption of 5-ASA in the stomach and the proximal small intestine. In commercially available 5-ASA preparations, the acrylic resins, Eudragit S (Asacol®) or Eudragit L, in combination with sodium bicarbonate/glycine buffering (Salofalk®, Claversal®), are used. Preparations with Eudragit S permit disintegration at pH > 7; those with Eudragit L permit disintegration at about pH 6[11]. 5-ASA preparations coated with acrylic resins are available in tablet form.

On the other hand, 5-ASA can be packed in microgranules and coated with ethylcellulose (Pentasa®). This preparation is available as a capsule which releases acid-stable microgranules of 5-ASA within the stomach. The ethylcellulose coating disintegrates gradually during small intestinal transit and releases active 5-ASA.

The release patterns of slow-release preparations of 5-ASA are substantially different. The luminal liberation of 5-ASA from different preparations can be studied by various approaches which include measuring of urinary or oral excretion, plasma appearance and disappearance rates of 5-ASA and its main metabolite acetyl-5-ASA in order to estimate kinetics and extent of its intraluminal release[7,12–14]. In addition, radiographic tracings of barium sulphate marker, scintigraphic tracings of radioactive isotopes released from coated tablets or the recovery of 5-ASA from the ileostomy effluent of patients are utilized in order to study the luminal liberation of 5-ASA[15]. The described approaches provide rather indirect methods to study the global delivery of 5-ASA into the colon. However, the availability of 5-ASA within individual levels of the small bowel, which is of interest because of the potential value of 5-ASA in the treatment of ileal Crohn disease, cannot be characterized by these indirect methods. In order to determine the luminal release and fate of different oral slow-release preparations of 5-ASA, we recently studied the luminal release and fate of 5-ASA from two different galenic preparations (Salofalk and Pentasa) by direct luminal measurement in healthy human volunteers. Volunteers were intubated with an integrated multilumen oro-ileal tube which allowed marker perfusion, aspiration of luminal contents from the duodenum, mid-jejunum and terminal ileum, and recording of intestinal motility[16–20]. These studies demonstrated significantly different release patterns of the two studied oral slow-release forms of 5-ASA (Salofalk and Pentasa). Both preparations predominantly release 5-ASA into the colon, but significantly different patterns of gastric emptying, small intestinal transit, and intraluminal bioavailability in the small intestine could be demonstrated.

Salofalk, 5-ASA encapsulated in a pH-sensitive release matrix (Eudragit L), is emptied from the stomach about 3 h after emptying of a co-administered test meal together with the first phase III of interdigestive motility. Increasing quantities of 5-ASA are released during the passage of the tablet through the small intestine. Thus, concentrations of 5-ASA and acetylated 5-ASA increase continuously from the duodenum to the distal ileum over 3 h and decrease over the next 3 h. The cumulative delivery of free 5-ASA to the duodenum is less than 2% of the total dose; approximately 6% is released in the jejunum and about 13% in the ileum. In parallel, increasing concentrations of acetylated 5-ASA are detected in the small intestine, averaging about 1.5% in the duodenum, 12% in the jejunum and 18% in the ileum. This simultaneous and approximately parallel appearance of 5-ASA and acetylated 5-ASA suggests mucosal generation and back-defusion of 5-ASA into the lumen rather than enteric–biliary recirculation. About 30% of the total dose passes the ileum in solution and another 10% is excreted in urine within 10 h after eating. Thus, about 60% of the total dose reaches the colon unreleased from tablets and another 30% is in solution[16].

In contrast, 5-ASA in microsphere preparations (Pentasa) is emptied simultaneously with a meal in the digestive period out of the stomach. 5-ASA from the Pentasa preparation is emptied roughly simultaneously with a meal and appears in the duodenum between 20 and 60 min after administration of the test meal[18]. Small intestinal transit times are similar to those of Salofalk. Cumulative delivery of free 5-ASA to the duodenum, jejunum and ileum is each approximately 10% of the total dose, reflecting significant pharmacokinetic differences compared with Salofalk. Cumulative amounts of acetylated 5-ASA tend to be slightly greater at distal intestinal sites. In contrast to Salofalk, plasma concentrations of 5-ASA are significantly lower than those of acetylated 5-ASA. Only traces of 5-ASA were present in urine; the cumulative excretion of acetylated 5-ASA amounts to approximately 5% of the total dose. Overall analysis suggests that about 20% of the total dose is released during small-intestinal transit and reaches the colon dissolved in luminal juice. Another 70% reaches the colon unreleased as microspheres and about 5% is absorbed.

The different release patterns of 5-ASA from Salofalk and Pentasa reflect the physiological gastric emptying mechanisms in humans. In the digestive period, gastric emptying of solid particles only occurs together with meal nutrients if their diameter does not exceed 1–2 mm. During the antral contractions, the pyloric lumen narrows to 1–2 mm. Bigger solid particles cannot pass the pylorus and remain in the stomach until they are further digested. Thus, only micro-granule preparations (Pentasa) can be emptied simultaneously with a meal, i.e. in the digestive period. 5-ASA coated with Eudragit is not released simultaneously with the meal but 3–5 h after a meal together with the first phase III of interdigestive motility which permits the emptying of bigger particles from the stomach.

Anyhow, both preparations produce considerable luminal concentrations of free 5-ASA in the small intestine. Thus, these preparations may also be effective in small intestinal Crohn disease provided that sufficient doses are administered. The specific release patterns of these compounds suggest that Salofalk may be favourably utilized in predominantly terminal ileal disease, while Pentasa may be particularly effective in extensive (including proximal) small intestinal involvement. So far, these assumptions are rather speculative and have not been confirmed in clinical trials.


## MECHANISMS OF ACTION OF 5-ASA

The landmark studies by Azad Khan and colleagues[1] have revealed that the anti-inflammatory activity of sulphasalazine is attributable to the 5-ASA moiety, while the sulphapyridine residue has few or no therapeutic effects in inflammatory bowel disease. Because of several important side-effects, the application of sulphasalazine has been limited and modern 5-ASA preparations have been developed. These different 5-ASA preparations have several mechanisms to attenuate intestinal inflammation. The precise mechanism of action of 5-ASA is obscured by a failure to understand the aetiopathogenesis of IBD. It seems that several mediators, identified in the inflammatory cascades and activated in IBD, are somehow modulated by 5-ASA, thus obscuring a single pivotal therapeutic effect. 5-ASA is a potent inhibitor of several inflammatory mediators, such as leukotrienes (e.g. $LTB_4$), prostaglandins and platelet activating factor (PAF) which may play an important role in inflammatory bowel diseases as chemo-attractive compounds that activate neutrophils and other constituents of the inflammatory response[21–23]. 5-ASA also affects immunoglobulin production by B cells, thus modulating the immune response. The production and binding of several cytokines (IL-1, TNF-$\alpha$, IFN-$\alpha$) is also modulated by 5-ASA[3]. In addition, 5-ASA appears to block the chemotactic activity of formylated bacterial peptides (FMLP), compounds that are assumed to recruit polymorphonuclear cells to the bowel. Other studies have demonstrated that 5-ASA can act as a scavenger of oxygen free radicals[24]. Reduction of superoxide radicals by 5-ASA is assumed to reduce increased intestinal permeability[25]. Furthermore, 5-ASA appears to inhibit the expression of HLA-antigens and the production of antibodies by B cells, thus modulating immune modulatory functions of the intestinal mucosa[26,27].

## ADVERSE EFFECTS OF 5-ASA AND DERIVATIVES

The new formulations of 5-ASA have significantly improved the armamentarium for the treatment of IBD because of their improved tolerance compared with sulphasalazine, whose side-effects, largely related to sulphapyridine, cause the discontinuation of treatment in a significant number of patients. Virtually all comparison studies have demonstrated better tolerability of non-sulphapyridine-containing aminosalicylates with sulphasalazine. Nevertheless, several side-effects have been reported for new formulations of 5-ASA which clearly implicate 5-ASA as a potent toxic agent in susceptible individuals in the absence of sulphapyridine. The most commonly reported adverse effects of 5-ASA are headache (up to 13%) and nausea (up to 8%), while itching, dizziness, indigestion, muscular ache and fever occur usually in fewer than 5% of patients. However, these effects were observed with similar frequency in patients with ulcerative colitis who received placebo. Furthermore, they did not appear to increase when the dose of 5-ASA was increased[11]. A large general practice study with 1730 patients treated with oral 5-ASA (1.5 g/d) revealed epigastric discomfort (8.0%), nausea (0.4%) and allergy (0.5%) as the most frequently observed side-effects[28]. An ileal secretory reaction to 5-ASA with apparent worsening of symptoms presenting with increased stool frequency, rectal bleeding and occasionally fever may occur infrequently within the first few days of administration[11]. These reactions resolve on discontinuation of 5-ASA and recur immediately after reintroduction of 5-ASA. There have also been rare case reports of perimyocarditis, bronchospasm, lupus-like syndrome, hepatitis, retrosternal chest pain, neutropenia, acute pancreatitis, accelerated hair loss and acute alveolitis following 5-ASA therapy[11,29,30]. In general, 5-ASA preparations are very well tolerated. Overall, 80–90% of patients intolerant of or allergic to sulphasalazine are able to tolerate 5-ASA[31]. However, 10–20% of patients intolerant of sulphasalazine will experience a reaction to 5-ASA. The most frequent and disturbing side-effect of olsalazine is the secretory watery diarrhoea, which has been reported in 15–35% of patients[32] and necessitates discontinuation of the drug in 5–10%[33]. The incidence of this watery diarrhoea is dose dependent and also depends on the extent of the colitis. The diarrhoea appears to result from stimulated ileal secretion related to anion secretagogue properties of olsalazine. Lowering the dose of olsalazine may reduce or eliminate the diarrhoea. Indeed, a recent study suggests that maintenance therapy with 1 g/d of olsalazine is well tolerated in > 90% of patients with a low incidence of diarrhoea (< 5%)[34].

## THERAPEUTIC EFFICACY OF 5-ASA AND DERIVATIVES IN IBD

5-ASA and derivatives can be administered orally or topically, as retention enemas, suppositories or foam preparations, for the treatment of IBD. There is unequivocal evidence that 5-ASA preparations are effective as both acute-phase therapy for mild to moderately active chronic inflammatory bowel disease and as maintenance therapy in quiescent inflammatory bowel disease. The benefits of the available topical and oral aminosalicylate preparations are not easy to summarize because of different formulations, doses, study duration and end-points. In maintenance trials, oral aminosalicylates (e.g. 750 mg/d) were as effective as sulphasalazine with less side-effects when provided in equimolar doses for different preparations. The equivalence between different 5-ASA preparations has been independent of the delivery system for 5-ASA, e.g. azo-bond (olsalazine, balsalazide), encapsulation with Eudragit (Claversal, Salofalk, Asacol), or continuous-release microgranule preparations (Pentasa). Therefore, it has to be assumed that differences between preparations may be trivial for the treatment of IBD within the applied doses[3]. In order to establish optimal doses for the treatment of active IBD and maintaining remission in quiescent IBD, further dose-finding studies are required.

## Ulcerative colitis

Topical 5-ASA is currently firmly established as therapy for the treatment of acute disease and maintenance of remission in left-sided ulcerative colitis or ulcerative proctitis[35]. Topical preparations of 5-ASA include 5-ASA enemas, suppositories or foam. 5-ASA enemas have been shown to reach up to the splenic flexure in most patients (approximately 92%), while the enema is spread in the sigmoid colon in 100% of patients[36]. The distribution of 5-ASA foam is similar to the distribution of 5-ASA enemas in about 90% of patients tested via scintigraphic evaluation[37]. 5-ASA foam seems to be advantageous because of a more uniform distribution and longer persistence in the descending and sigmoid colon. A recent study suggested that 5-ASA foam may provide prompter remission of symptoms compared with liquid enemas and significantly improve the quality of topical therapy in ulcerative colitis[38]. Patients with left-sided colitis using 5-ASA enemas have a typical response rate of 80% during treatment of active disease[38]. The typical onset of action for 5-ASA enemas in patients with new uncomplicated ulcerative colitis is 3–21 days and usually the treatment time for an acute flare of ulcerative colitis requires 3–6 weeks[38]. Patients who cannot tolerate retention enemas or cannot retain the fluid for a sufficient amount of time may be treated with 5-ASA suppositories which have been demonstrated to be an effective alternative for the treatment of proctitis ulcerosa[39]. Topical 5-ASA has also proved to be effective in patients who did not respond to conventional therapy with sulphasalazine and cortico-steroids[40–42].

Oral 5-ASA preparations have proved to be as effective as sulphasalazine in the treatment of mild to moderately active ulcerative colitis causing less side-effects than sulphasalazine. Larger doses of 5-ASA (3–4.8 g/d) seem to be more effective than lower doses (0.8–2.4 g/d) but smaller doses are also effective[40–44].

5-ASA preparations have also proved to be effective in maintaining remission for quiescent ulcerative colitis[45–47]. It seems to be sufficient in most cases to use 750–1500 mg 5-ASA or 1000 mg of diazo-bonded 5-ASA (olsalazine). A maintenance therapy should be initiated if the frequency of active phases exceeds 1/year and/or if disease activity reduces the quality of life. A maintenance therapy should be continued for a 2-year interval in the absence of recurrence of active disease.

## Crohn disease

Recent data provide significant evidence that 5-ASA may also be effective in the treatment of active Crohn disease and in maintaining remission in quiescent Crohn disease. The failure of 5-ASA preparations in earlier studies is most probably attributable to insufficient doses of 5-ASA utilized in these studies. A comparative trial of 5-ASA with sulphasalazine showed similar effectiveness of both compounds in mild to moderately active Crohn disease but a significant reduction of side-effects under 5-ASA medication[48]. Another study using 1.5 g/d 5-ASA failed to show differences in efficacy between 5-ASA and placebo[49]. More recent studies using higher doses of 5-ASA (up to 4.5 g/d) revealed that oral mesalazine preparations are effective in the treatment of active Crohn disease of the ileum and the colon[50,51] and may induce similar rates of remission as the standard acute-phase treatment regimen using corticosteroids[52]. Furthermore, it appears that patients with ileal involvement may profit more significantly from therapy with 5-ASA. These differences are probably caused by different pharmacokinetic profiles of various oral formulations (as discussed above) but so far there has been no direct comparison of these different formulations in larger clinical trails.

Recent studies have also demonstrated that 5-ASA is a safe and effective substance for the maintenance treatment of Crohn disease[51,53–55]. These studies indicate that higher doses of 5-ASA (> 2 g/d) are probably more effective in maintaining remission than the previously utilized low-dose regimen (< 2 g/d). Maintenance therapy should be initiated within 3 months of achieving remission. Furthermore, oral 5-ASA preparations seem also to be effective in preventing postoperative recurrence of Crohn disease if initiated soon after surgery[56].

## References


1. Azad Khan AK, Piris J, Truelove SC. An experiment to determine the active therapeutic moiety of sulphasalazine. Lancet. 1977;1:892–5.
2. Azad Khan AK, Truelove SC, Aronson R. The disposition and metabolism of sulphasalazine (salicylazosulphapyridine) in man. Br J Pharmacol. 1982;3:523.
3. Hanauer SB. Evolving medical therapies for inflammatory bowel disease. Prog Inflamm Bowel Dis. 1994;15:1–6.
4. Peppercorn MA, Goldman P. Distribution studies of salicylazosulphapyridine and its metabolites. Gastroenterology. 1973;64:240–5.
5. Shafi A, Chowdhury JR, Das KM. Absorption, enterohepatic circulation and excretion of 5-aminosalicylic acid in rats. Am J Gastroenterol. 1982;77:297–9.
6. Nielson OH, Bondesen S. Kinetics of 5-aminosalicylic acid after jejunal instillation in man. Br J Clin Pharmacol. 1983;16:738–40.
7. Klotz U, Maier KE, Fischer C, Bauer KH. A new slow-release form of 5-aminosalicylic acid for the oral treatment of inflammatory bowel disease. Biopharmaceutic and clinical pharmacokinetic characteristics. Arzneimittel Forschung/Drug Res. 1985;35:636–9.
8. Bondesen F, Bronn-Schou J, Pedersen V, Rafiolsadat Z, Hansen S, Huidberg EF. Absorption of 5-aminosalicylic acid from colon and rectum. Br J Clin Pharmacol. 1988;25:269.
9. Bachrach WH. Sulphasalazine. An historical perspective. Am J Gastroenterol. 1988;83:487–96.
10. Ewe K. Differentialtherapie von chronisch entzündlichen Darmerkrankungen mit oralen Aminosalizylaten. Dtsch Ärztebl. 1994;91:B2223–5.
11. Brogden RN, Sorkin EM. Mesalazine. A review of its pharmacodynamic and pharmacokinetic properties, and therapeutic potential in chronic inflammatory bowel disease. Drugs. 1989;38:500–23.

12. Myers B, Evans DNW, Rhodes J et al. Metabolism and urinary excretion of 5-aminosalicylic acid in healthy volunteers when given intravenously or released for absorption at different sites in the gastrointestinal tract. Gut. 1987;28:196–200.

13. Rijk MCM, van Schaik A, van Tongeren JHM. Disposition of 5-aminosalicylic acid by 5-aminosalicylic acid-delivering compounds. Scand J Gastroenterol. 1988;23:107–12.

14. Rasmussen SN, Bondesen S, Huidberg EF et al. 5-Aminosalicylic acid in a slow release preparation: bioavailability, plasma level and excretion in humans. Gastroenterology. 1982;83:1062–70.

15. Christensen LA, Fallingborg J, Jacobsen BA, Rasmussen SN. Pharmakokinetik der oral verabreichten 5-Aminosalizylsäure (Mesalazin)-Präparate: Unterschiede und mögliche klinische Auswirkungen. Chirurg Gastroenterol. 1993;9(Suppl.1):38–43.

16. Goebell H, Klotz U, Nehlsen B, Layer P. Oro-ileal transit of slow release 5-aminosalicylic acid. Gut. 1993;34:669–75.

17. Goebell H, Layer P, Nehlsen B, Klotz U. Oro-ileal transit and intestinal delivery of 5-aminosalicylic acid in humans. Gastroenterology. 1990;98:A172.

18. Layer PH, Goebell H, Keller J, Dignass A, Klotz U. Delivery and fate of oral mesalamine microgranules (Pentasa®) within the human small intestine. Gastroenterology. 1995;108:1427–33.

19. Layer P, Chan ATH, Go VLW, DiMagno EP. Human pancreatic secretion during phase II antral motility of the interdigestive cycle. Am J Physiol. 1988;254:G249–53.

20. Layer P, Peschel S, Schlesinger T, Goebell H. Human pancreatic secretion and intestinal motility: effects of ileal nutrient perfusion. Am J Physiol. 1990;258:G196–201.

21. Nielsen OH, Bukhave K, Elmgreen J, Ahnfelt-Ronne I. Inhibition of 5-lipoxygenase pathway of arachidonic acid metabolism in human neutrophils by sulphasalizine and 5-aminosalicylic acid. Dig Dis Sci. 1987;32:577–82.

22. Lauritsen K, Hansen J, Bytzer P, Bukhave K, Rask-Madsen J. Effects of sulphasalazine and disodium azodisalicylate on colonic $PGE_2$ concentrations determined by equilibrium in vivo dialysis of faeces in patients with ulcerative colitis and healthy controls. Gut. 1984;25:1271–8.

23. Greenfield SM, Punchard NA, Teare JP, Thompson RPH. Review article: The mode of action of the aminosalicylates in inflammatory bowel disease. Aliment Pharmacol Ther. 1993;7:369–83.

24. Miyachi Y, Yoshioka A, Imamura S, Niwa Y. Effect of sulphasalazine and its metabolites on the generation of reactive oxygen species. Gut. 1987;28:190–5.

25. Hiller KO, Willson RL. Hydroxyl free radicals and anti-inflammatory drugs: biological inactivation studies and reaction rate constants. Biochem Pharmacol. 1973;13:2109–11.

26. Mahida YR, Lamming CED, Gallagher A et al. 5-Aminosalicylic acid is a potent inhibitor of interleukin 1 beta production in organ culture of colonic biopsy specimens from patients with inflammatory bowel disease. Gut. 1991;32:50.

27. MacDermott RP, Schloemann SR, Bertovich MJ et al. Inhibition of antibody secretion by 5-aminosalicylic acid. Gastroenterology. 1989;96:442–8.

28. May B. Behandlung chronisch entzündlicher Darmerkrankungen. Studie über Mesalazin (5-Aminosalizylsäure) an mehr als 1700 Patienten unter Praxisbedingungen. Münchener Med Wochenschr. 1987;129:786–9.

29. Dent MT, Ganapathy S, Holdsworth CD, Channer KC. Mesalazine induced lupus-like syndrome. Br Med J. 1992;305:159.

30. Largler U, Schulthess HK, Kuhn M. Akute Alveolitis unter Mesalazin. Schweiz Med Wochenschr. 1992;122:1332–4.

31. Rao SS, Cann PA, Holdswarth CD. Clinical experience of the tolerance of mesalazine and olsalazine in patients intolerant of sulphasalazine. Scand J Gastroenterol. 1987;22:332–6.

32. Meyers S, Sachar DB, Present DH, Janowitz HD. Olsalazine sodium in the treatment of ulcerative colitis among patients intolerant of sulfasalazine. A prospective, randomized, placebo-controlled, double-blind, dose-ranging clinical trial. Gastroenterology. 1987;93:1255–62.

33. Jarnerot G. Clinical tolerance of olsalazine. Scand J Gastroenterol. 1988;23(Suppl.):21–3.

34. Courtney MG, Nunes DP, Bergin CF et al. Randomised comparison of olsalazine and mesalazine in prevention of relapse in ulcerative colitis. Lancet. 1992;339:1279–81.

35. Lichtenstein GR. Medical therapies for inflammatory bowel disease. Curr Opin Gastroenterol. 1994;10:390–403.

36. Chapman NJ, Brown NL, Phillips SF et al. Distribution of mesalamine enemas in patients with active distal ulcerative colitis. Mayo Clin Proc. 1992;67:245–8.

37. Campieri M, Corbelli C, Gionchetti P et al. Spread and distribution of 5-ASA colonic foam and 5-ASA enemas in patients with ulcerative colitis. Dig Dis Sci. 1992;37:1890–7.
38. Campieri M, Paoluzzi P, D'Albasio G, Brunetti G, Pera A, Barbara L. Better quality of therapy with 5-ASA colonic foam in active ulcerative colitis: a multicenter comparative trial with 5-ASA enema. Dig Dis Sci. 1993;38:1843–50.
39. Campieri M, DeFranchis R, Porto B. Mesalazine (5-aminosalicylic acid) suppositories in the treatment of ulcerative proctitis or distal proctosigmoiditis. A randomized controlled trial. Scand J Gastroenterol. 1990;25:663–8.
40. Rachmilewitz D on behalf of an international study group. Coated mesalazine (5-aminosalicylic acid) vs. sulphasalazine in the treatment of active ulcerative colitis: a randomized trial. Br Med J. 1989;298:82–6.
41. Schröder KW, Tremaine WJ. Oral 5-aminosalicylic acid (Asacol®) for treatment of symptomatic chronic ulcerative colitis. Gastroenterology. 1986;90:A1620.
42. Schröder KW, Tremaine WJ, Ilstrup DM. Coated oral 5-aminosalicylic acid therapy for mildly to moderately active ulcerative colitis. N Engl J Med. 1987;317:1625–9.
43. Siniski CA, Cort DH, Shanahan F et al. Oral mesalamine (Asacol) for mildly to moderately active ulcerative colitis. Ann Intern Med. 1991;115:350–5.
44. Hanauer S, Schwartz J, Robinson M and the Pentasa® Study Group. Mesalamine capsules for treatment of active ulcerative colitis: results of a controlled trial. Am J Gastroenterol. 1993;88:1188–97.
45. Azad Khan AK, Howes DT, Piris J, Truelove SC. Optimum dose of sulphasalazine for maintenance treatment in ulcerative colitis. Gut. 1980;21:232–40.
46. Riley SA, Mani V, Goodman MJ, Herd ME, Dutt S, Turnberg LA. Comparison of delayed release 5-aminosalicylic acid (Mesalazine) and sulfasalazine as maintenance treatment for patients with ulcerative colitis. Gastroenterology. 1988;94:1383–9.
47. Travis SPL, Tysk C, de Silva HJ, Sandberg-Gertzén H, Jewell DP, Järnerot G. Optimum dose of olsalazine for maintaining remission in ulcerative colitis. Gut. 1994;35:1282–6.
48. Maier K, Frühmorgen P, Bode JCH, Heller T, Gaisberg U, Klotz U. Erfolgreiche Akutbehandlung chronisch-entzündlicher Darmerkrankungen mit oraler 5-Aminosalizylsäure. Dtsch Med Wochenschr. 1985;110:363–8.
49. Rasmussen SN, Lauritsen K, Tage-Jensen U et al. 5-Aminosalicylic acid in the treatment of Crohn's disease. Scand J Gastroenterol 1987;22:877–88.
50. Singleton JW, Hanauer SB, Gitnick GL and the Pentasa Crohn's Disease Study Group. Mesalamine capsules for the treatment of active Crohn's disease: results of a 16 week trial. Gastroenterology. 1993;104:1293–301.
51. Hanauer SB, Krawitt EL, Robinson M and the Pentasa Crohn's Disease Compassionate Use Study Group. Long term management of Crohn's disease with mesalamine capsules (Pentasa®). Am J Gastroenterol. 1993;88:1343–51.
52. Gross V, Schölmerich J, Roth M et al. Vergleich zwischen hoch dosierter 5-Aminosalizylsäure (5-ASA) und 6-Methylprednisolon (6-MP) bci aktiver Ileocolitis. Crohn Med Klin. 1994;89(Suppl. 1):158.
53. Brignola C, Iannone P, Pasquali S et al. Placebo-controlled trial of oral 5-ASA in relapse prevention of Crohn's disease. Dig Dis Sci. 1992;37:29–32.
54. Gendre J-P, Mary J-Y, Florent C and the Groupe d'Études Thérapeutiques des affections inflammatoires digestives. Oral mesalamine (Pentasa) as maintenance treatment in Crohn's disease: a multicenter placebo-controlled study. Gastroenterology. 1993;104:435–9.
55. Messori A, Brignola C, Trallori G et al. Effectiveness of 5-aminosalicylic acid for maintaining remission in patients with Crohn's disease: a metaanalysis. Am J Gastroenterol. 1994;89:692–8.
56. Caprilli R, Andreoli A, Capurso L et al. Oral mesalazine (5-aminosalicylic acid; Asacol) for the prevention of postoperative recurrence of Crohn's disease. Aliment Pharmacol Ther. 1994;8:35–43.

# 21
# Old and new steroids

## J. SCHÖLMERICH and T. ANDUS

## INTRODUCTION

Since the aetiology of chronic inflammatory bowel disease (IBD) has not been illuminated and the pathophysiology is only partly understood, so far no specific causal treatment exists. As in most diseases with chronic inflammation, glucocorticoids have been successfully used in the treatment of symptoms and inflammation[1,2]. IBD can be divided into ulcerative colitis (UC) and Crohn disease (CD) although both diseases probably do not represent uniform entities.

In this chapter, the use of glucocorticosteroids in the treatment of IBD will be discussed, based on a short review of their anti-inflammatory actions. Since treatment with conventional steroids is hampered by a large number of side-effects, the use of newly developed 'non-systemic' steroids will be discussed in particular.

## MECHANISMS OF ANTI-INFLAMMATORY GLUCOCORTICOID ACTIONS

The actions of the natural glucocorticoid cortisol and of all its synthetic modifications, such as prednisolone and many others, are mediated by specific glucocorticoid receptors[3,4]. These receptors are present in most cells of the human organism at a concentration between 2000 and 30 000 binding sites per cell and their concentration is autoregulated[5,6]. After entrance of the glucocorticoid into the cell and binding to the cytoplasmic glucocorticoid receptor, the dissociation of the glucocorticoid receptor, the heat shock protein HSP 90 and the 59-kDa protein occurs. Homodimers of glucocorticoid receptors enter the nucleus and bind to a glucocorticoid-responsive element, thereby inducing the transcription of target genes (figure 1). The combination of interaction between the activated glucocorticoid receptor and glucocorticoid-responsive elements and cell-specific protein interactions determines which particular genes are activated or repressed by glucocorticoids in different cells. This allows for the upregulation of a gene in one cell type and the downregulation of the same gene in another cell type[7].

Since most cells express glucocorticoid receptors, glucocorticoids affect the function of many different cell types. Therefore, the therapeutic effect of glucocorticoids is multifactorial and cannot be explained by a single mechanism. Glucocorticoids impair specific and non-specific immune reactions. They suppress early events of inflammation, such as release of inflammatory mediators, vasodilatation, enhanced vascular permeability and leukocyte infiltration. They furthermore inhibit late inflammatory events, such as fibroblast activation, collagen deposition and vascular proliferation. Glucocorticoids affect many different inflammatory cells and regulate numerous functions of these cells[8,9] (Table 1). Many of these cells are involved in the pathogenesis of IBD[2,10,11]. The local inflammatory response in UC and CD is characterized by a mixed cellular infiltrate composed of lymphocytes, plasma cells, macrophages, eosinophils, mast cells and neutrophils[12,13].

## Lymphocytes and plasma cells

The cellular infiltrates of IBD lesions contain a considerably increased number of lymphocytes, the majority of which are memory T cells of the helper inducer type and the cytolytic type. A marked polyclonal activation of lamina propria T cells was found in IBD[14]. Activated lamina propria T lymphocytes produce high levels of interleukins and play a key role in antibody-dependent cell-mediated cytotoxicity. The number of immunoglobulin-producing cells is also strongly augmented in the mucosa of patients with IBD.

The anti-inflammatory effects of glucocorticoids on lymphocytes are numerous (Table 1). Their administration results in a marked but transient decrease in

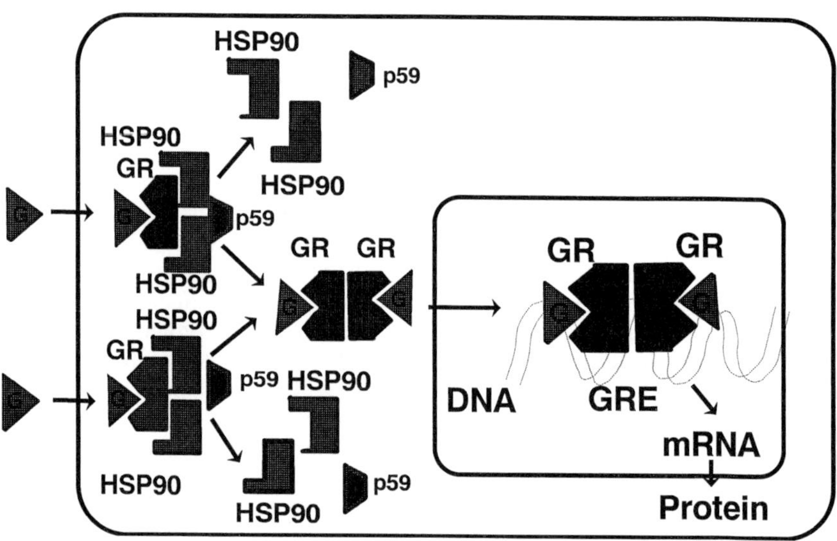


**Figure 1**   Glucocorticoid signal transduction

**Table 1**  Anti-inflammatory effects of steroids – possible influences on IBD

| | |
|---|---|
| Lymphocytes: | Redistribution ↑; T-cell proliferation ↓; cytotoxicity ↓; B-cell proliferation and differentiation ↓ |
| Macrophages: | Redistribution ↑; chemotaxis ↓; PG and LT production ↓; proinflammatory cytokines ↓; phagocytosis ↓; proteinase secretion ↓ |
| Endothelial cells: | Adhesion molecules ↓; vascular permeability ↓ |
| Neutrophils: | Migration ↓; activation ↓ |
| Eosinophils: | Differentiation and growth ↓; survival ↓; chemotactic activity ↓; migration ↓ |
| Basophils and mast cells: | Differentiation and growth ↓; migration ↓; secretion of histamine, PAF, $LTC_4$ ↓ |

the number of peripheral lymphocytes. Lymphocytopenia is maximal at 4–6 h, involves all subpopulations of lymphocytes, and is followed by a return to normal levels after 24 h[15]. These changes are caused by a redistribution of the lymphocytes from the blood to other lymphoid compartments due to a decreased eflux of circulating lymphocytes from the lymphoid organs, such as spleen, lymph nodes and others. Lymphocytes are very susceptible to the action of glucocorticoids. The latter inhibit lymphocyte proliferation and activation[16,17], and suppress the proliferation of lymphocytes by inhibiting lymphocytic production of IL-2 and IL-2 receptors. In addition, they inhibit the synthesis of IL-1 by monocytes and thus impair the synthesis of IL-2 by lymphocytes indirectly as well. They also suppress the production of lymphokines, such as interferon-γ, TNFα, and several other interleukins, thereby impairing the helper and cytotoxic functions of lymphocytes and reducing the activation of other cell types of the immune system[18].

## Macrophages

In IBD, antigen-presenting and scavenger macrophages are increased in the mucosa and activated[19,20]. In the granulomas of CD, they represent the most prominent cell type. The macrophages secrete inflammatory mediators, such as prostaglandins, leukotrienes, platelet activating factor, IL-1 and IL-6[21–25]. The expression of the intercellular adhesion molecule-1 (ICAM-1) by mucosal mononuclear phagocytes is significantly increased suggesting an augmented cell adhesiveness and interaction with T cells[26].

Administration of glucocorticoids markedly diminishes the number of circulating monocytes in blood by redistribution[27]. Monocytes and macrophages are functionally among the cells most sensitive to the anti-inflammatory effects of glucocorticoids. The latter inhibit the release of arachidonic acid metabolites, suppress the synthesis and secretion of many cytokines, including IL-1, IL-6, TNFα and monocyte chemotactic activator factor[24,28–32]. This effect impairs most of the inflammatory functions of the monocytes and macrophages. By reducing the synthesis of collagenase, elastase and tissue plasminogen activator, glucocorticoids also inhibit the degradation of the extracellular matrix and of fibrin by monocytes[33].

## Eosinophils

Eosinophils are present in increased numbers in the lamina propria and submucosa of patients with IBD[34]. They cause tissue damage by releasing their granule-associated proteins, major basic proteins, eosinophil cationic protein, peroxidase and eosinophil-derived neurotoxin. In IBD, eosinophils are activated and an increased release of these proteins has been found[35]. Glucocorticoids cause a marked fall in circulating and tissue eosinophil numbers[36] and reduce their chemotactic activity[37]. Survival, chemotaxis, and function of eosinophils is strongly controlled by cytokines[38,39]. The survival of eosinophils is promoted by GM-CSF, the release of which and the survival of eosinophils are inhibited by glucocorticoids[40]. Tissue infiltration starts with adherence of eosinophils to endothelial cells. This process is regulated by an induced expression of ICAM-1 and other adhesion molecules. This expression of these adhesion molecules is induced by IL-1[41]. The synthesis of the latter is blocked by glucocorticoids[42]. Therefore, glucocorticoids strongly impair survival and migration of eosinophils.

## Basophils and mast cells

The numbers of intestinal mast cells and basophils are increased in the submucosa of patients with IBD[34,43]. The degranulation of mast cells is a prominent feature in CD and UC[44,45].

Glucocorticoid treatment reduces the number of circulating basophils and inhibits the IgE-induced release of histamine and leukotriene C4[46]. As is the case with eosinophils, endothelial adherence of basophils is mediated by ICAM-1 and other adhesion molecules. Again, glucocorticoids can interfere with this process[47]. Mucosal mast cells need the cytokines, IL-3 and IL-4, for their presence and expansion[48]. They release a large number of immune regulatory mediators, including histamine, serotonin, prostaglandins, leukotrienes, platelet activating factor and proteases[45]. The release of these mediators is regulated by IgE and cytokines such as IFN$\gamma$ and IL-3[49]. Corticosteroid treatment reduces mucosal mast cell numbers[49,50], probably by inhibiting T-lymphocyte cytokine production[51].

## Neutrophils

Neutrophils are a major component of active lesions in both UC and CD[13,52]. Large numbers of neutrophils leave the circulation and enter the inflamed mucosa and submucosa of the bowel, indicating the presence of chemotactic agents in the inflamed lesions. In-vivo studies by scintigraphy have demonstrated a migration of radioactive-labelled neutrophils into the inflamed gut of patients with IBD, indicating a stimulated transmigration of neutrophils from the blood to the site of inflammation[53]. These neutrophils are activated and release proteinases, such as neutrophil elastase, cathepsins and myeloperoxidase, into the blood and gut lumen of patients with IBD[54]. The release of proteinases and respiratory burst products, such as superoxide, hydrogen peroxide and hydroxyl radicals, strongly contributes to the local destruction of the mucosa[55,56].

Glucocorticoids induce a neutrophilic leukocytosis that reaches a peak 46 h after glucocorticoid administration[8]. This is due to an increased release from the bone marrow and a reduced migration from the blood to the site of inflammation. The reduced migration of neutrophils to the site of inflammation is a very important factor in the reduction of inflammation in IBD by glucocorticoids. The reduction of adherence of neutrophils may be caused by a reduction of CR3, a member of the leukocyte adherence glycoprotein family[57]. Most probably, the transmigration of neutrophils is impaired by glucocorticoids in vivo due to inhibition of the local release of neutrophil attracting factors, such as IL-1, IL-8 and leukotriene B4.

## Endothelial cells

In order to reach the site of inflammation, inflammatory cells such as neutrophils, lymphocytes, mononuclear phagocytes or eosinophils have to cross the endothelial wall. The interactions between leukocytes and endothelial cells are regulated by specific cell adhesion molecules such as ICAM-1 and others. The expression of these adhesion molecules is inhibited by glucocorticoids[26,47,58]. Peptides produced by micro-organisms in the gut lumen and mast cell mediators, directly and via increasing adhesion and activation of neutrophils, open inter-endothelial cell junctions leading to an increased vasopermeability and formation of oedema in the gut mucosa[59]. Glucocorticoids are important inhibitors of the increased microvascular permeability by inhibiting histamine release from human basophils[60], blocking the synthesis of leukotrienes and platelet activating factor and suppressing the accumulation of leukocytes at the site of inflammation[60,61]. In addition, they are effective vasoconstrictors[62].

## Arachidonic-acid-derived mediators

Several mediators derived from arachidonic acid, such as prostaglandins, leukotrienes and platelet activating factor, are important soluble mediators of inflammation. Their concentration is raised in the mucosa of patients with IBD[63,64] and these levels decrease in patients responding to treatment with glucocorticoids. This is at least in part due to the inhibition of the protein lipocortine which inhibits the rate-limiting enzyme, phospholipase A2[65].

## Summary

As shown in Table 1, glucocorticoids can influence the inflammatory process in IBD at multiple sites. They may act directly on inflammatory cells at the site of inflammation and, in addition, inhibit the formation of cytokines and other proinflammatory mediators[66–69] which control the recruitment, proliferation and activation of inflammatory cells. It is not known to what extent each effect contributes to the therapeutic action of glucocorticoids in IBD.

## PHARMACOLOGY

Plasma concentrations of glucocorticoids vary considerably after oral ingestion of the same dose by normal subjects or patients with IBD[70]. Some studies found an impaired absorption of prednisolone in IBD patients[70,71], in particular in patients with extensive small bowel CD[72], whereas others found a normal absorption compared with healthy controls[73–75]. The biological half-life is 18–36 h, while the plasma half-life is only 2–4 h[76]. Glucocorticoids bind to plasma proteins, in particular to albumin. This allows further control of the biological activity of glucocorticoids by regulating these proteins and has implications for dosage calculations[77].

## ULCERATIVE COLITIS

### Classical treatment

More than 50 years ago, the first uncontrolled trials indicated that glucocorticoids and adrenocorticotropic hormone (ACTH) might be beneficial in the treatment of UC[78–84]. Controlled studies showed that 70–90% of patients with UC treated with cortisone[85,86] or prednisolone[87] improved while only 30–40% of patients treated with placebo did so. These studies clearly demonstrated the efficacy of glucocorticoids for the treatment of ulcerative colitis. Several further studies compared the use of glucocorticoids with ACTH[88–91]. In some of these studies, ACTH was found to be slightly superior to glucocorticoids while, in other studies, this effect was not found. Since ACTH has to be administered intravenously and is expensive, it is rarely used in clinical practice.

Dose-finding studies are rare[92–94]. A daily dose of 40–60 mg prednisolone was found to be optimal for patients with mildly to moderately active UC. There was no difference between the application of this dose as a single vs a divided dosage (Table 2)[94].

**Table 2**  Comparison of single vs multiple doses of oral prednisolone in active UC[94]

|  | 4 × 10 mg (n = 22) | 1 × 40 mg (n = 23) |
|---|---|---|
| Remission (n) | 5 | 3 |
| Improved (n) | 12 | 14 |
| No change (n) | 3 | 5 |
| Worse (n) | 2 | 1 |
| No side-effects (n) | 10 | 9 |

In severe disease, the benefit of intravenous application of glucocorticoids (60 mg prednisolone equivalent) has been shown in several studies. Remission rates of 60–80% were obtained[95,96]. In toxic megacolon, however, treatment should only be applied for short periods. If no improvement occurs, surgery is required[2].

It has to be mentioned that the use of glucocorticosteroids in mild and moderately active UC is not often necessary, since 5-aminosalicylic-acid-releasing preparations have been found to be as effective and have fewer side-effects[2,97].

The majority of patients with UC shows only distal involvement of the large bowel. In this situation, rectal treatment with steroids has been found to be superior to oral treatment (Table 3)[98]. Retention enemas of hydrocortisone[99], hydrocortisone hemisuccinate[100–102], prednisolone 21-phosphate[103–107], and

**Table 3**  Comparison of oral or rectal treatment with prednisolone in distal UC[98]

| | Prednisolone | |
| --- | --- | --- |
| | Oral<br>(*n*=18) | Rectal<br>(*n*=18) |
| Subjective improvement (*n*) | 7 | 14 |
| Cross-over effective | 3/4 | 9/11 |

betamethasone[108] have been found to be effective. The combination of oral and rectal glucocorticoids resulted, in some studies, in a more rapid remission than oral treatment alone[109,110]. The retrograde spread of glucocorticoid-containing enemas increases with increasing volume of the enemas[111] and with severity of the disease[112]. Similar results were obtained with hydrocortisone foam[113–118]. The development of these foams led to a further subjective improvement in the quality of life for patients since the instillation of 5 ml foam is much less troublesome than a 100-ml retention enema. Foams are much better tolerated by patients and lead to less impairment of daily activities (Table 4)[119]. Colitis limited to the rectum can also be treated effectively by suppositories of prednisolone phosphate[99]. Despite the local application of enemas with hydrocortisone, hemisuccinate, or prednisolone 21-phosphate, a considerable amount of the glucocorticoids is absorbed and causes unwanted side-effects[107,120,121]. It has to be mentioned again, that treatment with 5-ASA-releasing preparations by the rectal route is very effective in most patients with distal UC and the use of steroid enemas, foams or suppositories is only rarely necessary[122].

**Table 4**  Comparison of rectal steroids as foam or enema in patients with UC – influence on daily life[119]

| | Foam | Enema |
| --- | --- | --- |
| Work | 4 | 23* |
| Sex life | 1 | 18* |
| Leisure activity | 2 | 12* |

No difference with regard to efficacy
Score: 0–100 (increased score corresponds to increased disturbance); $*p < 0.05$

## Maintenance treatment

While glucocorticoids are very effective in the treatment of acute attacks of UC, they were not very effective for relapse prevention in some studies[88,100,123,124]. However, alternate-day prednisolone seems to be effective in patients with continuously active disease or unusually frequent relapses[125] (Figure 2). Relapses were reduced to 20% of those occurring with placebo in a controlled trial.

Again, it has to be mentioned that 5-ASA enemas are as effective as prednisolone enemas in mild-to-moderate proctosigmoiditis[126,127]. Furthermore, 5-ASA enemas as maintenance treatment can even achieve improvement or remission in patients not responding to hydrocortisone enemas[128]. 5-ASA prep-

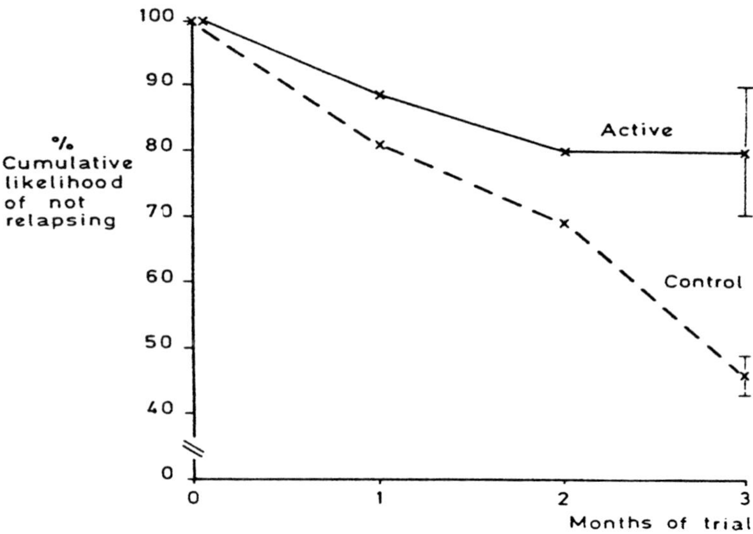


**Figure 2**   Alternate-day prednisolone for maintenance in UC[125]

arations are very effective in maintenance of remission in distal UC as are suppositories for proctitis[129]. Therefore, the use of glucocorticosteroid enemas for maintenance treatment is probably rather limited as well.

## New steroids

Due to the ubiquitous presence of steroid receptors on practically all cells of the human body during systemic glucocorticoid steroid treatment, unwanted effects on other organs are unavoidable (Table 5)[1]. In order to minimize these side-effects, in particular in patients needing long-term steroid treatment, 'non-systemic' steroids have been developed, primarily for pulmonary diseases[130]. These synthetic steroids are mainly substituted in the C17 position. They normally have a higher receptor affinity and a much higher relative activity than the conventional steroids[130]. Recently, such steroids have also been used in IBD. The substances which have been studied have either a low resorption or a high first-pass metabolism, either in the bowel mucosa or preferably in the liver (Figure 3), and therefore have a relatively low systemic bioavailability (Figure 4). These substances have been used primarily as enemas in distal ulcerative colitis. Initial studies of volunteers showed that the hypothalamus–pituitary–adrenal (HPA) axis was much less suppressed by using these steroids, as measured by the plasma cortisol levels[131]. The first clinical trial using beclomethasone dipropionate showed identical therapeutic activity and less suppression of the HPA axis as compared with conventional steroid enemas[132] (Table 6).

**Table 5**  Side-effects of glucocorticoids

Weight gain with redistribution of fat to the truncal areas
'Moon face', 'buffalo hump'
Striae, plethorae, acne
Adrenal atrophy
Impaired glucose tolerance, diabetes mellitus
Hypercholesterolaemia
Hypertension
Osteoporosis
Aseptic necrosis of bone
Increased incidence of peptic ulcers
Electrolyte imbalance, hypokalaemia
Posterior subcapsular cataract, glaucoma
Insomnia, psychosis
Neuropathy
Negative nitrogen balance, proximal myopathy
Increased susceptibility to infections
Growth retardation

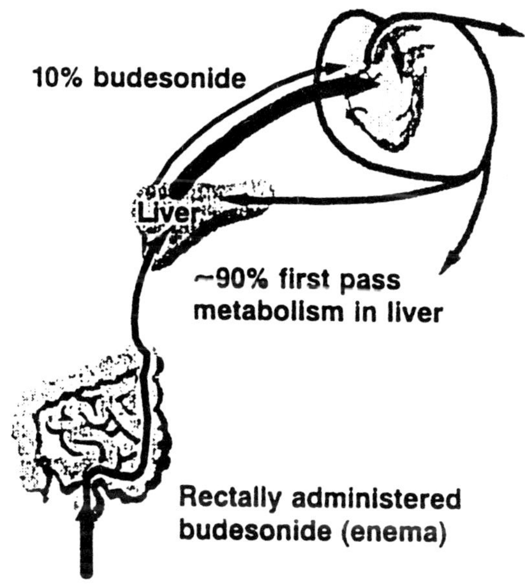


**Figure 3**  Metabolism of rectally administered budesonide[130]

In the case of beclomethasone dipropionate, the lower systemic bioavailability is probably due to decreased absorption and first-pass elimination in the liver. The substance has been studied in several further trials[133–135] with similar results (Table 7).

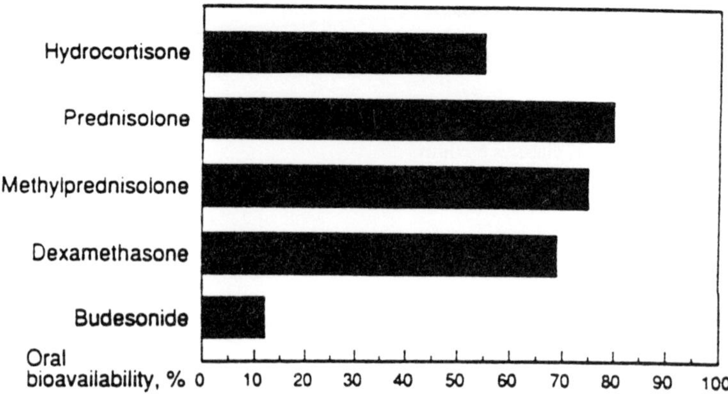


**Figure 4**   Oral bioavailability of several steroids[130]

**Table 6**   Comparison of beclomethasone vs betamethasone enemas in distal UC – efficacy and influence on the HPA axis[132]

|  | Beclomethasone dipropionate (0.5 mg) ($n = 9$) | Betamethasone (5 mg) ($n = 9$) |
|---|---|---|
| Subjective improvement | 8 | 7 |
| Objective improvement | 8 | 5 |
| $\Delta$ Plasma cortisone (nmol/L) | –53 | –329* |
| $\Delta$ Stimulation of cortisol (nmol/L) | +65 | –501* |

* $p < 0.01$

**Table 7**   Comparison of beclomethasone dipropionate and hydrocortisone enemas in active distal UC[135]

|  | Beclomethasone dipropionate (2 mg, $n = 20$) | Hydrocortisone (100 mg, $n = 20$) |
|---|---|---|
| **Clinical** |  |  |
| Remission (%) | 60 | 80 |
| Partial remission (%) | 15 | 5 |
| **Endoscopic** |  |  |
| Remission (%) | 45 | 50 |
| Partial remission (%) | 30 | 35 |

Results after 16 weeks

A number of studies has been performed using tixocortol enemas; remission rates and improvement were similar to those with hydrocortisone enemas as shown in a review of three trials[136].

Most studies have been performed using budesonide enemas. In particular, Scandinavian investigators have compared budesonide enemas with prednisolone enemas, where doses of 2 mg budesonide and 31 mg prednisolone were used[137]. Remission and improvement rates were superior with budesonide, and

**Table 8** Comparison of budesonide and prednisolone enemas in distal active UC: remission rates and plasma cortisol[137]

| | Budesonide (2 mg) (n = 28) | Prednisolone (31 mg) (n = 28) |
|---|---|---|
| Complete remission (%) | 52 | 24[*] |
| Objective improvement (%) | 93 | 75[*] |
| $\Delta$ Plasma cortisol (nmol/L) | +11 | − 127[*] |

[*] $p < 0.05$

plasma cortisol was much less suppressed (Table 8). The comparison of budesonide with placebo enemas revealed much higher therapeutic efficacy (20% failure vs 80% in the placebo group) while plasma cortisol was not different in both groups[138]. A dose-finding study found that 2 mg given as an enema was an optimal dose[139,140]. Several other studies have meanwhile confirmed these data[141]. It has, however, to be mentioned that one study did not find an increased efficacy compared with enemas containing 4 g 5-ASA (Table 9)[142]. A recent study comparing budesonide with 1 g 5-ASA, however, found better efficacy with budesonide[143].

**Table 9** Comparison of budesonide and 5-ASA enemas in active proctitis[142]

| | Budesonide (2 mg) (n = 32) | 5-ASA (4 g) (n = 30) |
|---|---|---|
| Endoscopic remission (%) | 34 | 37 |
| Endoscopic improvement (%) | 70 | 87 |

Results after 4 weeks

At this time, foam preparations containing budesonide are developed and undergoing clinical testing.

At the present state it can be concluded that enemas containing non-systemic steroids, such as budesonide or beclomethasone dipropionate, are as effective as conventional steroid enemas in active distal UC. They cause less or no suppression of the HPA axis compared with conventional steroid enemas. They may not be superior to 5-ASA enemas in most patients and should probably be reserved for those 10–20% of patients with distal UC needing steroid treatment. It is most probable that foams will be better tolerated and accepted by patients; these should therefore be developed.

## CROHN DISEASE

### Classical treatment

Several uncontrolled trials between 1950 and 1970 have demonstrated that glucocorticoids and ACTH might be helpful in the treatment of Crohn disease[144–148]. It took several years until controlled trials were performed. The first large trial, the National Cooperative Crohn's Disease Study (NCCDS) in the

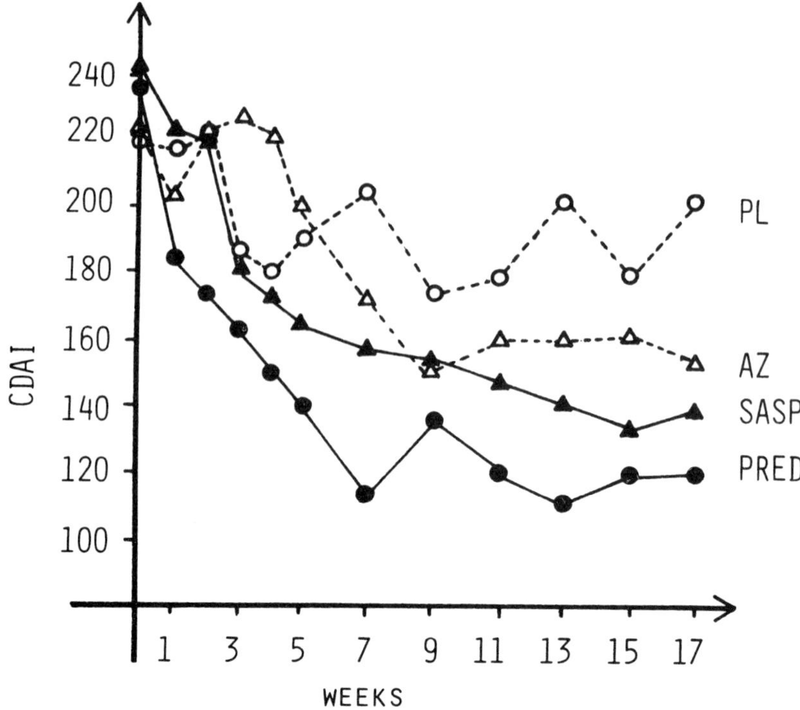


**Figure 5**  Results of treatment in the National Cooperative Crohn's Disease Study[149]. AZ = azathioprine, SASP = sulphasalazine, PRED = prednisone, CDAI = Crohn's Disease Activity Index

United States showed, in 1979, in a randomized prospective double-blind placebo-controlled study, that treatment with prednisolone (0.25–0.75 mg kg$^{-1}$ d$^{-1}$) led to an improvement in 60% of treated patients compared with 30% in the placebo group[149] (Figure 5). Similar or even better results were found for 6-methylprednisolone (48 mg/d initially, tapered weekly to 8 mg) by the European Cooperative Crohn's Disease Study (ECCDS) in 1984[150] (Table 10). Since then, a standard treatment regimen for active CD has been widely used (Table 11). Two other ECCDS studies showed that glucocorticoid treatment is better than nutritional therapy in active CD[151,152] (Table 12).

**Table 10**  Remission rates with different drugs in the treatment of active CD in the European Crohn's Disease Study I[150]

|  | Remission (%) |
| --- | --- |
| Placebo | 37.9 |
| SASP (3 g/d) | 50.0 |
| Methylprednisolone (48→ 8 mg) | 82.9 |
| SASP + methylprednisolone | 78.5 |

SASP = sulphasalazine

**Table 11**  Classical treatment with glucocorticosteroids in active CD given as prednisolone doses

| | |
|---|---|
| Week 1 | 60 mg |
| Week 2 | 40 mg |
| Week 3 | 30 mg |
| Week 4 | 25 mg |
| Week 5 | 20 mg |
| Week 6 | 15 mg |
| Weeks 7–14 | 10 mg |
| Thereafter, 10 mg alternate days for 3–6 months | |

**Table 12**  Comparison of enteral nutrition and treatment with steroids and sulphasalazine in active CD. (From ECCDS IV[152])

| | Enteral nutrition (n = 55) | Drug treatment (n = 52) |
|---|---|---|
| Percentage in remission[a] at 6 weeks | 53 | 79* |
| Time to remission (median, days) | 30.7 | 8.2* |

[a] CDAI 40%, $\leq$ 100 points; * $p < 0.01$

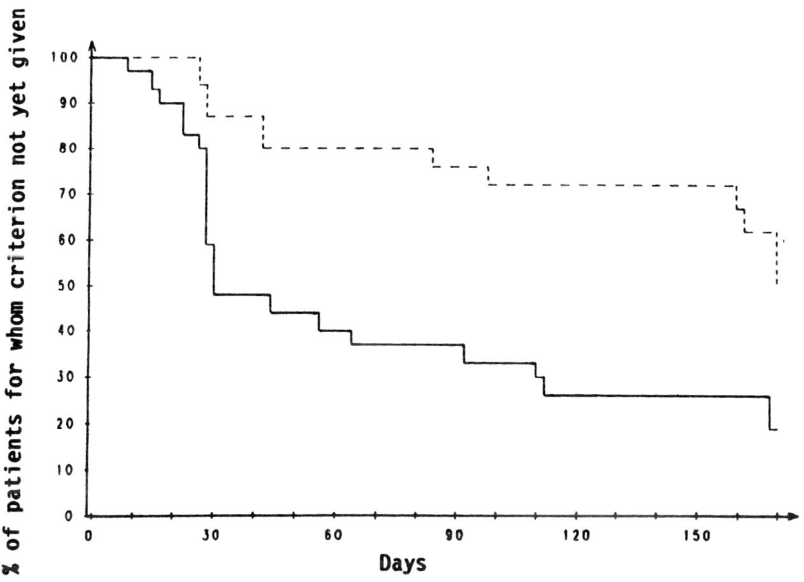


**Figure 6**  Cumulative probability of continuation of the study in the treatment of active CD. Solid line indicates 5-ASA (n = 30), dashed line indicates methylprednisolone (n = 32). Significant (p < 0.002) difference between the treatment groups[153]

6-Methylprednisolone was superior to 2 g 5-ASA in a recent trial where 34% of patients were not treated sufficiently with the steroid and 74% with 5-ASA (Figure 6)[153]. In this study, the time course of 6 methylprednisolone effects on

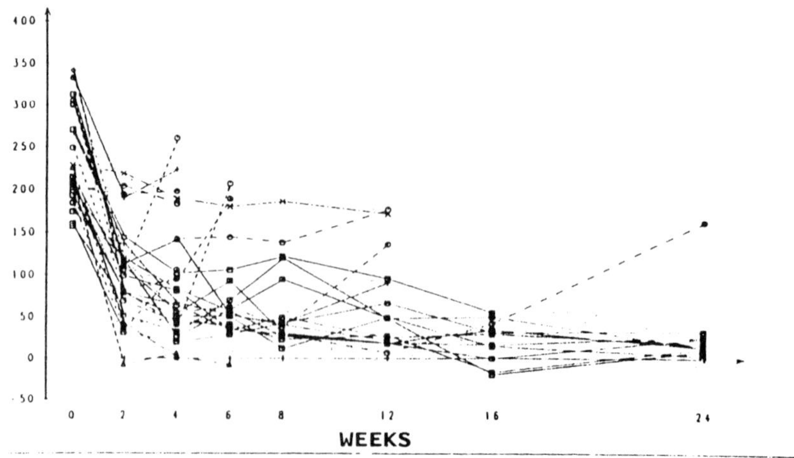

**Figure 7** Time course of the CDAI in 32 patients with active CD treated with 6-methylpred-nisolone, indicating a very rapid decrease in the first 2 weeks[153]

the Crohn disease activity index (CDAI) could be seen well, indicating that the major effect occurs during the first 2 weeks (Figure 7). A more recent trial comparing standard treatment with 6-methylprednisolone with the daily application of 4.5 g 5-ASA using a small number of patients found no significant difference between the treatments. It is noteworthy that, in most recent trials, only about 60–70% of patients with active CD treated with conventional steroids came into remission[153–156]. This is probably due to the predominant inclusion of patients from tertiary referral centres.

## Maintenance treatment

The role of glucocorticoids in maintenance treatment of CD has been studied in several trials. No benefit has been found for such treatment in patients with inactive CD or in patients with CD after bowel resection with or without residual disease[146,147,157–159]. However, the ECCDS I[150] and another recent trial[160] showed that low-dose glucocorticoid therapy, in patients brought into remission with glucocorticoids, reduced the rate of relapses. A similar trend was found in the NCCDS[149]. It was also found that glucocorticosteroids reduce relapse frequency in patients in clinical remission but with abnormal laboratory values[161] (Figure 8). It is of importance, however, to note that prolonged steroid treatment is not useful in patients who are in clinical but not endoscopic remission after conventional steroid treatment[162] (Figure 9).

In summary, it can be stated that steroids are the mainstay of drug treatment in active CD and induce remission in 60–80% of patients. The reduced efficacy in later trials may be due to selection of more severely ill patients in centres participating in those trials.

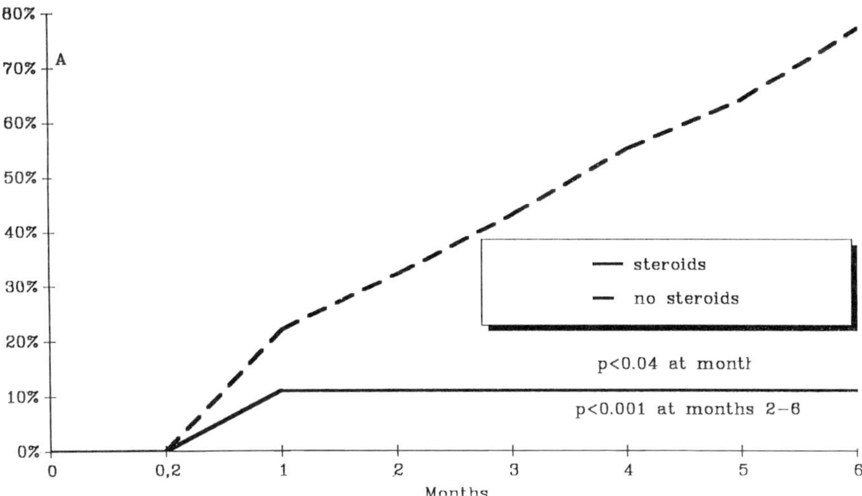


**Figure 8**  Relapse prevention in CD in remission using 2.5 mg methylprednisolone/10 kg per day compared with placebo[161]

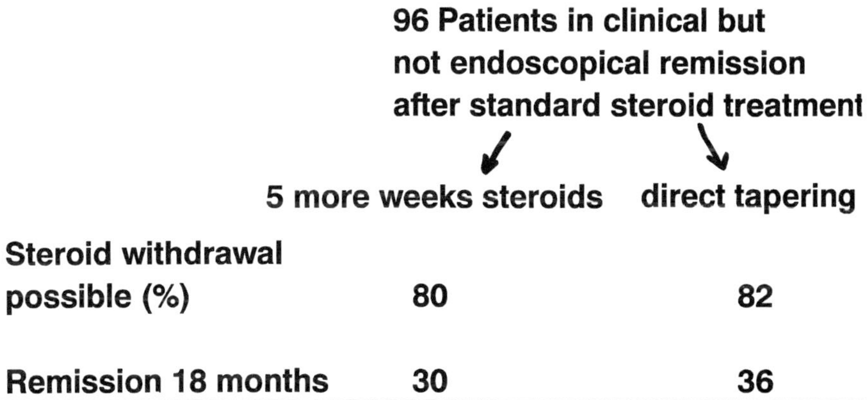


**Figure 9**  A lack of effect of continued steroid treatment for patients in clinical, but not endoscopic, remission after standard steroid treatment[162]

## New steroids

When the positive effects of the newly developed steroids, such as beclomethasone dipropionate and budesonide, were observed in enema treatment in distal UC, it was an obvious idea to develop galenic preparations releasing the active drug at the place of inflammation for patients with CD. In order to achieve this, 'slow-release' preparations, in analogy to modern 5-ASA-liberating systems, had to be developed[163]. Alternatively, poorly absorbed substances with extensive first-pass metabolism, such as fluticasone propionate, have been tested. It

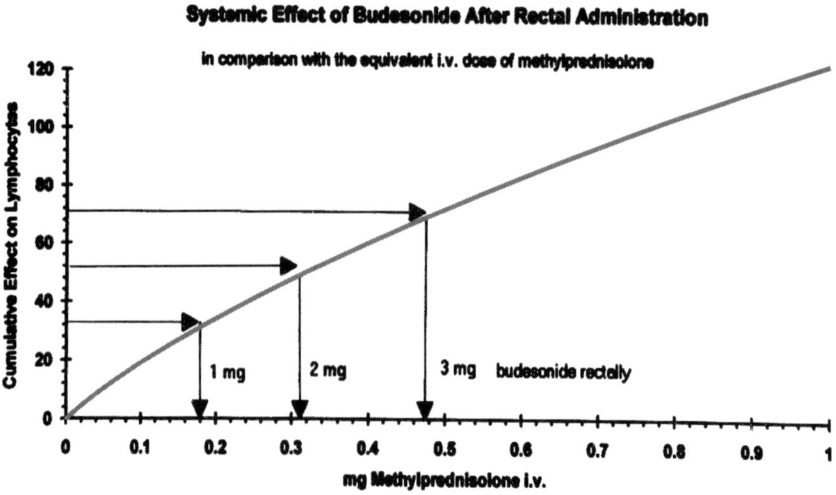

**Figure 10**   Dose equivalency of budesonide (BUD) and 6-methylprednisolone (MP) using the systemic effect of lymphocytes after rectal administration: 3 mg budesonide is equivalent to 0.48 mg 6-methylprednisolone[164]. The authors thank Prof. H. W. Möllmann for provision of this figure

has been shown that Eudragit-coated budesonide capsules can be delivered to the terminal ileum, inducing very few systemic changes as measured by lymphocyte counts and effects on the HPA axis[164]. Figure 10 shows the comparison of oral doses of budesonide in such a preparation and 6-methylprednisolone in relation to the systemic effects. It is obvious that the oral application of 3 mg budesonide has the same systemic effect as very low doses of 6-methylprednisolone (i.e. 0.6 mg). Several pilot trials using this preparation have been performed[165–167]. Our study showed that most patients had a decrease in their CDAI into the normal range during the first 2 weeks. It was, however, noted that patients with extraintestinal manifestations or with involvement of the upper intestinal tract, where the preparation did not release active substance, showed a re-increase after a short period of time (Figure 11)[167]. Although the basal cortisol levels were reduced to some extent, stimulation by corticotropin-releasing factor was still possible, indicating a non-disturbed HPA axis.

Following this pilot study, an open study with a large number of patients has been performed. Two thirds of patients came into remission and the number of steroid-typical side-effects was rather low[168]. It was of interest to note that all subjective components of the CDAI, such as abdominal pain, stool frequency and general well-being, responded to a similar extent. When looking at the responders and non-responders, it was obvious that non-responders had a much longer duration of disease than those responding (Figure 12).

Since most patients with active CD are already being treated with conventional steroids, a further study was initiated to assess the effect of switching treatment from conventional steroids to 9 mg budesonide. Of those patients with active disease (CDAI > 150) at the time of switching, 40% could be brought into

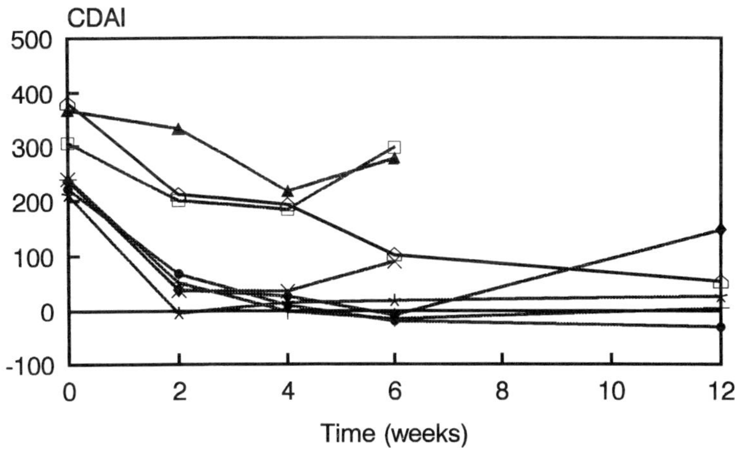



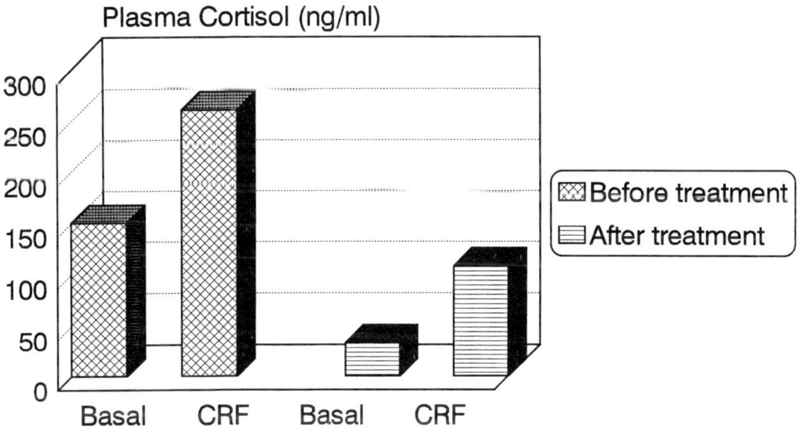



**Figure 11**　CDAI in patients with active CD treated with $3 \times 3$ mg budesonide in a pilot trial[167]. The lower panel demonstrates the results of the corticotropin releasing factor (CRF) test before and after 6 weeks treatment, indicating that plasma cortisol is suppressed but CRF test is unaffected

remission. Of those patients with a CDAI below 150, the situation was maintained in 81%. However, the most important finding of this study was that the number of steroid-related side-effects decreased significantly over time under

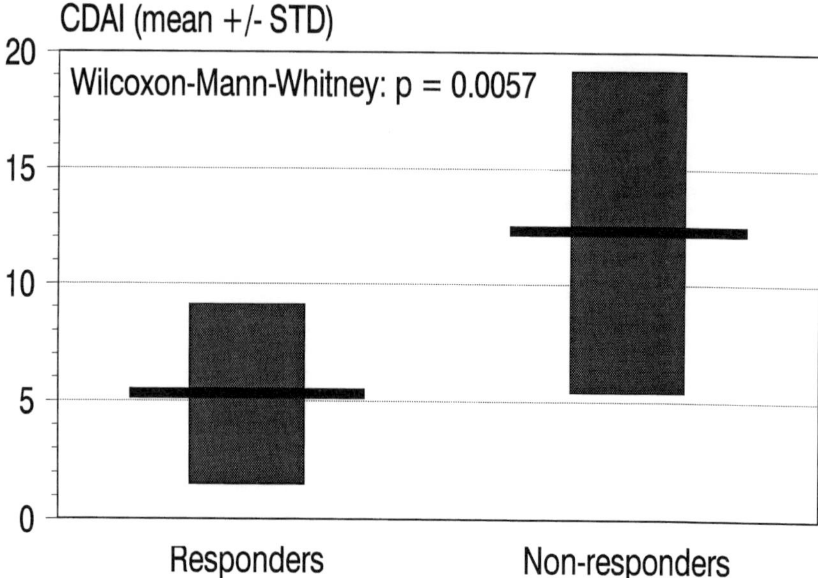


**Figure 12**  Duration of disease of successfully treated patients ($n = 20$) and treatment failures ($n = 10$). The duration of disease is the only parameter significantly different between patients responding and not responding to $3 \times 3$ mg oral budesonide

continuous treatment with $3 \times 3$ mg budesonide (Table 13). This was true for the percentage of patients having such side-effects as well as for the total number of side-effects observed in the whole group[169].

In the meantime, several control trials using oral budesonide in active CD have been completed. The European multicentre trial found that 53% of patients could be brought into remission with budesonide while this was the case for 66% with prednisolone using a conventional regimen[155]. Again, the number of

**Table 13**  Switch from standard steroid treatment to budesonide ($3 \times 3$ mg) in steroid-treated patients with CD – influence on side-effects[169]

|  | Week | | | | |
|---|---|---|---|---|---|
|  | 0 | 2 | 4 | 6 | 8 |
| Treatment | S | S+B($3 \times 3$ mg) | B($3 \times 3$ mg) | B($3 \times 3$ mg) | B($3 \times 3$ mg) |
| Side-effects (% of patients) | 68 | 53 | 52 | 45 | 38 |
| Side-effects (total number) | 88 | 47 | 43 | 35 | 29 |

S = conventional steroid treatment; B = budesonide

**Table 14** Comparison of budesonide vs prednisolone in active ileocaecal CD – remission and side-effects[155]

|  | Budesonide (9 mg) ($n = 88$) | Prednisolone (40 mg tapered after 2 weeks) ($n = 88$) |
|---|---|---|
| Remission (at 10 weeks, %) | 53 | 66 |
| Δ CDAI | 100 | 143 |
| Side-effects ($n$) | 12 | 27* |
| Δ Plasma cortisol (%) | 40 | 84 * |

* Significant

side-effects was much lower in the budesonide group (Table 14). The German trial using a very similar approach, and comparing 3 × 3 mg budesonide with conventional treatment with 6-methylprednisolone (Table 11), found surprisingly similar results. Fifty-six per cent in the budesonide group and 73% in the 6-methylprednisolone group were brought into remission; the difference was, as in the study by Rutgeerts et al.[155], not significant (Figure 13). The time course of the treatment effect was rather similar, as was the decrease in the CDAI (Figure 14). The most interesting finding was that the number of side-effects was reduced to 50%. In particular, the number of typical steroid-related side-effects decreased from 70% to 29% in the budesonide group (Figure 15). Interestingly, parameters of systemic inflammation, such as C-reactive protein, were less

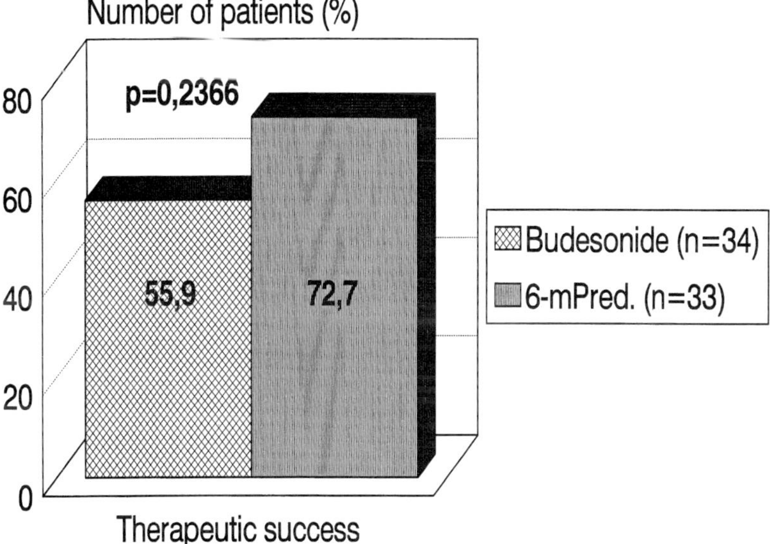


**Figure 13** Patients brought into remission by 8 weeks treatment with 3 × 3 mg oral budesonide or standard treatment with 6-methylprednisolone (6-mPred.)[154] (Success rates of intention-to-treat analysis)

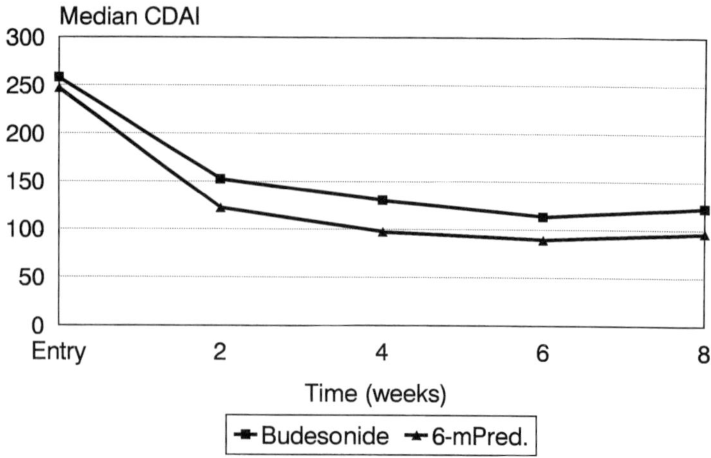



**Figure 14**  Similar degrees of median CDAI were obtained during the trial of 3 × 3 mg oral budesonide and standard treatment with 6-methylprednisolone (intention-to-treat analysis)

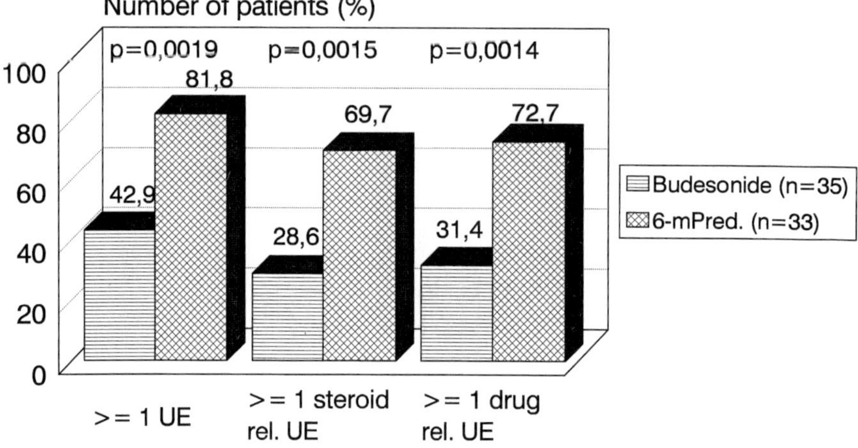



**Figure 15**  Side-effects during the trial comparing 3 × 3 mg oral budesonide and standard treatment with 6-methylprednisolone (6-mPred.) in active CD[154]. UE = unwanted event

influenced by budesonide than 6-methylprednisolone, indicating, again, the topical character of this treatment[156].

A dose-finding study in Canada revealed that 9 mg of budesonide seems to be the optimal dose; the treatment efficacy was again in the region of 50%, and side-effects were observed in about 27%, which was not different from placebo[170]. As in the pilot study mentioned, plasma cortisol was decreased to some extent in this study as well as in the study by Rutgeerts[155] (Table 15). It can be summarized that treatment with Eudragit-coated oral budesonide is somewhat less effective than conventional steroid treatment in active CD but the difference does not reach statistical significance in several trials and the results of these trials are surprisingly similar. However, all trials found that the number of side-effects, and in particular of steroid-related side-effects, was much lower under budesonide treatment. This is in accordance with the results of the open trials.

**Table 15**  Dose-finding study of oral budesonide in active CD[170]

|  | Placebo (n = 66) | Budesonide | | |
| --- | --- | --- | --- | --- |
|  |  | 3 mg (n = 67) | 9 mg (n = 61) | 15 mg (n = 64) |
| Remission (% at 8 weeks) | 20 | 30 | 45 | 42 |
| Side-effects (%) | 27 | 15 | 27 | 35 |
| Δ Plasma cortisol (nmol/L) | 0 | 60 | 200 | 250 |

As mentioned before, maintenance of remission is a major problem in CD. Two studies have been performed using lower doses of budesonide to maintain remission induced by steroid treatment. A European trial on a smaller number of patients found that the length of remission was prolonged using 3 mg budesonide and even more using 6 mg budesonide per day. However, after 1 year, the number of patients still in remission was similar to placebo. In the group treated with 6 mg, side-effects and adrenal suppression were observed to some extent[171]. A large trial comparing 3 mg budesonide given as 3 × 1 mg found no difference as compared with placebo in patients who had been brought into remission by conventional steroid treatment (Figure 16)[172]. Most treatment failures occurred during the first 3 months after initiation of the study and this was so for both treatment groups.

Fluticasone propionate has been compared with prednisolone in active CD in one large trial. Remission was obtained in 47% under prednisolone and in 39% with fluticasone propionate, the difference being significant. It was of interest that, in patients having ileal involvement, identical remission rates of 75% and 80% respectively, were obtained; the difference in the whole study group was due to those patients with colonic involvement. Again, the number of side-effects was much lower in patients treated with the non-systemic steroid than in patients treated with prednisolone (Table 16)[173].

In summary, it can be stated that oral Eudragit coated budesonide, at a dose of 9 mg/d, is effective in active CD although to a somewhat lesser extent than conventional steroids. It causes significantly fewer side-effects than conventional

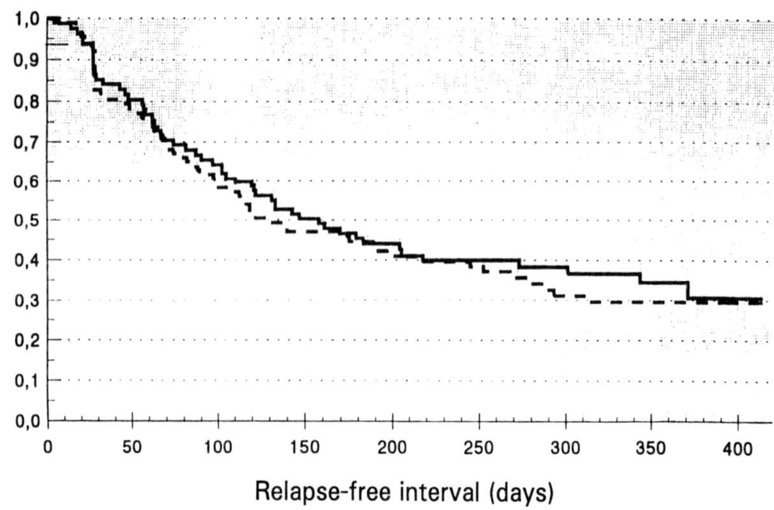



**Figure 16**  Cumulative probability for maintenance of remission in patients with CD brought into remission by conventional steroid treatment under budesonide (solid line, $n$ = 85) and placebo (dashed line, $n$ = 93) – no significant difference[172]

**Table 16**  Comparison of fluticasone propionate and prednisolone in active CD[153]

|  | Fluticasone propionate<br>($n = 177$) | Prednisolone<br>($n = 167$) |
|---|---|---|
| Remission (at 4 weeks, %) | 39 | 47* |
| Improved (at 4 weeks, %) | 24 | 39 |

For ileitis effects identical (75% vs 80% remission). Side-effects: fluticasone propionate < prednisolone (2 vs 17 patients). * Significant.

steroid treatment. Furthermore, it could be shown that budesonide reduces pre-existing steroid side-effects when treatment is switched from conventional steroid treatment while the therapeutic effect can be maintained. A dose of 3 mg budesonide per day has no relapse-preventive effect; a dose of 6 mg has a slight effect although its clinical relevance is unclear. Fluticasone propionate may be useful in ileal CD[173,174].

## SPECIAL PROBLEMS OF GLUCOCORTICOID TREATMENT IN IBD

### Glucocorticoids in pregnancy

Several studies have shown that glucocorticoids can be given during pregnancy without increasing the risks for the mother or the child[175–177]. In a case of acute exacerbation during pregnancy, remission should be induced using standard medical treatment. This results in the best outcome.

## Glucocorticoids in childhood

The strategy of therapy with glucocorticoids in childhood is similar to that used in adults[10]. However, the dosage has to be adjusted to the body weight. The most important side-effect of glucocorticoid therapy in childhood is growth retardation[178]. Alternate-day treatment has been shown to reduce this effect[179]. Furthermore, growth retardation may be worse if UC or CD in particular is not treated adequately and malnutrition occurs. Thus, steroid treatment must be initiated in active IBD in childhood, when surgery is not advised or not possible.

## Extraintestinal manifestations

Patients with UC or CD often (10–30%) have extraintestinal manifestations, such as arthritis, erythema nodosum, pyoderma gangrenosum, uveitis or stomatitis[180,181]. Extraintestinal manifestations usually correlate well with disease activity and most of them respond to treatment with glucocorticoids[182]. Non-systemic steroids are, for obvious reasons, not useful in this context. The presence of severe extraintestinal manifestations seems to be a contraindication for their use.

## Side-effects

Long-term use of glucocorticoids frequently causes side-effects which are the major factors limiting their use in the treatment of IBD[10]. The iatrogenic Cushing syndrome includes adrenal atrophy, osteoporosis, aseptic necrosis of the head of the femur, weight gain with redistribution of fat to the truncal areas, 'moon face', 'buffalo hump', striae, plethorae, acne and many other symptoms (Table 5)[10,149,150,183].

Osteoporosis is the most common and potential detrimental side-effect of long-term glucocorticoid therapy[10,184,185]. Bone fractures and vertebral compression can occur. Glucocorticoids diminish bone formation and enhance resorption by inhibiting intestinal calcium absorption and inducing parathormone secretion in all patients treated with glucocorticoids[10]. Osteoporosis can be diminished by supplementation with calcium (> 1.5 g/d) and vitamin D. Furthermore, exercise is recommended.

The suppression of the hypothalamic–pituary–adrenal axis by long-term treatment with glucocorticoids requires the gradual reduction of glucocorticoid therapy. Steroid-related osteonecrosis, particularly of the femoral heads, is less common but represents a serious complication which can lead to severe disability in relatively young patients[186].

Subcapsular cataracts and glaucoma occur quite frequently during long-term glucocorticoid treatment. Periodic ophthalmological examinations should be performed. Steroid-induced myopathy is also a rare but significant problem. Here, use of the new non-systemic steroids seems to be helpful[187].

The suppressive effect of glucocorticoids also weakens resistance against infections. Therefore, a possible infectious complication indicated, for example, by a palpable mass increases the risk for treatment with steroids[150]. In addition, the presence of abscesses should be excluded before treatment with glucocorticosteroids is started.

## RECOMMENDATIONS FOR THERAPY

At the present time, conventional glucocorticosteroids are still the mainstay of treatment of IBD. However, uncomplicated proctitis and left-sided UC can be treated locally with 5-ASA enemas. More active diseases require additional steroids which should be given preferably as foam; the non-systemic steroids seem to be advantageous. In pancolitis, steroids have to be used after failure of treatment with 5-ASA. Here, conventional steroids should be used since little or no clinical experience exists of using non-systemic steroids up to now. In severe or toxic UC, the intravenous application of steroids is standard. However, it should be mentioned that, in particular in toxic colitis, surgery is indicated when conventional treatment has failed after several days.

In CD, classical treatment with conventional steroids is standard up to now. Most probably, treatment with budesonide in oral formulations will become a major alternative for patients with classical ileocaecal disease but no proximal involvement or extraintestinal manifestations. In severe CD, intravenous application of steroids, together with parenteral or enteral nutrition, can be used successfully.

The application of glucocorticoids in the treatment of IBD has improved prognosis of these patients. Life expectancy is, meanwhile, almost identical to that of the general population. In order to improve quality of life, the side-effects have to be minimized and the non-systemic steroids seem to be the first step in this direction although they certainly do not represent a 'magic bullet'[188].

## References


1. Andus T. Corticosteroids. In: Targan S, Shanahan F, eds. Inflammatory bowel disease: From bench to bedside. Baltimore, MD, USA: Williams and Wilkins;1993:487–502.
2. Gross V, Schölmerich J. Morbus Crohn und Colitis ulcerosa. Fortschritte in der Therapie. Deutsches Ärzteblatt. 1993;90:3160–68.
3. Podolsky DK. Medical progress: Inflammatory bowel disease. N Engl J Med. 1991;325:928–37.
4. Muller M, Renkawitz R. The glucocorticoid receptor. Biochim Biophys Acta. 1991;1088:171–82.
5. Distelhorst CW. Recent insight into the structure and function of the glucocorticoid receptor. J Lab Clin Med. 1989;113:404–12.
6. Venkatesh VC, Ballard PL. Glucocorticoids and gene expression. Am J Resp Cell Mol Biol. 1991;4:301–3.
7. Nechushtan H, Benvenisty N, Brandeis R, Reshef L. Glucocorticoids control phospho-enolpyruvate carboxykinase gene expression in a tissue specific manner. Nucleic Acids Res. 1987;15:6405–17.
8. Fauci AS. Glucocorticosteroid therapy: Mechanisms of action and clinical considerations. Ann Intern Med. 1976;84:304–15.
9. Schleimer RP. Effects of glucocorticosteroids on inflammatory cells relevant to their therapeutic applications in asthma. Am Resp Dis. 1990;141:S59–S69.
10. Kuritzkes R, Shanahan F. Corticosteroid therapy. In: Gitnick G, ed. Steroids and inflammatory bowel disease: Diagnosis and treatment. New York, Tokyo: Igaku-Shoin;1990:299–321.
11. MacDermott RP. Cell-mediated immunity in gastrointestinal disease. Hum Pathol. 1986;17:219–33.

12. Truelove SC, Richards LG. Biopsy studies in ulcerative colitis. Br Med J. 1956;3:1315–18.
13. vHerbay A, Gebbers J-O, Otto HF. Immunopathology of ulcerative colitis: A review. Hepato-Gastroenterology. 1990;37:99–107.
14. Schreiber S, MacDermott RP, Raedler A, Pinnau R, Bertovich MJ, Nash GS. Increased activation of isolated intestinal lamina propria mononuclear cells in inflammatory bowel disease. Gastroenterology. 1991;101:1020–30.
15. Bloemena E, Weinreich S, Schellekens PT. The influence of prednisolone on the recirculation of peripheral blood lymphocytes in vivo. Clin Exp Immunol. 1990;80:460–6.
16. Nowell PC. Inhibition of human leukocyte mitosis by prednisolone in vitro. Cancer Res. 1961;21:1518–21.
17. Gillis S, Crabtree, GR, Smith KA. Glucocorticoid-induced inhibition of T-cell growth factor production. I. The effect on mitogen-induced lymphocyte proliferation. J Immunol. 1979;123:1624–31.
18. Raghavachar A, Fleischer S, Frickhofen N, Heimpel H, Fleischer B. T lymphocyte control of human eosinophilic granulopoiesis. J Immunol. 1987;139:3753–8.
19. Tanner AR, Arthur MJP, Wright R. Macrophage activation, chronic inflammation, and gastrointestinal disease. Gut. 1984;25:760–83.
20. Mahida YR, Sarla Patel, Wu K, Jewell DP. Interleukin 2 receptor expression by macrophages in inflammatory bowel disease. Clin Exp Immunol. 1988;74:382–6.
21. Donowitz M. Arachidonic acid metabolites and their role in inflammatory bowel disease. An update requiring addition of a pathway. Gastroenterology. 1985;88:580–7.
22. Eliakim R, Karmelli F, Razin E, Rachmilewitz D. Role of platelet-activating factor in ulcerative colitis. Gastroenterology. 1988;95:1167–72.
23. Mahida YR, Wu K, Jewell DP. Enhanced production of interleukin 1-beta by mononuclear cells isolated from mucosa with active ulcerative colitis or Crohn's disease. Gut. 1989;30:835–8.
24. Andus T, Gross V, Cäsar I et al. Activation of monocytes during inflammatory bowel disease. Pathobiology. 1991;59:166–70.
25. MacDonald TT, Hutchings P, Choy M-Y, Murch S, Cooke A. Tumor necrosis factor-alpha and interferon-gamma production measured at the single cell level in normal and inflamed human intestine. Clin Exp Immunol. 1990;81:301–5.
26. Malizia G, Calbrese A, Cottone M et al. Expression of leukocyte adhesion molecules by mucosal mononuclear phagocytes in inflammatory bowel disease. Gastroenterology. 1991;100:150–9.
27. Thompson J, vanFurth R. The effect of glucocorticosteroids on the kinetics of mononuclear phagocytes. J Exp Med. 1970;131:429–42.
28. Mier JW, Vachino G, Klempner MS et al. Inhibition of interleukin-2-induced tumor necrosis factor release by dexamethasone: prevention of an acquired neutrophil chemotaxis defect and differential suppression of interleukin-2-associated side effects. Blood. 1990;76:1933–40.
29. Waage A, Slupphaug G, Shalaby R. Glucocorticoids inhibit the production of IL6 from monocytes, endothelial cells and fibroblasts. Eur J Immunol. 1990;20:2439–43.
30. Hart PH, Whitty GA, Burgess DR, Croatto M, Hamilton JA. Augmentation of glucocorticoid action on human monocytes by interleukin-4. Lymphokine Res. 1990;9:147–53.
31. Goode HF, Rathbone BJ, Kelleher J, Walker BE. Monocyte zinc and in vitro prostaglandin E2 and interleukin-1 beta production by cultured peripheral blood monocytes in patients with Crohn's disease. Dig Dis Sci. 1991;36:627–33.
32. Mukaida N, Zachariae CC, Gusella GL, Matsushima K. Dexamethasone inhibits the induction of monocyte chemotactic-activating factor production by IL-1 or tumor necrosis factor. J Immunol. 1991;146:1212–15.
33. Werb Z. Biochemical actions of glucocorticoids on macrophages in culture. Specific inhibition of elastase, collagenase, and plasminogen activator secretion and effects on other metabolic functions. J Exp Med. 1978;147:1695–712.
34. Sarin SK, Malhotra V, Sen Gupta S, Karol A, Gaur SK Anand BS. Significance of eosinophil and mast cell counts in rectal mucosa in ulcerative colitis. A prospective controlled study. Dig Dis Sci. 1987;32:363–67.
35. Choy MY, Walker Smith JA, Williams CB, MacDonald TT. Activated eosinophils in chronic inflammatory bowel disease. Lancet. 1990;336:126–7.

36. Saunders RH, Adams E. Changes in circulating leukocytes following the administration of adrenal cortex extract (ACE) and adrenocorticotropic hormone (ACTH) in infectious mononucleosis and chronic lymphatic leukemia. Blood. 1950;5:732–41.

37. Altman LC, Hill JS, Hairfield WM, Mullarkey MF. Effects of corticosteroids on eosinophil chemotaxis and adherence. J Clin Invest. 1981;67:28–36.

38. Rothenberg ME, Owen WF, Silberstein DS, Gasson JC, Stevens RL, Ausen KF. Regulation of human eosinophil viability, density, and function by granulocyte/macrophage colony-stimulating factor in the presence of 3T3 fibroblasts. J Exp Med. 1987;166:129–41.

39. Lamas AM, Marcotte GV, Schleimer RP. Human endothelial cells prolong eosinophil survival. Regulation by cytokines and glucocorticoids. J Immunol. 1989;142:3978–84.

40. Lamas AM, Leon OG, Schleimer RP. Glucocorticoids inhibit eosinophil responses to granulocyte-macrophage colony-stimulating factor. J Immunol. 1991;147:254–9.

41. Bochner BS, Luscinskas FW, Gimbrone MA Jr et al. Adhesion of human basophils, eosinophils, and neutrophils to interleukin 1-activated human vascular endothelial cells: contributions of endothelial cell adhesion molecules. J Exp Med. 1991;173:1553–7.

42. Snyder DS, Unanue ER. Corticosteroids inhibit murine macrophage Ia expression and interleukin-1 production. J Immunol. 1982;129:1803–5.

43. Dvorak AM. Ultrastructural evidence for release of major basic protein-containing crystalline cores of eosinophil granules in vivo: cytotoxic potential in Crohn's disease. J Immunol. 1980;125:460–2.

44. Fox CC, Lazenby AJ, Moore WC, Yardley JH, Bayless TM, Lichtenstein LM. Enhancement of human intestinal mast cell mediator release in active ulcerative colitis. Gastroenterology. 1990;99:119–24.

45. Befus D, Fujimaki H, Lee TD, Swieter M. Mast cell polymorphisms. Present concepts, future directions. Dig Dis Sci. 1988;33:16S–24S.

46. Schleimer RP, Lichtenstein LM, Gillespie E. Inhibition of basophil histamine release by antiinflammatory steroids. Nature. 1981;292:454–5.

47. Sawyerr AM, Wakefield AJ, Hudson M, Dhillon AP, Pounder RE. Review article: the pharmacological implications of leucocyte–endothelial cell interactions in Crohn's disease. Aliment Pharmacol Ther. 1991;5:1–14.

48. Irani-A-MA, Craig SS, DeBlois G et al. Deficiency of the tryptase-positive, chymase-negative mast cell type in gastrointestinal mucosa of patients with defective T lymphocyte function. J Immunol. 1987;138:4381–6.

49. Bissonnette, EY, Benyon RC, Befus AD. Mast cells as targets for the therapy of inflammatory bowel disease. Can J Gastroenterol. 1990;4:285–8.

50. Goldsmith P, McGarity B, Walls AF, Church MK, Millward Sadler GH, Robertson DA. Corticosteroid treatment reduces mast cell numbers in inflammatory bowel disease. Dig Dis Sci. 1990;35:1409–13.

51. Levo Y, Livni N. Mast-cell degranulation in Crohn's disease. Lancet. 1978,1:1262.

52. MacDermott RP, Stenson WF. Inflammatory bowel disease. In: Targan S, Shanahan F, eds. Immunology and immunopathology of the liver and gastrointestinal tract. New York, Tokyo: Igaku-Shoin; 1990:459–86.

53. Schölmerich J, Schmidt E, Schümichen C, Billmann P, Schmidt H, Gerok W. Scintigraphic assessment of bowel involvement and disease activity in Crohn's disease using technetium-99m-HM-PAO as leukocyte label. Gastroenterology. 1988;95:1287–98.

54. Andus T, Gross V, Caesar I et al. PMN-elastase in the assessment of patients with inflammatory bowel disease. Dig Dis Sci. 1993;38:1638–44.

55. Ritter C, Grisham MB, Hollwarth M, Inauen W, Granger DN. Neutrophil-derived oxidants mediate formyl-methionyl-leucyl-phenylalanine-induced increases in mucosal permeability in rats. Gastroenterology. 1989;97:778–80.

56. Grisham MB, Granger DN. Neutrophil-mediated mucosal injury. Role of reactive oxygen metabolites. Dig Dis Sci. 1988;33:6S–15S.

57. Schleimer RP, Freeland HS, Peters SP, Brown KE, Derse CP. An assessment of the effects of glucocorticoids on degranulation, chemotaxis, binding to vascular endothelium and formation of leukotriene B4 by purified human neutrophils. J Pharmacol Exp Ther. 1989;250:598–605.

58. Sawyerr AM, Wakefield AJ, Hudson M, Dhillon AP, Pounder RE. Review article: the pharmacological implications of leucocyte–endothelial cell interactions in Crohn's disease. Aliment Pharmacol Ther. 1991;5:1–14.

59. Lewis RE, Granger HJ. Diapedesis and the permeability of venous microvessels to protein macromolecules: the impact of leukotriene B4 (LTB4). Microvasc Res. 1988;35:27–47.
60. Williams TJ, Yarwood H. Effect of glucocorticoids on microvascular permeability. Am Rev Respir Dis. 1990;141:S39–S43.
61. Watanabe M, Yagi M, Omata M et al. Stimulation of neutrophil adherence to vascular endothelial cells by histamine and thrombin and its inhibition by PAF antagonists and dexamethasone. Br J Pharmacol. 1991;102:239–45.
62. Allison F Jr, Smith MR, Wood WB Jr. Studies on the pathogenesis of acute inflammation. II. The action of cortisone on the inflammatory response to thermal injury. J Exp Med. 1955;102:669–79.
63. Lauritsen K, Laursen LS, Bukhave K, Rask-Madsen J. Effects of topical 5-aminosalicylic acid and prednisolone on prostaglandin $E_2$ and leukotriene $B_4$ levels determined by equilibrium in vivo dialysis of rectum in relapsing ulcerative colitis. Gastroenterology. 1986;91:837–44.
64. Lauritsen K, Laursen LS, Bukhave K, Rask-Madsen J. In vivo effects of orally administered prednisolone on prostaglandin and leukotriene production in ulcerative colitis. Gut. 1987;28:1095–9.
65. Peers SH, Flower RJ. The role of lipocortin in corticosteroid actions. Am Rev Respir Dis 1990;141:S18–S21.
66. Mahida YR, Lamming CED, Gallagher A, Hawthorne AB, Hawkey CJ. 5-Aminosalicylic acid is a potent inhibitor of interleukin $1\beta$ production in organ culture of colonic biopsy specimens from patients with inflammatory bowel disease. Gut. 1991;32:50–4.
67. Pullman WE, Elsbury S, Kobayashi M, Hapel AJ, Doe WF. Enhanced mucosal cytokine production in inflammatory bowel disease. Gastroenterology. 1992;102:529–37.
68. Lauritsen K, Staerk Laursen L, Bukhave K, Rask-Madsen J. In vivo effect of orally administered prednisolone on prostaglandin and leukotriene production in ulcerative colitis. Gut. 1987;28:1095–9.
69. Rachmilewitz D, Karmeli F, Eliakim R. Platelet-activating factor – A possible mediator in the pathogenesis of ulcerative colitis. Scand J Gastroenterol. 1990;25(suppl 172):19–21.
70. Pickup ME. Clinical pharmacokinetics of prednisone and prednisolone. Clin Pharmacokinet. 1979;4:111–28.
71. Elliott PR, Powell-Tuck J, Gillespie PE et al. Prednisolone absorption in acute colitis. Gut. 1980;21:49–51.
72. Rodrigues CA, Nabi EM, Spiliadis C et al. Prednisolone absorption in inflammatory bowel disease: correlation with anatomical site and extent. Aliment Pharmacol Ther. 1987;1:391–9.
73. Tanner AR, Halliday JW, Powell L. Serum prednisolone levels in Crohn's disease and coeliac disease following oral prednisolone administration. Digestion. 1981;21:310–15.
74. Olivesi A. Normal absorption of oral prednisolone in children with active inflammatory bowel disease, including cases with proximal to distal small bowel involvement. Gastroenterol Clin Biol. 1985;9:564–71.
75. Milsap RL, George DE, Szefler SJ, Murray KA, Lebenthal E, Jusko WJ. Effect of inflammatory bowel disease on absorption and disposition of prednisolone. Dig Dis Sci. 1983;28:161–8.
76. Swartz S, Dluhy R. Corticosteroids: Clinical pharmacology and therapeutic use. Drugs. 1978;16:238–55.
77. Barth J, Möllmann HW, Wagner T, Hochhaus G, Derndorf H. Problematik des Äquivalenzbegriffes bei der Therapie mit Glucocorticoiden. Dtsch Med Wschr. 1994;119:1671–6.
78. Kirsner JB, Palmer WE, Merimen SH et al. Clinical course of chronic nonspecific ulcerative colitis. JAMA. 1948;137:922–8.
79. Dearing WH, Brown PW. Experiences with cortisone and ACTH in chronic ulcerative colitis. Proc Mayo Clin. 1950;25:486–8.
80. Elliott JM, Kiefer ED, Hurxthal LM. Treatment of chronic ulcerative colitis with pituitary adrenocorticotrophic hormone (ACTH): Clinical study of 28 cases. N Engl J Med. 1951;245:288–92.
81. Kirsner JB, Palmer WE. Effect of corticotropin (ACTH) in chronic ulcerative colitis: Observations in 40 patients. JAMA. 1951;147:541–9.
82. Halsted JA, Adams WS, Sloan S et al. Clinical effects of ACTH in ulcerative colitis. Gastroenterology. 1951;19:698–721.
83. Elliot J, Giansiracusa J. ACTH and cortisone in the treatment of ulcerative colitis. An evaluation of their prolonged administration. N Engl J Med. 1954;250:969–76.

84. Gray SJ, Reifenstein RW, Benson JA Jr, Gordon Young JC. Treatment of ulcerative colitis and regional enteritis with A.C.T.H. Arch Intern Med. 1951;87:646–62.
85. Truelove SC, Witts LJ. Cortisone in ulcerative colitis. Preliminary report on a therapeutic trial. Br Med J. 1954;2:375–8.
86. Truelove SC, Witts LJ. Cortisone in ulcerative colitis. Final report on a therapeutic trial. Br Med J. 1955;2:1041–8.
87. Lennard-Jones JE, Longmore AJ, Newell AC, Wilson CWE, Avery Jones F. An assessment of prednisone, salazopyrin, and topical hydrocortisone hemisuccinate used as out-patient treatment of ulcerative colitis. Gut. 1960;1:217–22.
88. Truelove SC, Witts LJ. Cortisone and corticotrophin in ulcerative colitis. Br Med J. 1959;1:387–94.
89. Kaplan H, Portnoy B, Binder HJ, Amatruda T, Spiro H. A controlled evaluation of intravenous adrenocorticotropic hormone and hydrocortisone in the treatment of acute colitis. Gastroenterology. 1975;69:91–5.
90. Powell-Tuck J, Buckell N, Lennard-Jones JE. A controlled comparison of corticotropin and hydrocortisone in the treatment of severe proctocolitis. Scand J Gastroenterol. 1977;12:971–5.
91. Meyers S, Sachar DB, Goldberg JD, Janowitz HD. Corticotropin versus hydrocortisone in the intravenous treatment of ulcerative colitis. A prospective, randomized, double blind clinical trial. Gastroenterology. 1983;85:351–7.
92. Baron JH, Connell AM, Kanaghinis TG, Lennard-Jones JE, Avery Jones F. Out-patient treatment of ulcerative colitis. Comparison between three doses of oral prednisone. Br Med J. 1962;2:441–3.
93. Lennard-Jones JE. Toward optimal use of corticosteroids in ulcerative colitis and Crohn's disease. Gut. 1983;24:177–81.
94. Powell-Tuck J, Brown R, Lennard-Jones JE. A comparison of oral prednisolone as single or multiple daily doses for active proctocolitis. Scand J Gastroenterol. 1987;13:833–7.
95. Truelove SC, Jewell DP. Intensive intravenous regimen for severe attacks of ulcerative colitis. Lancet. 1974;1:1067–70.
96. Margolin ML, Krumholz MP, Fochios SE, Korelitz BI. Clinical trials in ulcerative colitis. II: Historical review. Am J Gastroenterol. 1988;83:227–43.
97. Sutherland LR, Robinson M, Onstad G et al. A double blind, placebo controlled multicentric study of the efficacy and safety of 5-aminosalicylic acid tablets in the treatment of ulcerative colitis. Can J Gastroenterol. 1990;4:463–7.
98. Hamilton I, Pinder IF, Dickinson RJ, Ruddell WSJ, Dixon MF, Axon ATR. A comparison of prednisolone enemas with low-dose oral prednisolone in the treatment of acute distal ulcerative colitis. Dis Colon Rectum. 1984;27:701–2.
99. Truelove SC. Treatment of ulcerative colitis with local hydrocortisone. Br Med J. 1956;2:1267–72.
100. Truelove SC. Treatment of ulcerative colitis with local hydrocortisone hemisuccinate sodium. A report on a controlled therapeutic trial. Br Med J. 1959;2:1072–7.
101. Truelove SC. Treatment of ulcerative colitis with local hydrocortisone hemisuccinate sodium. Br Med J. 1957;1:1437–43.
102. Watkinson G. Treatment of ulcerative colitis with topical hydrocortisone hemisuccinate sodium. A controlled trial employing restricted sequential analysis. Br Med J. 1958;2:1077–82.
103. Matts S. Local treatment of ulcerative colitis with prednisolone-21-phosphate enemata. Lancet. 1960;1:517–19.
104. Matts SGF. Intrarectal treatment of 100 cases of ulcerative colitis with prednisolone 21-phosphate retention enemata. Br Med J. 1961;1:165.
105. Lennard-Jones JE, Baron JH, Connell AM, Jones FA. A double blind controlled trial of prednisolone-21-phosphate suppositories in the treatment of idiopathic proctitis. Gut. 1962;3:207–10.
106. Macdougal I. Treatment of ulcerative colitis with rectal steroids. Lancet. 1963;1:826–7.
107. Powell-Tuck J, Lennard-Jones JE, May CS, Wilson CG, Paterson JW. Plasma prednisolone levels after administration of prednisolone 21-phosphate as a retention enema in colitis. Br Med J. 1976;1:193–5.
108. Matts S. Betamethasone enemata in ulcerative colitis. Gut. 1962;3:312–14.
109. Truelove SC. Systemic and local corticosteroid therapy in ulcerative colitis. Br Med J. 1960;1:464–7.

110. Truelove SC. Local corticosteroid treatment in severe attacks of ulcerative colitis. Br Med J. 1960;2:102–8.
111. Swarbick E, Loose H, Lennard-Jones JE. Enema volume as an important factor in successful topical corticosteroid treatment of colitis. Proc R Soc Med. 1974;67:753–4.
112. Jay M, Digenis GA, Foster TS, Antonow DR. Retrograde spreading of hydrocortisone enema in inflammatory bowel disease. Dig Dis Sci. 1986;31:139–44.
113. Kratzer G. Conference on chronic ulcerative colitis and clinical experience with cortifoam. AJCR. 1970;1:111–14.
114. Scherl M, Scherl B. Adjunctive use of a steroid rectal foam in the treatment of ulcerative colitis. Dis Colon Rectum. 1973;16:149–51.
115. Clark M. A local foam aerosol in ulcerative colitis. Practitioner. 1977;219:103–4.
116. Hay D, Sharma H, Irving M. Spread of steroid-containing foam after intrarectal administration Br Med J. 1979;1:1751–3.
117. Farthing M, Rutland M, Clark M. Retrograde spread of hydrocortisone containing foam given intrarectally in ulcerative colitis. Br Med J. 1979;2:822–4.
118. Ruddel WSJ, Dickinson RJ, Dixon MF, Axpon ATR. Treatment of distal ulcerative colitis (proctosigmoiditis) in relapse: comparison of hydrocortisone enemas and rectal hydrocortisone foam. Gut. 1980;21:885–9.
119. Somerville KW, Langman MJS, Kane SP, MacGilchrist AJ, Watkinson G, Salmon P. Effect of treatment on symptoms and quality of life in patients with ulcerative colitis: comparative trial of hydrocortisone acetate foam and prednisolone-21-phosphate enemas. Br Med J. 1985;291:866–7.
120. Liddle G. 9α-Fluorohydrocortisone: A new investigative tool in adrenal physiology. J Clin Endocrinol. 1956;16:557–9.
121. Multicenter Trial. Betamethasone 17-valerate and prednisolone 21-phosphate retention enemata in proctocolitis. Br Med J. 1971;3:84–6.
122. Campieri M, Lanfranchi GA, Bazzocchi G et al. Treatment of ulcreative colitis with high-dose 5-aminosalicylic acid enemas. Lancet. 1981;2:270–1.
123. Lennard-Jones JE, Misiewitcz JJ, Connel AM, Baron JH, Avery Jones F. Prednisone as maintenance treatment for ulcerative colitis in remission. Lancet. 1965;1:188–9.
124. Cocco A, Mendeloff A. An evaluation of intermittent corticosteroid therapy in the management of ulcerative colitis. Johns Hopkins Med J. 1967;120:162–9.
125. Powell-Tuck J, Brown RL, Chambers TJ, Lennard-Jones JE. A controlled trial of alternate day prednisolone as a maintenance treatment of ulcerative colitis in remission. Digestion. 1981;22:263–70.
126. Bondesen S, Rasmussen SN, Rask Madsen I et al. 5-Aminosalicylic acid in the treatment of inflammatory bowel disease. Acta Med Scand. 1987;221:227–42.
127. Danish 5-ASA Group. Topical 5-aminosalicylic acid versus prednisolone in ulcerative proctosigmoiditis: a randomized double-blind multicenter trial. Dig Dis Sci. 1987;2:598–602.
128. Friedmann LS, Ritcher JM, Kirkhan SE, DeMonaco HJ, May RJ. 5-Aminosalicylic acid enemas in refractory distal ulcerative colitis: a randomized, controlled trial. Am J Gastroenterol. 1986;6:412–18.
129. Williams CN. Role of rectal formulations: suppositories. Scand J Gastroenterol Suppl. 1990;172:60–62.
130. Brattsand R. Overview of newer glucocorticosteroid preparations for inflammatory bowel disease. Can J Gastroenterol. 1990;4:407–14.
131. Kumana CR, Seaton T, Meghji M, Casteli M, Benson R, Sivakumaran T. Beclomethasone dipropionate enemas for treating inflammatory bowel disease without producing Cushing's syndrome or hypothalamic–pituitary–adrenal suppression. Lancet. 1982;1:579–83.
132. Bansky G, Buhler H, Stamm B, Häcki WH, Buchmann P, Müller J. Treatment of distal ulcerative colitis with beclomethasone enemas: high therapeutic efficacy without endocrine side effects. A prospective, randomized, double-blind trial. Dis Colon Rectum. 1987;30:288–92.
133. Heide Hvd, Brandt-Gradel Vvd, Tytgat GNJ et al. Comparison of beclomethasone dipropionate and prednisolone 21-phosphate enemas in the treatment of ulcerative proctitis. J Clin Gastroenterol. 1988;10:169–72.
134. Mulder CJJ, Endert E, Heide Hvd et al. Comparison of beclomethasone dipropionate (2 and 3 mg) and prednisolone sodium phosphate enemas (30 mg) in the treatment of ulcerative proctitis. An adrenocortical approach. Neth J Med 1989;35:18–24.

135. Vignotti D, Ranzi T, Campanini MC, Lisciandrano D, Monti GB, Bianchi PA. Topical treatment of active distal ulcerative colitis with beclomethasone dipropionate. Curr Ther Res. 1992;52:659–65.
136. Hanauer S. Clinical experience with tixocortol pivalate. Can J Gastroenterol. 1988;2:156–8.
137. Danielsson A, Hellers G, Lyrenäs E et al. A controlled randomized trial of budesonide versus prednisolone retention enemas in active distal ulcerative colitis. Scand J Gastroenterol. 1987;22:987–92.
138. Danielsson A, Löfberg R, Persson T et al. A steroid enema, budesonide, lacking systemic effects for the treatment of distal ulcerative colitis or proctitis. Scand J Gastroenterol. 1992;27:9–12.
139. Matzen and the Danish budesonide study group. Budesnoide enema in distal ulcerative colitis. A randomized dose–response trial with prednisolone enema as positive control. Scand J Gastroenterol. 1991;26:1225–30.
140. Löfberg R, Ostergaard T, Komsen O et al. Budesonide vs prednisolone enema in active distal ulcerative colitis. A comparative eight week study. Gut. 1993;34(Suppl. 1):40(abstract).
141. Bianchi-Porro G, Campieri M, Bianchi P et al. Comparative trial of budesonide and methylprenisolone enemas in the treatment of ulcerative colitis. Eur J Gastroenterol Hepatol. 1994;6:125–30.
142. Lamers C, Meijer J, Engels L et al. Comparative study of the topically acting glucocorticosteroid budesonide and 5-aminosalicylic acid enema therapy of proctitis and proctosigmoiditis. Gastroenterology. 1991;101:A223(abstract).
143. Leman M, Rutgeerts P, van Heuverzwijn R et al. Comparison of budesonide enema and 5-ASA enema in the treatment of active distal ulcerative colitis. Hellenic J Gastroenterol. 1995;5:194.
144. Standley M, Rosenberg I, Cleroux A. The use of corticotropin (A.C.T.H.) in the treatment of chronic regional enteritis. Med Con N Am. 1951;35:1255–65.
145. Kirsner JB, Palmer WE, Klotz A. A.C.T.H. in severe chronic regional enteritis. Gastroenterology. 1952;20:229–33.
146. Sparberg M, Kirsner JB. Long-term corticosteroid therapy for regional enteritis. An analysis of 58 courses in 54 patients. Am J Dig Dis. 1966;11:865–80.
147. Jones J, Lennard-Jones JE. Corticosteroids and corticotrophin therapy in Crohn's disease. Gut. 1966;7:181–7.
148. Cooke W, Fielding J. Corticosteroid or corticotrophin therapy in Crohn's disease (regional enteritis). Gut. 1970;11:921–7.
149. Summers RW, Switz DM, Sessions Jr JT et al. National Cooperative Crohn's Disease study: Results of drug treatment. Gastroenterology. 1979;77:847–69.
150. Malchow H, Ewe K, Brandes JW et al. European Cooperative Crohn's Disease Study (ECCDS): Results of drug treatment. Gastroenterology. 1984;86:249–66.
151. Malchow H, Steinhardt HJ, Lorenz Meyer H et al. Feasibility and effectiveness of a defined-formula diet regimen in treating active Crohn's disease. European Cooperative Crohn's Disease Study III. Scand J Gastroenterol. 1990;25:235–44.
152. Lochs H, Steinhardt HJ, Klaus-Wentz B et al. Comparison of enteral nutrition and drug treatment in active Crohn's disease. Results of the European Cooperative Crohn's Disease Study IV. Gastroenteroogy. 1991;101:881–8.
153. Schölmerich J, Jenss H, Hartmann F, the German 5-ASA Study Group. Oral 5-aminosalicylic acid versus 6-methylprednisolone in active Crohn's disease. Can J Gastoenterol. 1990;4:446–51.
154. Gross V, Andus T, Fischbach W and the German 5-ASA Study Group. Comparison between high dose 5-aminosalicylic acid and 6-methylprednisolone in active Crohn's ileocolitis. A multicenter randomized double-blind study. Z Gastroenterol. [In press].
155. Rutgeerts P, Löfberg R, Malchow H et al. A comparison of budesonide with prednisolone for active Crohn's disease. N Engl J Med. 1994;331:842–5.
156. Gross V, Andus T, Caesar I et al. Oral pH-modified release budesonide vs 6-methylprednisolone in active Crohn's disease. Gastroenterology. 1995;108:A828(abstract).
157. Lefton H, Farmer R, Fazio V. Ileorectal anastomosis for Crohnis disease of the colon. Gastroenterology. 1975;69:612–17.
158. Bergmann L, Krause U. Postoperative treatment with corticosteroids and salazosulphapyridine (Salazopyrin) after radical resection for Crohn's disease. Scand J Gastroenterol. 1976;II:651–6.

159. Smith RC, Rhodes J, Heatley RV et al. Low dose steroids and clinical relapse in Crohn's disease: A controlled trial. Gut. 1978;19:606–10.

160. Bello C, Goldstein F, Thornton JJ. Alternative-day prednisone treatment and treatment maintenance in Crohn's disease. Am J Gastroenterol. 1991;86:460–6.

161. Brignola C, Campieri M, Farruggio P et al. The possible utility of steroids in the prevention of relapses of Crohn's disease in remission. J Clin Gastroenterol. 1988;10:631–4.

162. Landi B, Anh TN, Cortot A et al. Endoscopic monitoring of Crohn's disease treatment: a prospective, randomized clinical trial. The Groupe d'Etudes Therapeutiques des Affections Inflammatoires Digestives. Gastroenterololgy. 1992;102:1647–53.

163. Levine DS, Raisys VA, Ainardi V. Coating of oral beclomethasone dipropionate capsules with cellulose acetate phthalate enhances delivery of topically active antiinflammatory drug to the terminal ileum. Gastroenterology. 1987;92:1037–44.

164. Möllmann HW, Hochhaus G, Tromm A et al. Topical use of steroids in gastoenterology. In: Schölmerich J, Gross V, Goebel H, Hohenberger W, eds. Inflammatory bowel dieases. Pathophysiology as a basis for therapy. Lancaster, UK: MTP Press; 1993:343–9.

165. Löfberg R, Danielsson A, Salde L. Oral budesonide in active Crohn's disease. Aliment Pharmacol Therap. 1993;7:611–16.

166. Wolman SL, Greenberg GR. Oral budesonide in active Crohn's disease. An initial experience [abstract]. Gastroenterology. 1991;100:A263.

167. Roth M, Gross V, Schölmerich J, Überschaer B, Ewe K. Treatment of active Crohn's disease with an oral slow release budesonide formulation. Am J Gastroenterol. 1989;88:968–9.

168. Caesar I, Gross V, Roth M et al. Budesonide study group. Treatment of active Crohn's ileocolitis with an oral slow release Eudragit-coated budesonide formulation. Z Gastroenterol. 1995;33:247–50.

169. Andus T, Gross V, Caesar I and the German Budesonide Study Group. Replacement of conventional steroids by budesonide in active or inactive Crohn's disease. Interim analysis of an open, prospective, multicenter trial. Gastroenterology. 1995;108:A771(abstract).

170. Greenberg GR, Feagan BG, Martin F and the Canadian inflammatory bowel disease study group. Oral budesonide for active Crohn's disease. N Engl J Med. 1994;331:836–41.

171. Löfberg R, Rutgeerts P, Malchow H and the European Budesonide Study Group. Budesonide C/R for maintenance of remission in ileocaecal Crohn's disease. A European multicenter placebo controlled trial for 12 months. Gastroenterology. 1994;106:A722.

172. Gross V, Andus T, Ecker KW et al. Oral pH-modified release budesonide for maintenance of steroid induced remission in Crohn's disease – an interim analysis. Gastroenterology. 1995;105:A828(abstract).

173. Wright JP, Jarnum S, Schaffalitzky de Muckadell O, Keech ML, Lennard-Jones JE. Oral fluticasone propionate compared with prednisolone in treatment of active Crohn's disease. Gastroenterology. 1993;104:A803(abstract).

174. Carpani de Kaski M, Peters AM, Lavender JP, Hodgson HJF. Fluticasone propionate in Crohn's disease. Gut. 1991;32:657–61.

175. Warsof SL. Medical and surgical treatment of inflammatory bowel disease in pregnancy. Clin Obstet Gynecol. 1983;26:822–31.

176. Mogadam M, Dobbins WO, Korrelitz BJ, Ahmed SW. Pregnancy in inflammatory bowel disease: the effect of sulphasalazine and corticosteroids of fetal outcome. Gastroenterology. 1981;80:72–6.

177. Rasenack J, Schölmerich J. Inflammatory bowel disease and pregnancy. Gynäkologe. 1990;23:11–17.

178. Daum F. Management of pediatric inflammatory bowel disease. In: MacDermott RP, Stenson WF, eds. Inflammatory bowel disease. Amsterdam: Elsevier; 1992.

179. Whittington PF, Barnes HV, Bayless TM. Medical management of Crohn's disease in adolescence. Gastroenterology. 1977;72:1338–44.

180. Schölmerich J. Pathophysiology and treatment of extraintestinal symptoms in Crohn's disease. Clin Res Gastroenterol. 1989;2:65–86.

181. Greenstein AJ, Janowitz HD, Sachar DB. Extraintestinal manifestations of Crohn's disease and ulcerative colitis: a study of 700 cases. Medicine. 1976;55:401–12.

182. Janowitz HD. Extraintestinal manifestations. In: Bayless TM, ed. Current management of inflammatory bowel disease. Toronto, Philadelphia: Decker Inc.; 1989:157–60.

183. Jewell DP. Corticosteroids for the management of ulcerative colitis and Crohn's disease. Gastroenterol Clin N Am. 1989;18:21–34.

184. Hahn TJ, Biseau VC, Avioli LV. Effect of chronic corticosteroid administration on diaphyseal and metaphyseal bone mass. J Clin Endocrinol Metab. 1974;39:274–82.
185. Compston JE, Judd D, Crawley EO et al. Osteoporosis in patients with inflammatory bowel disease. Gut. 1987; 28:410–15.
186. Vakil N, Sparberg M. Steroid-related osteonecrosis in inflammatory bowel disease. Gastroenterology. 1989;96:62–7.
187. Caesar I, Gross V, Roth M, Schölmerich J. Steroidinduzierte Myopathie bei linksseitiger Colitis ulcerosa–erfolgreiche Behandlung und Therapiefortsetzung mit dem topischen Steroid Budesnoid. DMW, eingereicht.
188. Sacchar DB. Budesonide for inflammatory bowel disease. Is it a magic bullet? N Engl J Med. 1994;331:873–4.

# 22
# An update of immunosuppressive therapy in IBD

E. F. STANGE

It has been estimated that approximately 20% of patients with Crohn disease do not respond satisfactorily to standard conservative treatment with corticosteroids and aminosalicylates. It is this problematic patient cohort, especially those with chronic active disease, which requires more aggressive immunosuppressive therapy. Particular interest has also been paid to an eventual steroid-sparing effect and fistula healing as well as the role of therapeutic agents in maintaining remission. In comparison with Crohn disease, the data base concerning immunosuppression in ulcerative colitis is much more scanty.

The standard immunosuppressive agents in inflammatory bowel disease are azathioprine and 6-mercaptopurine. More recently, methotrexate and cyclosporin A have been introduced in refractory disease. The rationale for the use of these drugs lies in the multiple immunological abnormalities described in both types of disease[1]. The role of these treatment alternatives will be reviewed in the present chapter.

## AZATHIOPRINE AND 6-MERCAPTOPURINE

The precise mechanism of action of both azathioprine and 6-mercaptopurine remains enigmatic although some progress has been made in this regard. Azathioprine has been demonstrated to be converted to 6-mercaptopurine in vivo, suggesting that there is no major difference in action between the agents. 6-Mercaptopurine is subsequently metabolized to 6-thioinosinic acid, the presumed active metabolite which becomes incorporated into developing strands of DNA[2]. In lymphocytes, this substitution blocks critical gene activation of effector lymphocyte clones, thus inhibiting their proliferation.

In Crohn disease, eight reports of controlled trials of azathioprine or 6-mercatopurine either in active disease[3-8] or as maintenance treatment[6,9,10] have been fully published. An overview of these studies is given in Table 1. The two initial small trials[3,4] failed to show a significant benefit, probably due to insufficient statistical power ($\beta$-error) and the short treatment course. In the

**Table 1**  Azathioprine and 6-mercaptopurine: controlled trials

| Study | Dose (mg/kg per day) | Duration (months) | $n$ | Overall result |
|---|---|---|---|---|
| **Crohn disease** | | | | |
| *Active disease* | | | | |
| Rhodes et al.[3] | 2–4 | 2 + 2 | 16 | A = P |
| Klein et al.[4] | 3 | 4 + 4 | 26 | A = P |
| Rosenberg et al.[5] | 2 | 6.5 | 20 | A > P ($p < 0.05$) |
| Summers et al.*[6] | 2.5 | 4 | 136 | A = P |
| Present et al.[7] | 1.5 | 12 + 12 | 83 | 6MP > P ($p < 0.001$) |
| Ewe et al.[8] | 2.5 | 4 | 42 | A > P ($p = 0.0.3$) |
| *Maintenance* | | | | |
| O'Donoghue et al.[9] | 2 | 12 | 51 | A > P ($p < 0.01$) |
| Willoughby et al.[10] | 2–4 | 6 | 22 | A > P ($p < 0.01$) |
| Summers et al.*[6] | 1 | 12–24 | 155 | A = P |
| **Ulcerative colitis** | | | | |
| *Acute active disease* | | | | |
| Caprilli et al.*[12] | 2.5 | 3 | 20 | A = S |
| Jewell and Truelove[13] | 2.5 | 1 | 80 | A = P |
| *Chronic active disease* | | | | |
| Kirk and Lennard-Jones[14] | 2–2.5 | 6 | 44 | A > P ($p < 0.001$) |
| Rosenberg et al.[15] | 1.5 | 6 | 30 | A > P ($p < 0.05$) |
| *Maintenance* | | | | |
| Jewell and Truelove[13] | 1.5–2.5 | 12 | 80 | A = P |
| Hawthorne et al.[16] | Variable | 12 | 79 | A > P ($p < 0.01$) |

A: azathioprine; 6MP: 6-mercaptopurine; P: placebo; *no concomitant steroids

study by Present et al.[7], 83 chronically ill patients were entered into a 2-year double-blind study comparing 6-mercaptopurine with placebo. Cross-over data showed that improvement occurred in 26 of 39 courses of drug (67%) compared with 3 of 39 courses of placebo (8%; $p < 0.0001$). Non-crossover data also confirmed the superiority of 6-mercaptopurine. The drug was more effective in closing fistulae (31% vs 6%) and in permitting discontinuation or reduction of steroid dosage (75% vs 36%). It is important to note that the onset of response was often delayed, with 32% of the patients taking longer than 3 months to respond, and 19% taking longer than 4 months. The National Cooperative Crohn's Disease Study[6] was biased against azathioprine for several reasons: first, corticosteroids were withdrawn in a significant proportion of the patients immediately before the start of the trial so that many patients experienced an early relapse. Since azathioprine requires several months for its action to begin this design probably doomed the azathioprine arm of the trial. Also for this reason, the treatment period of 4 months may simply have been too short and the data do actually indicate an improved action after 7 weeks of treatment[6].

A more recent study examined whether azathioprine combined with standard prednisolone therapy improved the therapeutic outcome compared with monotherapy with prednisolone in active Crohn disease[8]. At the end of the 4 months trial, 16 of 21 patients (76%) with combined therapy vs 8 of 21 patients

(38%) treated with corticosteroids alone were in remission ($p = 0.03$). The differences in activity indices became significant after 8 weeks. In addition, the average steroid dose was significantly lower in the combined treatment group. A recent uncontrolled study also supports a corticoid-sparing effect in 76% of patients, control of refractory disease in 73%, lessening of fistula formation in 63% and overall achievement of treatment goals in 72%[11]. Thus, although a synergistic effect of azathioprine and corticosteroids is not yet proven, the combination of the two agents, at low doses of the steroid, is probably wise.

Whether this also holds in the maintenance situation is unclear. Two[9,10] but not a third[6] trial suggested a significant superiority of azathiopirne in maintaining remission and many of the patients were treated in parallel with corticosteroids. Again, in the large negative study by Summers et al.[6], the patients did not receive comedication with steroids and the dose of azathioprine at 1 mg/kg body weight per day was lower than in most other treatment regimes (2–4 mg/kg body weight per day).

The trials using azathioprine in ulcerative colitis are fewer and less conclusive. Conspicuously, both studies in patients with acute relapse failed to detect a significant benefit[12,13] whereas two trials focusing on patients with chronic active disease reported significant improvement[14,15]. In an early report, azathioprine was ineffective in both achieving and maintaining a remission[13]. In contrast, patients who had been taking azathioprine for 6 months prior to another trial and who were in remission for at least 2 months displayed a significantly higher relapse rate when withdrawn from the drug (59%) compared with the group continued on the medication (36%)[16].

The benefit of these immunosuppressive agents, which is now generally accepted, has to be weighed against eventual toxicity. In the large experience of Present et al.[17] in 396 patients treated with 6-mercaptopurine based on a mean period of follow-up of 5 years, toxicity included pancreatitis (3.3%), bone marrow depression (2%), allergic reactions (2%) and drug hepatitis (0.3%). All complications were reversible with no mortality. Infectious complications were seen in 7.4% of patients, of which 1.8% were severe. Again, all infections were cured with no deaths. Of the cohort, 3.1% developed neoplasms but only 1 (0.3%), a diffuse histiocytic lymphoma of the brain, had a probable association with the drug.

It may be concluded that azathioprine and 6-mercaptopurine represent a reasonable and reasonably safe medication in otherwise intractable inflammatory bowel disease, provided that surgery is not indicated. However, the precise clinical setting ideal for the drugs is still ill defined and requires further studies. Most importantly, all patients must be carefully monitored to detect potential side-effects early.


## METHOTREXATE

Use of methotrexate, another cytotoxic immunosuppressant, in refractory Crohn disease has been suggested by Kozarek et al[18] in an uncontrolled trial of limited size (Table 2). Nevertheless, this study, reporting an improvement in the majority of patients with chronic active disease, formed the basis for a series of

**Table 2** Methotrexate: uncontrolled trials

| Study | Dose | Duration (months) | *n* | Response |
|---|---|---|---|---|
| **Crohn disease** | | | | |
| Kozarek et al.[18] | 25 mg per week | 3 | 14 | 79% |
| Chamiot-Prieur et al.[19] | 25 mg per week | 6 | 39 | 72% |
| **Ulcerative colitis** | | | | |
| Kozarek et al.[18] | 25 mg per week | 3 | 7 | 71% |

ongoing controlled trials. Methotrexate is administered as weekly intramuscular injections during a 12-week treatment period. Thereafter, the dosage is switched to oral medication in tapered fashion if remission is achieved. Other uncontrolled experience using the same protocol has been published in abstract form[19] and essentially confirmed the original observations. In these 39 French patients, the probability of achieving a remission after 6 months amounted to 72% (life-table analysis). However, 32 of these stopped taking methotrexate because of later treatment failure (51%), toxicity (10%), non-compliance (13%) or prolonged remission (5%). Since experience with the drug in ulcerative colitis is even more limited, a final evaluation of the role of methotrexate in chronic active inflammatory bowel disease clearly awaits full publication of controlled trials. Outside formal clinical studies, the use of this drug is not yet warranted.

## CYCLOSPORIN A

Despite its revolutionary role in transplantation medicine and its well-known mechanism of action, cyclosporin A has only recently been introduced in the field of inflammatory bowel diseases. This hydrophobic undecapeptide is obtained by extraction of the soil fungus, *Tolypocladium infatum gams*. After entering the target cell, the drug binds to cyclophilin, inactivates calcineurin and prevents the nuclear factor of activated T cells (NFAT)-induced transcription of messenger RNA encoding for interleukin-2 and its receptor[20]. In addition, cyclosporin interferes with B cell activation indirectly by suppressing the formation of activating factors by helper T cells. These molecular mechanisms are responsible for the unique selectivity of cyclosporin which acts only on lymphocytes but not on granulocytes, monocytes or macrophages. Since the T cell is currently believed to play a pivotal role in the mucosal inflammatory process[1], the rationale for the use of the drug in these diseases is obvious.

As reviewed recently by Sandborn and Tremaine[20], cyclosporin has been used extensively in uncontrolled trials in both Crohn disease and ulcerative colitis. The number of patients studied ranged from 1 to 32, the dose from 1 to 15 mg/kg body weight per day and the duration of therapy from 2 to 56 weeks. Overall, the impression of rapid clinical response within 1–3 weeks prevailed in the majority of patients and studies but many patients relapsed rapidly after discontinuation of treatment[20]. Our own early encouraging results on fistula treatment[21] are in agreement with several other trials reporting on rapid closure of fistulae in Crohn disease[20] but, again, the success was often not maintained. Of particular interest is the intravenous route which eliminates problems arising in some patients due to inconsistent or poor absorption in those with rapid intestinal transit[22].

The first fully reported controlled trial is that of Brynskov et al. in active chronic Crohn disease[23]. Following a 3-month study period, 59% of cyclosporin-treated but only 32% of placebo patients had improvement ($p$ = 0.032). The effect became evident after 2 weeks. However, during the subsequent 3 months, when the drug was gradually withdrawn, the proportion of patients with improvement dropped to 38%[23] and the benefit was essentially lost after 1 year[24]. The study was criticized because response was measured by a somewhat subjective grading score rather than the standard Crohn's Disease Activity Index (CDAI). In contrast, the other controlled trials were all negative, including the Canadian Crohn's Relapse Prevention Trial[25], the multicentre trial by the Cyclosporin Study Group of Great Britain and Ireland[26] and the European Trial of Cyclosporin in Chronic Active Crohn's Disease[27]. These disappointing results of long-term cyclosporin (3–18 months) in 3 out of 4 trials and the moderate effect of the single positive study do not support a role of cyclosporin in this indication (Table 3).

**Table 3** Cyclosporin A: controlled trials

| | Dose (mg/kg per day) | Duration (months) | $n$ | Overall result |
|---|---|---|---|---|
| **Crohn disease** | | | | |
| *Chronic active disease* | | | | |
| Brynskov et al.[23] | 5–7.5 (oral) | 3 | 71 | CA > P ($p$ = 0.032) |
| Feagan et al.[25] | 5–15 (oral) | 18 | 305 | CA = P |
| Jewell et al.[26] | 5 (oral) | 3 | 147 | CA = P |
| Stange et al.[27] | 5 (oral) | 12 | 182 | CA = P |
| **Ulcerative colitis** | | | | |
| *Severe disease* | | | | |
| Lichtiger et al.[28] | 4 (iv) | Variable | 20 | CA > P ($p$ < 0.001) |

CA: cyclosporin A

In ulcerative colitis, a small controlled trial suggests that intravenous cyclosporin is useful in severe disease[28]. It is still unclear whether this aggressive therapy may indeed avert colectomy or simply postpones and possibly delays the operation. As an alternative to standard therapy, cyclosporin enemas may be applied in treatment-resistant mildly to moderately active left-sided ulcerative colitis[29].

Side-effects are frequent but rarely serious[20]. Paraesthesia (30%) and hypertrichosis (14%) are common, followed in frequency by tremor, hypertension and nausea. Renal insufficiency may occur (7%) but is usually reversible.

Taken together, the data support the use of cyclosporin in very severe disease as a last resort, particularly in fistulating Crohn disease and severe ulcerative colitis. However, patient monitoring has to be very close, indicating that the drug should only be given in centres with particular experience in its prudent use.

## NEW DEVELOPMENTS

An altogether different approach is based on the concept of neutralizing excess local or systemic cytokines or T cells by appropriate monoclonal antibodies. The use of anti-CD4 antibodies has prompted apparent clinical and laboratory response in an uncontrolled study[30] but larger scale experience is missing. A clear-cut explanation concerning the mechanism of action of these antibodies against the CD4-helper cell epitope is lacking. Similarly, an anecdotal report[31] on the beneficial action of anti-TNF antibodies is interesting but the approach is still experimental. Nevertheless, since the number of infiltrating cells in the lamina propria of Crohn disease mucosa producing TNF is high[32], the blockage of this cytokine appears promising. It has to be postulated, however, that TNF plays a key role as an immune mediator and may not be substituted by other cytokines. A general problem limiting the repeated application of these mouse-derived monoclonal antibodies is the development of anti-mouse antibodies. It is hoped that the formulation of hybrid antibodies may help to solve this problem.

Possibly, newer drug developments, like FK 506[33] or rapamycin, may further expand the scope and enhance the effectiveness of immunosuppressive treatment in inflammatory bowel disease. However, the caveat holds that the potential benefit should always be considered in the light of known, and possibly unknown, untoward effects of these aggressive and often long-term treatments. Particularly, in the case of chronic active ulcerative colitis, many patients may prefer to have a definitive operation like a colectomy with ileo-anal pouch.

## References


1. Podolski DK. Inflammatory bowel disease (first of two parts). N Engl J Med. 1991;324:928–37.
2. Linn FV, Peppercorn MA. Drug therapy for inflammatory bowel disease: Part I and Part II. Am J Surg. 1992;164:85–9 and 178–85.
3. Rhodes J, Beck P, Bainton D, Campbell H. Controlled trial of azathioprine in Crohn's disease. Lancet. 1971;2:1273–6.
4. Klein M, Binder HJ, Mitchell M, Aaronson R, Spiro H. Treatment of Crohn's disease with azathioprine: a controlled evaluation. Gastroenterology. 1974;66:916–22.
5. Rosenberg JL, Levin B, Wall AJ, Kirsner JB. A controlled trial of azathioprine in Crohn's disease. Am J Dig Dis. 1975;20:721–6.
6. Summers RW, Switz DM, Sessions JT et al. National Cooperative Crohn's Disease Study: results of drug treatment. Gastroenterology. 1979;77:847–69.
7. Present DH, Korelitz BI, Wisch N, Glass JL, Sachar DB, Pasternack BS. Treatment of Crohn's disease with 6-mercaptopurine. A long-term, randomized, double-blind study. N Engl J Med. 1980;302:981–7.
8. Ewe K, Press AG, Singe CC et al. Azathioprine combined with prednisolone or monotherapy with prednisolone in active Crohn's disease. Gastroenterology. 1993;105:367–72.
9. O'Donoghue DP, Dawson AM, Powell-Tuck J, Bown RL, Lennard-Jones JL. Double-blind withdrawal trial of azathioprine as maintenance treatment for Crohn's disease. Lancet. 1978;2:955–7.
10. Willoughby JMT, Beckett J, Kumar P, Dawson AM. Controlled trial of azathioprine in Crohn's disease. Lancet. 1971;2:944–6.
11. O'Brien JJ, Bayless TM, Bayless JA. Use of azathioprine or 6-mercaptopurine in the treatment of Crohn's disease. Gastroenterology. 1991;101:39–46.
12. Caprilli R, Carratu R, Babbini M. A double-blind comparison of the effectiveness of azathioprine and sulphasalazine in idiopathic proctocolitis. Am J Dig Dis. 1975;20:115–20.
13. Jewell DP, Truelove SC. Azathioprine in ulcerative colitis: final report on a controlled therapeutic trial. Br Med J. 1974;4:627–30.

14. Kirk AP, Lennard-Jones JE. Controlled trial of azathioprine in chronic ulcerative colitis. Br Med J. 1982;284:1291–2.

15. Rosenberg JL, Wall AJ, Levin B, Binder HJ, Kirsner JB. A controlled trial of azathioprine in the management of chronic ulcerative colitis. Gastroenterology. 1975;69:96–9.

16. Hawthorne AB, Logan RFA, Hawkey CJ et al. Randomized controlled trial of azathioprine withdrawal in ulcerative colitis. Br Med J. 1992;305:20–2.

17. Present DH, Meltzer STJ, Krumholz MP, Wolke A, Korelitz BI. 6-Mercaptopurine in the management of inflammatory bowel disease: short- and long-term toxicity. Ann Intern Med. 1989;111:641–9.

18. Kozarek RA, Patterson DJ, Gelfand MD, Botoman VA, Ball TJ, Wilske KR. Methotrexate induces clinical and histologic remission in patients with refractory inflammatory bowel disease. Ann Intern Med. 1989;110:353–6.

19. Chamiot-Prieur C, Lémann M, Mesnard B et al. Treatment of refractory Crohn's disease (CD) with methotrexate (MTX) [abstract]. Gastroenterology. 1993;104:A2140.

20. Tremaine WJ, Sandborn WJ. Cyclosporine treatment of inflammatory bowel disease. Mayo Clin Proc. 1992;67:981–90.

21. Stange EF, Fleig W, Rehklau E, Dischuneit H. Ciclosporin A treatment in inflammatory bowel disease. Dig Dis Sci. 1989;34:1387–92.

22. Hanauer STB, Smith MB. Rapid closure of Crohn's disease fistulas with continuous intravenous ciclosporin A. Am J Gastroenterol. 1993;88:646–9.

23. Brynskov J, Freund L, Rasmussen SN et al. A placebo-controlled, double-blind, randomized trial of cyclosporine therapy in active chronic Crohn's disease. N Engl J Med. 1989;321:845–50.

24. Brynskov J, Freund L, Norby R et al. Final report on a placebo-controlled, double-blind, randomized, multicentre trial of cyclosporin treatment in active chronic Crohn's disease. Scand J Gastroenterol. 1991;26:689–95.

25. Feagan BG, McDonald JWD, Rochon J et al. for the Canadian Crohn's Relapse Prevention Trial Investigators. Low-dose cyclosporine for treatment of Crohn's disease. N Engl J Med. 1994;330:1846–51.

26. Jewell DP, Lennard-Jones JE and the Cyclosporin Study Group of Great Britain and Ireland. Oral cyclosporin for chronic active Crohn's disease: a multicentre controlled trial. Eur J Gastroenterol Hepatol. 1994;6:499–505.

27. Stange EF, Modigliani R, Peña AS et al. and the European Study Group. European trial of cyclosporin in chronic active Crohn's disease: a 12 month study. Gastroenterology. [in press].

28. Lichtiger S, Present DH, Kornbluth A et al. Cyclosporin in severe ulcerative colitis refractory to steroid therapy. N Engl J Med. 1994;330:1841–5.

29. Sandborne WJ, Tremaine WI, Schroeder KW, Steiner BL, Batts KP, Lawson GM. Cyclosporine enemas for treatment-resistant, mildly to moderately active, left-sided ulcerative colitis. Am J Gastroenterol 1993;88:640–5.

30. Emmrich J, Seyfarth M, Emmrich F. Anti-CD4-antibody therapy. In: Stange EF, ed. Chronic inflammatory bowel disease. Lancaster: Kluwer Academic Publishers; 1995:136–40.

31. Derkx B, Taminiau J, Radema S et al. Tumor-necrosis-factor antibody treatment in Crohn's disease. Lancet. 1993;342:173–4.

32. Woywodt A, Neustrock P, Kruse A et al. Cytokine expression in intestinal mucosal biopsies. In situ hybridisation of the mRNA for interleukin-1$\beta$, interleukin-6 and tumor necrosis factor-$\alpha$ in inflammatory bowel disease. Eur Cytokine Netw. 1994;5:387–95.

33. Bierer BE, Mattila PS, Standaert RF et al. Two distinct signal transmission pathways in T lymphocytes are inhibited by complexes formed between an immunophilin and either FK 506 or rapamycin. Immunology. 1990;87:9231–5.

# 23
# Nutrition and diet

## H. LORENZ-MEYER

---

Signs of malnutrition ranging from weight loss, cachexia, anaemia, hypovitaminosis (predominantly due to vitamin $B_{12}$, D and A deficiencies), hypalbuminaemia, growth retardation, electrolyte and trace-element deficiencies are relatively common in patients with Crohn disease. In contrast, they are rather rare in patients with ulcerative colitis.

The reasons for their development are, on the one hand, anorexia, nausea and vomiting, abdominal pain and restrictive diets prescribed by the physician, and, on the other hand, catabolic effects of inflammation and treatment.

Functional disorders of the gastrointestinal tract, such as bacterial overpopulation of the small bowel, atrophy of the intact absorption epithelium, pancreatic failure and loss of bile acids, are of particular importance. Also of importance is the loss of the absorbing surface, partly due to direct inflammation and partly as a result of surgical resections (see Table 1).

**Table 1**  Reasons for malnutrition in chronic inflammatory bowel disease

Insufficient intake
    Anorexia, disturbed sense of taste, aversion, abdominal pain, diarrhoea, nausea, vomiting, restrictive diets

Malabsorption
    Impaired digestive function as a result of loss of bile acids and bacterial proliferation
    Impaired absorbent surface as a result of bowel disease and/or after surgical resections
    Drug-induced malabsorption (steroids: calcium; SASP: folate; cholestyramine: vitamins A, D, E, K)

Increased gastrointestinal loss
    Exudative enteropathy
    Gastrointestinal bleeding
    Loss of electrolytes and trace elements

Increased nutritive requirements
    In fever, fistulae, infections
    Corticosteroid therapy
    Replacement of lost body reserves

After Perkal and Seashore[1]

Thus, nutritive deficiency is a result of insufficient oral intake, malabsorption, increased intestinal loss and increased requirements.

With regard to the various nutrients, the following occurs in Crohn disease:

*Carbohydrate-deficiency symptoms* are observed in 16–40% of adults and children suffering from Crohn disease; secondary lactose intolerance is seen in 35% of patients with active Crohn disease[1].

*Insufficient fat intake and absorption* are noticed above all from a caloric point of view and may also lead to deficiencies in fat-soluble vitamins (A, D, E, K). Clinically speaking, the absorption disorder may be accompanied by steatorrhoea, which is observed in 30–40% of those affected[1].

*Disorders in protein absorption* are caused, for example, by an exudative enteropathy which, in turn, is caused by inflammatory exudation of the diseased bowel wall. This disorder occurs in 50–70% of patients suffering from active Crohn disease and may be demonstrated by faecal $^{51}$Cr excretion or, now even better, by $\alpha_1$-antitrypsin excretion[1,2].

Malnutrition also leads to disturbed iron, electrolyte and trace-element uptake. The cause of this and the effects on the patients are as follows:

*Iron*: Loss occurs due to intestinal bleeding and expenditure in the inflammatory process and may best be recorded by serum ferritin determination ($< 18$ mg/ml)[1].

*Electrolytes*: Calcium deficiency is found in 13% of those affected, potassium deficiency in 6–20% and magnesium deficiency in 14–33%, caused by absorption disorders and diarrhoea; osteoporosis and neurological symptoms are the results of these conditions[1].

*Trace elements*: relevant above all is a developing zinc deficiency, observed in 40–50% of patients. $Cu^{2+}$ deficiency is more rare. These deficiencies lead to varied symptoms, such as anaemia and disorders in taste, growth and wound healing.

*Vitamin deficiency states* also develop with long-term nutritive deficiency. For example, vitamin $B_{12}$ deficiency is observed in 48% of cases, vitamin A deficiency in 11% and folic acid deficiency in 36–54%[1]. Characteristic haematological and neurological symptoms, mucosal damage accompanied by differentiation disorders of the epithelial cells and impaired immuno-competence result and affect the normal course of healing[3].

The question arises as to what role nutrition plays in the development of these conditions and whether a caloric deficiency alone essentially contributes towards the deterioration in the patient's clinical picture. To answer this question, let us first present data on the issue of calorie expenditure and requirements in patients with this consuming syndrome.

Thorough investigations of patients suffering from Crohn disease have shown that these patients do not deviate from standard calorie expenditure[4]. The authors could show that there is a close linear 1:1 correlation between resting energy expenditure (REE), measured using indirect calometry, and predicted

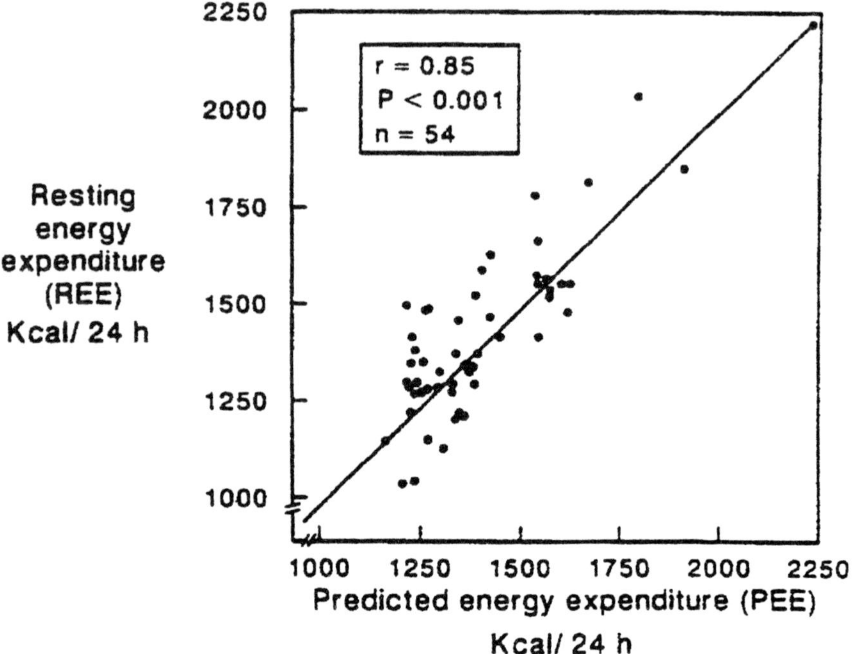



**Figure 1**   Resting energy expenditure (kcal/24 h), calculated using indirect calometry, and plotted against predicted energy expenditure (kcal/24 h), calculated using the Harris–Benedict formula[4]

energy expenditure (PEE), which was calculated for healthy controls (see Figure 1), i.e. an average of 25 ± 4 kcal/kg per 24 h. On the other hand, the patients showed an inverse relationship between the REE and the deviation in per cent from ideal body weight, i.e. patients with the highest weight deficiency also had the greatest energy expenditure. This fits in with the observation that patients suffering from Crohn disease show an elevated REE (when related to the fat-free mass (FFM))[5]. A significant correlation with CDA, C-reactive protein and oro-somucoid could be demonstrated.

More recent investigations of patients suffering from Crohn disease using the combined body scan technique show a total energy expenditure of 33 kcal/kg per day, 70% of which is used for REE, 10% for food-induced thermogenesis (irrespective of the type of calorie intake) and the remaining 20% for energy requirements for movement[6]. There is also an inverse relationship between the disease activity and the energy expenditure required for movement, making total expenditure appear stable, independent of the inflammatory activity.

Investigations carried out by Smith et al.[7] on underweight patients (including those with Crohn disease) showed that energy equilibrium on 2-week glucose substitution is reached with an intake of 40 kcal/kg and that 1.8 g/kg per day of protein is required to prevent loss of body proteins. Thus, the actual require-ment is 1.6 times higher than the calorie expenditure spontaneously measured on the patients (REE, see above). In the case of patients with an active episode who were successfully administered total parenteral nutrition, the resting energy expenditure (REE), related to the fat-free mass, normalized[5]. It thus appears to be an important therapeutic concept to bring patients with this disease picture into energy equilibrium by controlled intake of deficient nutrients, a measure which has led to the definition 'nutritional support'. This method of treatment is an alternative to the usual conservative drug treatment. It is also important in preoperative preparation for planned interventions as it contributes essentially to increasing the number of successful operations.

The principles of nutritional support are total parenteral nutrition (TPN) and total enteral nutrition (TEN) with elemental diets (oligopeptide diets) or with polymeric diets. Both procedures achieve nearly the same rates of remission, although TEN has the advantage of being easier to administer and having fewer side-effects while retaining the intestinal mucosa barrier[8].

## HOW CAN THE EFFECT OF NUTRITIONAL SUPPORTS BE EXPLAINED?

*Bowel rest*? This concept, which was developed at the beginning of the 1970s, is too mechanistic and has proven to be no longer sustainable.

*Do they affect the intestinal flora*? This is difficult to prove but does probably occur. The composition of stool micro-organisms, rather than their number, is affected[9].

*Do they cause a change in immunological reactions*? A reduced supply of intestinally active immunogens was the principle of the oligopeptide diets[9]. The success of polymeric diets with a high proportion of potential immunogens disproves the theory that this reduced supply plays an important role.

*Do they cause a change in intestinal permeability*? This was demonstrated experimentally in Crohn patients, particularly in the active episode[10–12]. Altered permeability possibly plays a role in the pathogenesis of Crohn disease. Thus, an increase in intestinal permeability precedes a relapse[12].

*Do they have purely dietary effects*? They are certainly of the utmost importance for the improvement of the clinical picture.

## WHAT TYPES OF DIETARY TREATMENT ARE SUITABLE FOR TREATMENT OF THE ACUTE SYMPTOMS?

The use of TPN as a supportive therapeutic concept has become established in the clinical sphere, particularly in the case of severe chronic inflammatory bowel disease. However, there are no good controlled studies in the literature on the effect of TPN alone, and relevant effects of a concomitant drug therapy have never been excluded in published studies. It can be demonstrated that

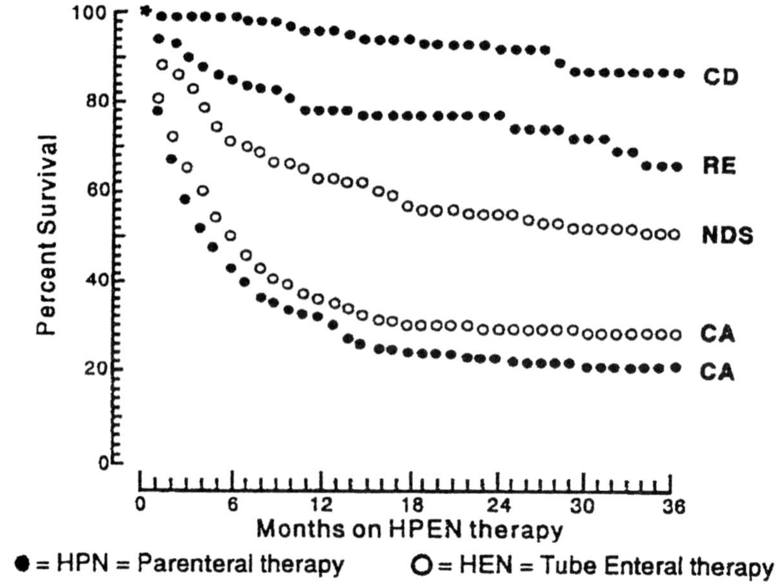


**Figure 2**   Survival curve on HPEN for 4 years. CD = Crohn disease, RE = radiation enteritis, NDS = neurological disturbances in swallowing, CA = cancer patients[13]

TPN causes an increase in weight, an improvement in anthromorphic values and nitrogen balance, and an increase in serum protein[1]. Retrospective studies have postulated that preoperative TPN reduces the risk of septic complications; however, no prospective studies are available on this subject. Some further positive effects of TPN may be seen as definite: comparative studies investigating the duration of remissions achieved by TPN indicate a nearly equally good effect with TPN as with TEN[8]. Home TPN was more successful in patients with Crohn disease than in comparable patients suffering from radiation enteritis, neurological disease and even cancer (see Figure 2)[13]. On the other hand, in the case of acute colitis (UC and Crohn disease), no relevant effect on the actual course of the disease could be found with TPN, although patients treated with TPN had better values of body protein than their controls[14].

It should be remembered that this type of nutritive support is particularly tricky and has an increased risk of complications due to the requirements of parenteral access and sterile supply.

The efficacy of total enteral nutrition (TEN) may be assessed as better than TPN, as demonstrated by a number of good, controlled studies on the subject[15–17]. According to these studies, this form of nutritive support is effective in treating Crohn disease, although it is not as good as steroids. Patients with small bowel involvement and who are suffering from stenosis profit the most[16]. In addition, long-term treatment with elemental diets leads to a clear improvement in intestinal permeability[10].

## DIETS IN THE REMISSION PHASE

Whereas nutrition therapy is of definite value in the acute phase of Crohn disease, this is not the case for the remission phase. In the past, two approaches have received particular attention and will be discussed here: the *elimination diet* and the *carbohydrate-reduced diet* or the *refined carbohydrate-reduced diet*.

In 1985, Jones et al.[18] presented the results of an individually balanced diet. After obtaining remission with TPN or TEN, each patient was examined to see whether various nutrients were tolerated or whether they triggered intolerance reactions. If the latter was the case, they were eliminated from the patient's diet and the patient was instructed to include only the tolerated foods in his diet. In this study, the patients given such advice showed much better results than the patients in a control group who had a high-fibre, refined-carbohydrate-reduced diet (see Figure 3). A study with the same design carried out by the Ulm Group could not confirm these findings[19]. In addition, it was seen in a detailed check of the tested intolerances that these did not remain stable over a long period of time. Rather, they disappeared, with the exception of intolerance to a few foods, such as citrus fruits which are known to be poorly tolerated by patients with this clinical picture[19] (see Figure 4). Thus, the individualized elimination diet could not fulfil expectations.

Great hope was placed on a reduction in carbohydrates, especially refined ones, in the diet of patients suffering from Crohn disease after a series of epidemiological studies in the mid-70s showed that patients suffering from Crohn disease had a particular preference for sweets, bread, cakes and pastries. A large multicentre study included Crohn patients of every degree of activity and super-

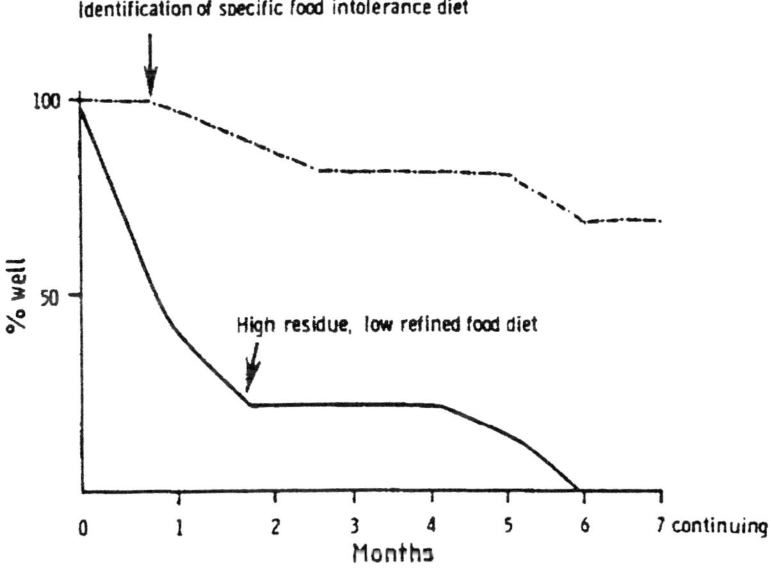


**Figure 3**  Length of remission, in months, of patients in a controlled trial[18]

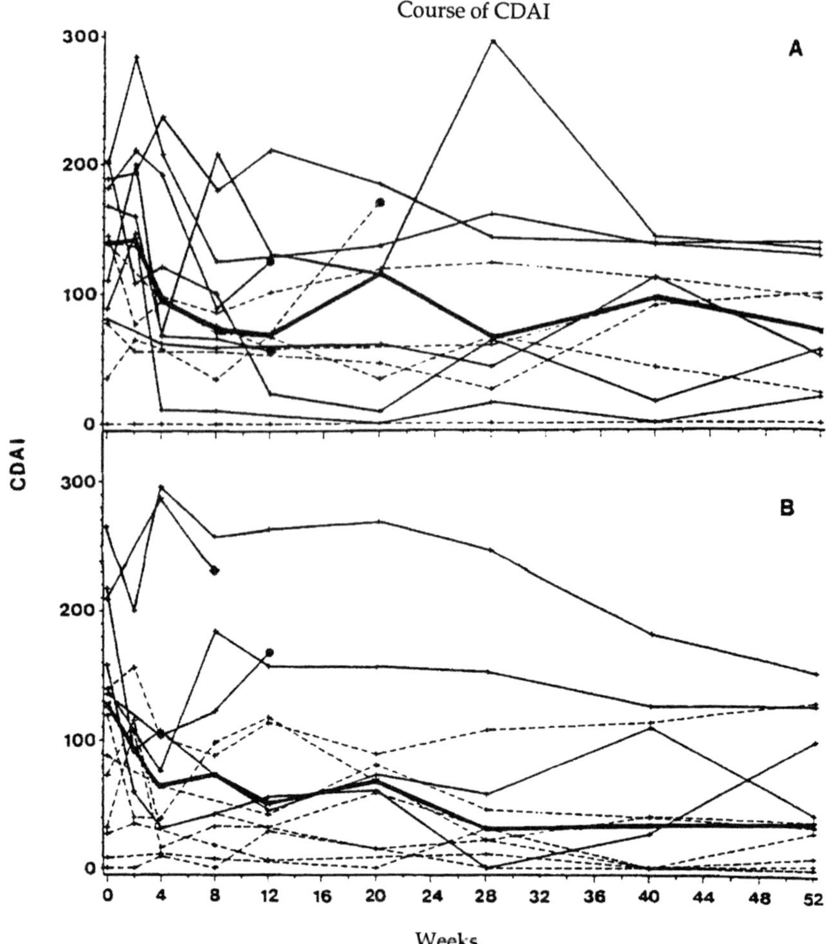



**Figure 4** Course of Crohn disease activity index (CDAI) in two dietary groups. A: Elimination diet. B: Low-sugar high-fibre diet. ● Remission (remission group, dotted line) or operation due to significant deterioration (chronic active group, continuous line). ♦ Discontinuation, emphasized line: median curve[19]

vised the diet of the two comparison groups over a period of 2 years. One group received a high-fibre diet with reduced intake of refined carbohydrates; the other group a diet with a clearly lower fibre proportion but with a greater amount of refined carbohydrates. The acceptability of the first diet was clearly poorer, and the clinical findings in patients with such a diet were no better. A dietary recommendation for patients in remission could not be deduced from the study's findings[20] (see Figure 5).

Another approach was used in the European Crohn Study V[21]. In this study, the effect of omega-3-FS was tested on Crohn disease in remission (and was disappointing). In a further arm of this multicentre study, patients were random-

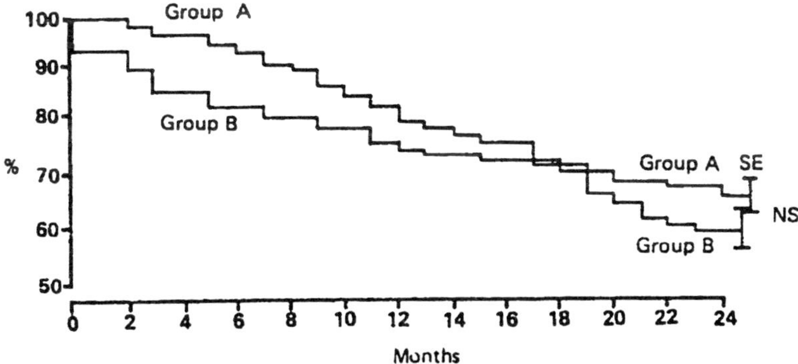



**Figure 5** Cumulative probability (%) of a deterioration in the disease due to reaching one of the end points defined in the trial protocol[20]. Group A: normal intake of refined carbohydrate, reduced intake of dietary fibre; Group B: reduced intake of refined carbohydrate, increased intake of dietary fibre

ized to a carbohydrate-reduced diet (if they came out of an acute phase of their disease with conventional steroid treatment), advised on their diet and monitored for a year in comparison with a control group which received a 'normal' diet. These patients showed better results than their controls when they adhered to the dietary recommendations but very rapidly experienced a new episode when they deviated from them, making differentiation from their controls then impossible. It proved to be difficult to persuade the patients to adhere to this regimen, even when they were in good health[21] (see Figure 6).

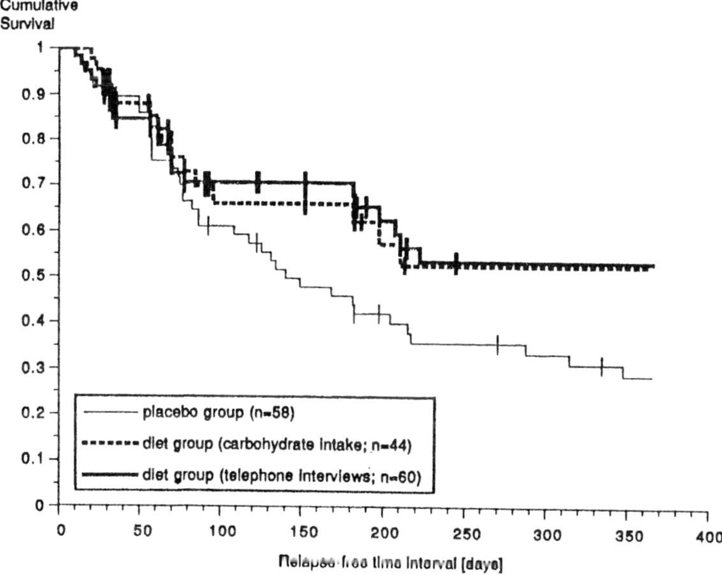



**Figure 6** Distribution of relapse-free time intervals of the diet group vs placebo group, cases in compliance with the protocol marked[21]

Thus, these observations cause us to question whether patients are willing to adhere to dietary recommendations even when they experience a positive response. Thus, one of the main problems of long-term dietary therapy is and will remain compliance, a fact we already know from other diseases which may be controlled by diet.

Ulcerative colitis appears to have drawn the short straw in this chapter. However, patients with this clinical picture usually have fewer nutritive problems, apart from those cases with a severe course, with catabolic situations which are refractory to therapy. In these cases, the same rule applies as for treatment of active Crohn disease. A dietary guideline for remission of ulcerative colitis cannot be explicitly given, apart from the recommendation to avoid food which is poorly tolerated, even by people with healthy bowels.

## References


1. Perkal MF, Seashore JH. Nutrition and inflammatory bowel disease. In: Fisher RL, ed. Malabsorption and nutritional status and support. Gastroenterology clinics of North America. Vol 18, No 3;1989:567–78.
2. Meyers S, Wolke A, Field SP, Feuer EJ, Johnson JW, Janowitz HJ. Fecal $\alpha_1$-antitrypsin measurements: an indicator of Crohn's disease activity. Gastroenterology. 1985;89:13–18.
3. Lorenz-Meyer H. Ist eine Substitution von Vitaminen und Spurenelenmenten notwendig? In: Kuris W, Feifel G, eds. Colitis ulcerosa, Morbus Crohn: interdisziplinäre Therapie in Klinik und Praxis. Berlin, New York: Acron-Verl.; 1990:61–71.
4. Chan ATH, Fleming CR, O'Fallon WM, Huigenza KA. Estimated versus measured basal energy requirements in patients with Crohn disease. Gastroenterology. 1986;91:75–8.
5. Rigaud D, Cerf M, Angel-Alberto L, Sobhani I, Carduner MJ, Mignon M. Increase of resting energy expenditure during flare-ups in Crohn disease. Gastroenterol Clin Biol. 1993;17:932–7.
6. Stokes MA, Hill GL. Total energy expenditure in patients with Crohn's disease: Measurements by the combined body scan techniques. J Parenteral Enteral Nutr. 1993;17:3–7.
7. Smith RC, Burkinshaw L, Hill GL. Optimal energy and nitrogen intake for gastroenterological patients requiring intravenous nutrition. Gastroenterology. 1982;82:445–52.
8. Greenberg GR. Nutritional support in inflammatory bowel disease: current status and future directions. Scand J Gastroenterol. Suppl. 1992;192:117–22.
9. Lorenz-Meyer H. Synthetische Diäten and Sondenernährung. In: Caspary W, ed. Handbuch der Inneren Medizin, Dünndarm. Berlin, Heidelberg, New York: Springer–Verlag; 1983:669–88.
10. Theahon K, Smethurst P, Pearson M, Levi AJ, Bjarnason I. The effect of elemental diet in intestinal permeability and inflammation in Crohn's disease. Gastroenterology. 1991,101:84–9.
11. Adenis A, Colombel JF, Lecouffe P et al. Increased pulmonary and intestinal permeability in Crohn's disease. Gut. 1992;33:678–82.
12. Wyatt J, Vogelsang H, Hübl W, Waldhöer T, Lochs H. Intestinal permeability and the prediction of relapse in Crohn's disease. Lancet. 1993;341:1437–9.
13. Howard L. Home parenteral and enteral nutrition in cancer patients. Cancer Suppl. 1993;72:3531–41.
14. Dickinson RJ, Ashton MG, Axon ATR, Smith RC, Yeung CH, Hill GL. Controlled trial of intravenous hyperalimentation and total bowel rest as an adjunct to the routine therapy of acute colitis. Gastroenterology. 1980;79:1199–204.
15. O'Morain C, Segal AW, Levi AJ. Elemental diets in treatment of acute Crohn's disease. A controlled trial. Br Med J. 1984;288:1859–62.
16. Malchow H, Steinhardt HJ, Lorenz-Meyer H et al. Feasibility and effectiveness of a defined formula diet regimen in treating active Crohn's disease. European Cooperative Crohn's disease Study III. Scand J Gastroenterol. 1990;25:235–44.
17. Lochs H, Steinhardt HJ, Klaus-Wentz B et al. Comparison of enteral nutrition and drug treatment in active Crohn's disease. Results of the European Cooperative Crohn's disease Study IV. Gastroenterology. 1991;101:881–8.
18. Jones VA, Dickinsons RJ, Workam E, Wilson AJ, Freeman AH, Hunter JO. Crohn's disease: maintenance of remission by diet. Lancet. 1985;2:177–80.

19. Stange EF, Schmid U, Fleig WE, Ditschuneit H. Ausschlußbdiät bei Morbus Crohn: eine kontrollierte, randomisierte Studie. Z Gastroenterol. 1990;28:561–4.
20. Ritchie JK, Wadsworth J, Lennard-Jones JE, Rogers E. Controlled multicentre therapeutic trial of an unrefined carbohydrate, fibre rich diet in Crohn's disease. Br Med J. 1987;295:517–20.
21. Lorenz-Meyer H, Purrmann J, Scheurlen C et al. Crohn Study V: Results of a trial with n-3 PUFAs or carbohydrate-reduced diet for maintenance of remission in Crohn's disease (Abstr). In: Schölmerich J, Goebell H, Kruis W, Hohenberger W, Gross V, eds. Inflammatory bowel diseases: Pathophysiology as basis of treatment. Dordrecht/Boston/London: Kluwer Academic Publishers; 1993:549.

# 24
# Efficacy of psychosomatic therapy in Crohn disease

**W. KELLER, W. OSBORN, P. SCHEIB, G. JANTSCHEK and THE GERMAN STUDY GROUP 'PSYCHOSOCIAL INTERVENTION IN CROHN'S DISEASE', BERLIN, FREIBURG, GIESSEN, LÜBECK***

## STATEMENT OF THE PROBLEM

The influence of psychological factors in the pathogenesis and course of Crohn disease is a matter of dispute[1-6].

The chronic course and sometimes very severe clinical symptomatology of Crohn disease have marked effects on the social interrelationships and life perception of patients with this disease, many of whom are young. This can lead to difficulties in managing and coping with the disease[7-11]. The extent to which concomitant psychotherapeutic measures can alter the course of disease in Crohn patients is still an open question.

The lack of prospective studies in this field is essentially due to methodological problems, but also to the occasionally serious difficulties in communication

***Medical University, Lübeck:**
Department of Psychosomatic Medicine and Psychotherapy: Prof. Dr. H. Feiereis, Dr. J.v. Wietersheim, PD Dr. F. Balck, PD Dr. Jantschek.
**Free University of Berlin, Benjamin Franklin Clinic:**
Department of Psychosomatic Medicine and Psychotherapy: Prof. H. H. Studt, Prof. H.-C. Deter, Dr. W. Keller, Dipl.Psych. R. Dilg. Medical Clinic: Prof. Dr. E. O. Riecken, Prof. Dr. M. Zeitz, Dr. M. Vallo-Wermes.
**Justus-Liebig University, Giessen:**
Centre for Psychosomatic Medicine: Dipl.Psych. E. Schmelz-Schumacher, Dipl.Psych. W. Osborn. Medical Polyclinic: Prof. H.-U. Klör.
**Albert-Ludwigs University, Freiburg:**
Department of Psychosomatic Medicine and Psychotherapy: Prof. Dr. M. Wirsching, Dipl.Psych. P. Scheib, T. Bay, Dr. C. Scheidt, Dr. K. Fritzsche, O. Rayki. Department of Internal Medicine II: PD Dr. J. Rasenack.
**Centre for methodological support of therapeutic studies (ZMBT) Heidelberg:**
Dipl.Math. M. Pritsch, M. Holzmeier.

between specialists in psychosomatic medicine and somatically oriented physicians[12].

Despite this, the treatment of patients with Crohn disease is often regarded as a 'chronic interdisciplinary problem'[13]. This is because difficulties often arise during treatment in relation to the way patients manage their disease, their behaviour in relation to the disease, and the psychological, social and interpersonal problems arising as reactions to the disease. In many cases, therefore, in association with additional predisposing personality factors, there is a clinical indication for psychotherapy despite the lack of satisfactory empirical confirmation. It cannot of course be generally assumed that the mere fact of suffering from Crohn disease represents an indication for psychotherapeutic treatment. A study by Andrews[4] demonstrated a correlation between the extent of psychopathology and an unfavourable disease course.

Kordy and Norman[11], in a prospective study, demonstrated a correlation between coping style and prolonged duration of acute episodes. There is, however, a lack of further studies on the significance of disease-coping strategies in Crohn disease.

The sometimes profound communication problems and reservations that separate gastroenterologists from specialists in psychosomatic medicine still stand in the way of an interdisciplinary approach to treatment combining internal medicine with psychosomatic treatment.

Despite this, combined medical and psychosomatic therapy has been given in the German Federal Republic for many years, based on clinical experience of inpatient treatment[14,15]. In most university departments of psychosomatic medicine, and in many rehabilitation clinics, selected patients with Crohn disease have received supplementary psychosomatic treatment with clinical success. Of course, the selection mechanisms operating in such institutions create a specialized patient population, so that these patients are not representative of the Crohn patients seen in a gastroenterological clinic[16].

The indication for psychosomatic diagnosis and (if appropriate) treatment, as derived from clinical experience, are shown in Table 1 (see also Reference 17).

Social problems, unusual behaviour in relation to the disease, psychological symptoms, disparity between subjective complaints and objective findings, a tendency to withdraw to the point of social isolation, lack of insight into the disease, impaired physician/patient relationships with problems in compliance, are the commonest indications for psychosomatic diagnosis and treatment.

Despite wide clinical experience of the interdisciplinary treatment of Crohn disease patients, no prospective controlled longitudinal studies have so far been

**Table 1**  Clinical indications for psychosomatic diagnosis and psychotherapy

- Clinical evidence of emotional disturbance
- 'Difficult' or behaviourally disturbed patients
- Problems of compliance
- Problems with the physician–patient relationship
- Indication of psychosocial conflicts
- Severe continuous underlying disease
- Serious causative events
- The patient wants psychotherapy

carried out that could have provided empirical confirmation of the efficacy of combined medical and psychosomatic treatment, and a differential indication for concomitant psychosomatic treatment. It also remains an open question whether the physical course of disease can be influenced by psychosomatic measures. The reason for this lack of research, in a disease with such a heterogeneous clinical course, lies partly in methodological problems, such as the operational adoption of target criteria or efficacy parameters that are both suitable and sensitive to change; or patient compliance problems in longer-term studies; and partly in the lack of adequate forms of co-operation between somatically and psychosomatically oriented physicians. Finally, mention should also be made here of the lack of adequate financial support for such longitudinal studies, which are demanding in terms of both staff and equipment.

There are, so far, only three prospective psychosomatic intervention studies in the literature[18–20]; and even these can only be regarded as pilot studies, in view of the small case numbers and also, to some extent, for methodological reasons.

The German Study Group "Psychosocial Intervention in Crohn's Disease" investigated some of these open questions in a prospective controlled multicentre study of 'The Efficacy of Psychotherapeutic Measures in Crohn's Disease'. This study, with its demanding design, was financially aided by the Federal Ministry of Research and Technology (BMFT). The study plan presented here follows the design of a drug study. Although such a design has methodological advantages and allows interdrug comparisons, it probably has a relatively adverse effect on the efficacy of psychotherapy, for instance because randomization causes the motivation factor to be lost, and randomization itself probably has a negative effect on the physician–patient relationship[21].

Publication of the principal results is in preparation. However, the study design and some aspects of this multicentre Crohn disease study will be described below.

The principal question addressed by the study was:

Do psychotherapeutic measures, when used together with standard somatic therapy, influence the course of disease in patients with Crohn disease?


## METHODS

For purposes of inference–statistical measurement, we defined one somatic and one psychosocial target criterion:

1.  A confirmatory evaluation of the somatic course of the disease, over a two-year observation period. For this purpose, the course of disease in all Crohn patients was ordered in ranked sequence using a ranking scheme.

2.  Confirmatory evaluation of the patients' psychosocial state, using a variety of measuring instruments, one year after randomization, after completion of psychotherapy.

The relevant hypotheses were formulated as follows:

1.  Patients who are treated with a combination of standardized somatic therapy and additional psychotherapeutic measures have a better disease course than patients in a control group receiving only standardized therapy.

2.   Patients receiving additional psychotherapy show a better psychosocial state after the first year (end of psychotherapy).

A patient's psychosocial state can only be assessed at several levels; at the same time, methodological problems affecting the confirmatory evaluation limit the possible number of variables. We defined the psychosocial state with the help of a total score obtained from the following measuring instruments:

Beck depression inventory[22]
Trait anxiety, measured by the STAI[23]
Life satisfaction questionnaire[24]
Psychological and social–communicative findings[25]

Details of all Crohn disease patients from each gastroenterological polyclinic in the four participating centres were recorded using a basic questionnaire. Table 2 shows the inclusion and exclusion criteria.

**Table 2**   Inclusion and exclusion criteria for participation in the study

Inclusion
    Substantiated diagnosis (endoscopy, X-ray, histology)
    Age: 18–55 years
    Active disease in the last 2 years
    Consent

Exclusion
    No episode within 2 years after surgery
    Planned resection
    Immunosuppressive therapy
    Psychotherapy in the last 2 years; thereafter no episode
    Colostomy or ileostomy

A total of 522 patients with Crohn disease were covered by the basic questionnaire. Of these 522 patients, 111 were eligible to be entered into the study and were randomized in accordance with the criteria described above. This represented approximately one fifth of the recorded Crohn disease patients. Eleven patients who insisted that they wished to receive psychotherapy were initially also entered in the study. The reasons for exclusion of the remaining patients not entered in the study are shown below. The most frequent exclusion criteria in rank order were: no acute episode in the last two years (87), refusal to participate in the study (77), and bowel resection followed by no further acute episodes (48), followed approximately equally by: a desire for psychotherapy (25), age over 55 years (25) and planned resection (23).

This therefore represented a selected patient population consisting predominantly of somatically oriented patients, whose attitude to psychotherapy was one of indifference, and who, in all probability, would not have tried to obtain psychotherapy, either of their own accord or at the suggestion of their physician.

The analysis of patients not entered in the study is shown in Table 3.

The original aim of entering and randomizing 200 patients could not be achieved in the time available to us.

**Table 3**  Selection and exclusion (broken down by reasons)

| | |
|---|---|
| Patients covered by a basic questionnaire | 522 |
| Patients not included | 400 |
|   No episode in the last 2 years | 87 |
|   Refusal to participate | 77 |
|   Resection; thereafter no episode | 48 |
|   Desire for psychotherapy | 25 |
|   Age > 55 years | 25 |
|   Planned resection | 23 |
|   No diagnostic confirmation | 21 |
|   Current psychotherapy | 19 |
|   Previous psychotherapy | 18 |
|   Refusal of psychotherapy | 13 |
|   Other drug therapy | 13 |
|   Other diseases | 12 |
|   Missing entries | 11 |
|   Colostomy or ileostomy | 8 |
| Patients included | 122 |
|   Fringe group psychotherapy | 11 |
|   Randomized patients | 111 |

**Table 4**  Standardized somatic therapy and psychotherapeutic measures

Standard somatic therapy
- During an episode (CDAI > 150), prednisolone 60 mg daily in decreasing dosage (according to ECCDS); thereafter, maintenance therapy with 10 mg daily over 4 months
- If no primary activity, no therapy.

Psychotherapeutic measures
- At least 20 therapy sessions, 50–100 min each, of which at least 10 verbal over the course of 1 year
- *Berlin*: Out-patient individual and disease-specific group therapy
  *Giessen* and *Freiburg*: In-depth psychologically oriented short-term therapy
  *Lübeck*: In-patient individual and group therapy, music and associative painting therapy
- At all centres: Additional non-verbal relaxation therapeutic procedures

Randomization: A : B = 1 : 2

Group A: somatic therapy only; group B: somatic therapy plus psychotherapy

## Standard somatic therapy

At the onset of an acute episode of their disease, patients received standard treatment with prednisolone on a reducing dosage schedule in accordance with the guidelines of the European Cooperative Crohn's Disease Study[26] starting with 60 mg prednisolone daily and reducing over the course of six weeks, followed by maintenance therapy with 10 mg daily for four months. As acute episode was defined by a CDAI of over 150 (Table 4).

## Psychotherapeutic measures

The aims of verbal psychotherapy procedures were, firstly, to inform patients about their disease and to support them in managing and coping with it, in order to achieve better adaptation to it; secondly, to address any associated psychological symptoms, such as depression, psychosocial stresses and conflicts, that might be related to the illness.

The psychotherapeutic measures in this study were much harder to standardize. Features common to all centres were a psychodynamic orientation and a short-term treatment concept, combined with a non-verbal relaxation procedure. But the study centres differed with respect to their treatment concepts and focal issues in treatment. This resulted in a difference in the frequency, duration and settings of treatments. A minimum of 20 treatment sessions, each lasting 50–100 min, had to be achieved for each patient, of which at least 10 sessions had to consist of verbal therapy. The total duration was not to exceed one year. In Berlin, out-patient disease-oriented group therapy with associated supportive individual therapy was given. Giessen and Freiburg had in-depth psychologically oriented short-term therapy and a family-therapy oriented approach. Lübeck had an integrated multidimensional in-patient treatment concept lasting some six weeks. The emphasis was on individual and group therapy, and, in addition, music and associative painting therapy were used.

Randomization was carried out using a balanced randomization procedure taking account of the main prognostic factors: acute episode at the time of randomization, previous intestinal resections, pattern of involvement, and patient age.

Allocation to the control group (A) or the psychotherapy group (B) was in a 1:2 ratio. Because of the better standardization of steroid medication, this randomization ratio was regarded as adequate.

The schedule of investigations at the different measurement times over the two years of observation is shown in Figure 1.

At the start and end of the two-year period, patients were subjected to a detailed somatic diagnostic investigation comprising a disease history, physical examination, laboratory tests, CDAI, etc., and diagnostic procedures to determine the extent of disease. Subsequent control investigations were then carried

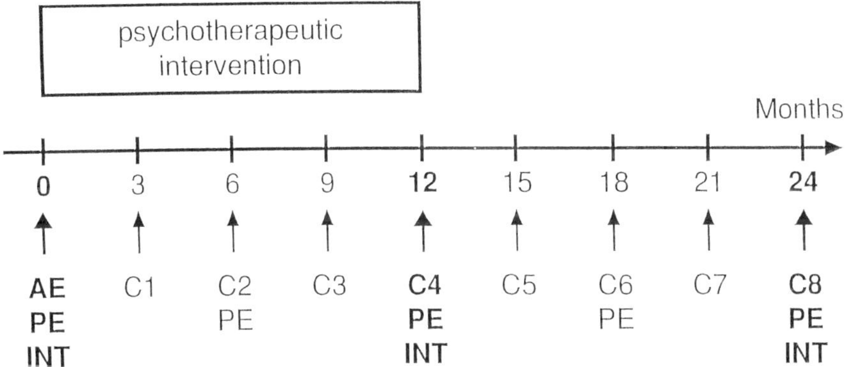


**Figure 1**  Timetable of investigations. AE: admission examination, PE: evaluation of psychosocial instruments; INT: interview; C: control investigations; C8: final examination. Additionally, weekly control examinations were performed during acute episodes

out every three months (physical examination, laboratory tests, CDAI). If an acute episode occurred in the interim, detailed tests were carried out at weekly intervals until the end of the episode. Psychosocial studies were carried out at the beginning of the study, and at one and two years, taking the form of an exhaustive in-depth psychologically oriented history and psychometric testing in order to obtain an assessment of the patient's psychosocial status. Changes in the patient's self-assessment were recorded at half-yearly intervals using a variety of psychometric investigation instruments.

A description of the two comparison groups is shown in Table 5. The control group contained somewhat more younger men, and there were somewhat more patients with large intestinal involvement in the psychotherapy group. Patients in the control group had undergone somewhat more resections. However, all the differences lay within the range of probability of chance occurrences. It can therefore be taken that the two groups were more or less balanced.

Due to the heterogeneous course characteristic of Crohn disease, it was not possible to define a single target criterion, e.g. time spent in acute episodes. We therefore decided to rank the randomized patients according to their disease course at the end of the two-year observation period (Figure 2).

Ranking was carried out blind by the gastroenterologists in the participating centres at the end of the two-year observation period. Four main groups were distinguished.

Category 1, with the worst course, contained patients who required surgery due to disease activity uncontrollable by conservative means, or who had failed on alternative conservative therapy.

Category 2 consisted of patients in whom standard therapy had failed and who had had to be changed to a different form of therapy, e.g. azathioprine.

**Table 5**  Characteristics of the two groups

|  | Group A | Group B |
|---|---|---|
| **Sex** | | |
| Male | 44.8 | 34.6 |
| Female | 55.2 | 65.4 |
| **Age** | | |
| < 25 years | 41.4 | 32.7 |
| 25–35 years | 34.5 | 34.6 |
| > 35 years | 24.1 | 32.7 |
| **Pattern of involvement** | | |
| Small intestine | 17.2 | 11.5 |
| Small and large intestine | 75.5 | 71.2 |
| Large intestine | 6.9 | 17.3 |
| **Previous resections** | | |
| Yes | 41.4 | 25.0 |
| No | 58.5 | 75.0 |

All figures are percentages. Group A: somatic therapy only; group B: somatic therapy plus psychotherapy

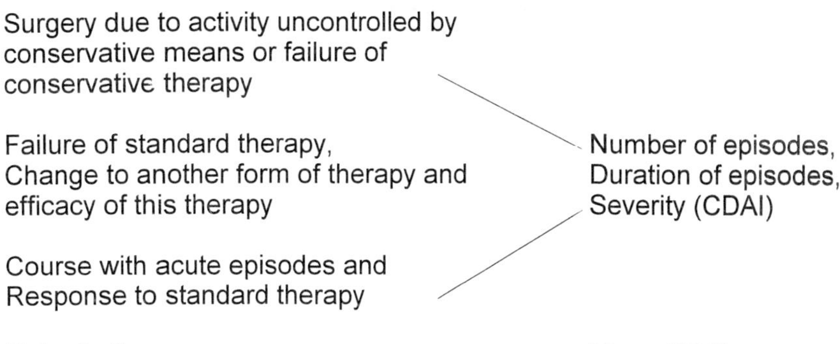


**Figure 2**  Main ranking and subranking for the physical course of the disease

Category 3 contained patients whose disease course showed acute episodes which responded to standard treatment with prednisolone.

Category 4 consisted of patients with an episode-free course.

In addition, disease course in all principal categories was subranked on the basis of the CDAI[27]. Each patient received a rank number depending on the number of acute episodes, their duration, and their severity as measured by the CDAI. At the end of two years, patients' rank numbers were compared between the psychotherapy and control groups.

## RESULTS

It is only possible here to give a descriptive presentation of the results. A full published report is in preparation.

### Principal somatic criteria

Eighty-four of 111 randomized patients were included in the evaluation of the principal somatic criteria. The confirmatory comparison between the psychotherapy and control group demonstrated a trend in favour of the psychotherapy group. Patients receiving psychotherapy had markedly fewer resections.

### Principal psychosocial criteria

The deciding factor with respect to the principal psychosocial criteria was the confirmatory comparison between the two groups at one year. At this point in time, no clear difference could be demonstrated for any of the four selected parameters of psychosocial state. Neither depression, trait anxiety, life satisfaction nor psychological/social communicative findings were different between the psychotherapy and control groups.

Generally speaking, these psychometric features were only expressed to a minor degree, and the question arises whether the selection of test instruments was excessively oriented towards psychopathology.

## Time-course of psychosocial results

Even when viewed longitudinally, the four total scores in the psychotherapy group did not show a clear superiority over the control group. Both groups showed a slight reduction in total scores over the course of time, so that the possibility of non-specific psychotherapeutic effects (a placebo effect) having an influence on the control group must be taken into account.

However, the number of Crohn-related hospital in-patient days over the period from one year before randomization to three years after randomization showed a significant reduction in the psychotherapy group as compared with the control group.

The results of the confirmatory comparison of the two groups are in contrast to the patients' own assessment of the efficacy of psychotherapy.

## Efficacy of psychotherapy as viewed by the patients

The results of self-assessment by the psychosomatically treated patients regarding the efficacy of psychotherapy two years after randomization are shown in Figure 3.

Patients assessed eleven different therapeutic goals. For purposes of presentation of the results, the six-point polar scales have been dichotomized to show two variables: improvement and deterioration. Between two thirds and three quarters of treated patients described an improvement in the physical course of the disease, their psychological health or their coping with their disease, thanks to psychotherapy. They also reported improved coping with conflicts and a good

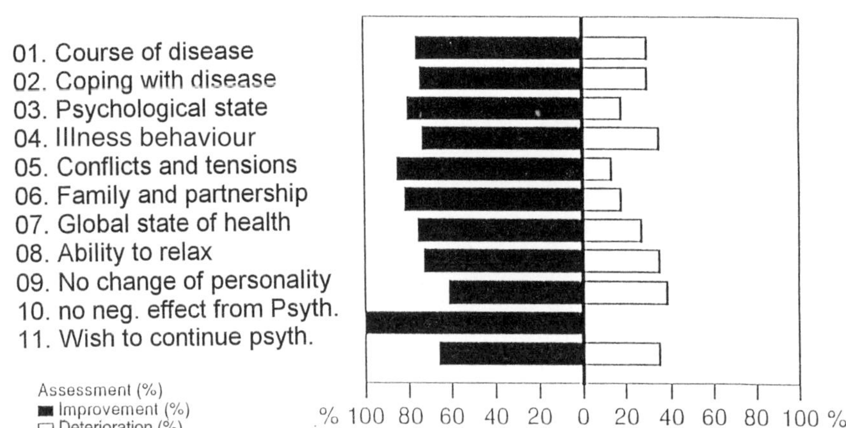


**Figure 3** Percentage of reported improvement or deterioration following psychotherapy, as assessed by patients with Crohn disease, related to eleven different treatment goals. This assessment was made two years after randomization and one year after the end of psychotherapy ($n = 56$)

effect on their interpersonal relationships. About two thirds of patients would have liked to continue psychotherapy. On average, over 70% of patients described beneficial effects of psychotherapy. This is in contrast to the results presented above, relating to the confirmatory comparison between the two groups. In relation to some of the eleven treatment goals, patients' assessments after two years (specifically relating to somatic treatment) reflected significant improvements in the psychotherapy group compared with the control group.

## DISCUSSION

The central result of this study can be summarized as follows: with psychotherapy, a trend towards a better disease course can be observed. The low frequency of surgery in the psychotherapy group led to a significant reduction in Crohn-related hospital in-patient days compared with the control group (Deter *et al.*, unpublished data).

Contrary to our expectations, psychotherapy had no influence worth mentioning on the patients' psychosocial status. This is in contrast with the high degree of satisfaction expressed by the patients receiving psychotherapy with their own perception of the efficacy of psychotherapy in a variety of psychosocial contexts. This might be interpreted as a phenomenon of avoidance of a cognitive dissonance in relation to each patient's experience of the aim and direction of his therapy. However, the different assessments, given by the two groups, of the therapies they experienced make this unlikely.

The present study is the only psychotherapeutic intervention study in Crohn disease to use improvement in the physical course of the disease as a somatic target criterion.

There have only been three prospective intervention studies, but the small numbers of cases involved and other methodological problems mean that these studies have only limited comparability with our own results.

In a pilot study on 31 randomized Crohn-disease patients, the psychotherapeutically treated group showed a trend towards a lower frequency of operations (three operations in the control group and none in the psychotherapy group), and significantly fewer in-patient days[18]. These results are similar to our own.

In another prospective randomized study, 21 patients with ulcerative colitis and Crohn disease were compared with an untreated control group of patients with the same disorders, with respect to the effects of stress management on the disease course[20]. Despite subjectively improved wellbeing, these patients showed no significant changes on the Beck depression inventory or the State-Trait Anxiety Inventory, either in the course of their disease or in comparison with the control group; these findings are comparable to our own results.

As mentioned above, however, the small size of the sample and the methodological limitations (e.g. the lack of standardization of drug treatment and lack of stratification at randomization) impose a limitation on comparability.

Only 84 out of 111 randomized patients were evaluable for the principal somatic criteria. It is possible that a larger sample might have been able to provide statistical confirmation of the trend we were able to demonstrate in favour of the psychotherapy group in respect of the principal somatic criteria. Prolongation of the follow-up period (we originally requested a five-year period) would also have been desirable. This, however, was refused by the sponsors on financial grounds. We still hope to be able to achieve this on a more limited scale at our own expense.

For methodological reasons, psychiatrically ill patients, for whom psychotherapy would have been particularly indicated and relevant, could not be entered into the study because of the exclusion criteria used. Thus, beneficial effects of psychotherapy were made less likely in the remaining patients, who had less-severe psychiatric problems. A relatively high variance in the psychosocial variables might indicate that a proportion of the psychotherapeutically treated group profited from psychotherapy. The literature contains repeated allusions to the need for such treatment, in particular patient subgroups (e.g. Reference 16).

## CONCLUSIONS

The following conclusions can be drawn:

1. Supplementary psychotherapeutic measures showed a trend towards a more favourable disease course in patients with Crohn disease over a two-year observation period. The results just failed to achieve statistical significance.

2. The Crohn-disease patients in this sample showed few psychopathological peculiarities. There was no difference in this respect between the psychotherapy and control groups.

3. The question of whether particular groups of patients profit from concomitant psychotherapy will be further clarified in a later evaluation.

4. Future studies must therefore address in particular the question of differential therapeutic indications, so as to clarify which patients need psychotherapy. In this respect, Crohn disease appears not to differ from other chronic diseases. In addition to quantitative investigations, qualitative aspects should also be taken into account for identification of subgroups that could profit from psychotherapy.

5. Until further results of prospective psychotherapeutic intervention studies in Crohn disease are available, decisions on concomitant psychotherapy should continue to be made on the basis of the clinical indication criteria mentioned at the outset.

## References


1. McKegney FP, Gordon RO, Levine St M. A psychosomatic comparison of patients with ulcerative colitis and Crohn's disease. Psychosom Med. 1970;32:153–66.
2. Latimer PR. Crohn's disease: a review of the psychological and social outcome. Psych Med. 1978;8:649–56.
3. Helzer JE, Chammas S, Norland Ch C, Stillings WA, Alppers DH. A study of the association between Crohn's disease and psychiatric illness. Gastroenterology. 1984;86:324–30.

4. Andrews H, Barczak P, Allan RN. Psychiatric illness in patients with inflammatory bowel disease. Gut. 1987;28:1600–4.

5. Mitchell CM, Drossman DA. Survey of the AGA membership relating to patients with functional gastrointestinal disorders. Gastroenterology. 1987;92:1282–4.

6. North CS, Alpers DH, Helzer JE, Spitznagel EL, Clouse RE. Do life events or depression exacerbate inflammatory bowel disease? Ann Intern Med. 1991;114:381–6.

7. Sørensen VZ, Olsen BC, Binder V. Life prospects and quality of life with Crohn's disease. Gut. 1987;28:382–5.

8. Drossman DA, Patrick DL, Mitchell CM et al. Health-related quality of life in inflammatory bowel disease. Dig Dis Sci. 1989;34:1379–86.

9. Drossman DA, Mitchell CM, Leserman J et al. Psychosocial and disease predictors of utilisation in IBD. Gastroenterology. 1990;98:A167.

10. Drossman DA. Psychosocial factors in inflammatory bowel disease. Pract Gastroenterol. 1993;16:24N-24-U.

11. Kordy H, Norman D. Psychische und somatische Faktoren des Krankheitsverlaufes bei Morbus Crohn. Psychother Psychosom Med Psychol. 1992;42:141–9.

12. Gerbert B. Psychological aspects of Crohn's disease. J Behav Med. 1980;8:649–56.

13. Huchzermeyer H, ed. Chronisch-entzündliche Darmerkrankungen. München: Dustri-Verlag;1983.

14. Feiereis H. Morbus Crohn. In: Uexkull T, Adler R, Herrmann JM, Köhle K, Schonecke OW, Wesiak W eds. Psychosomatische medizin. München: Urban & Schwarzenberg;1990:788–814.

15. Jantschek G. M. Crohn-Psychotherapie: Klinische Anwendung und Grundlagen. In: Gheorghiu Th, Kruis W, eds. Chronisch entzündliche Darmerkrankungen, aktuelle Therapiekonzepte. 3. Interdisziplinares Symposium über chronisch entzündliche Darmerkrankungen. Falk Foundation, Wiesbaden;1992.

16. Deter HC, Rapf M, Gladisch R, Rohner R. Psychodiagnostische Verlaufsuntersuchungen von Morbus-Crohn-Patienten während der internistischen Intensivbehandlung. Z Gastroenterol. 1993;31:703–10.

17. Kiss A, Ferenci P. Psychosomatische Behandlung von Patienten mit M. Crohn. In: Jenss H, ed. Morbus Crohn. Stuttgart–New York: Schattauer;1990.

18. Künsebeck HW, Lempa W, Freyberger H. Kurz- und Langzeiteffekte ergänzender Psychotherapie bei Patienten mit Morbus Crohn. In: Lamprecht F, ed. Spezialisierung und Integration in Psychosomatik und Psychotherapie. Berlin: Springer; 1987:253–62.

19. Milne B, Oachim G, Niedhardt J. A stress management programme for inflammatory bowel disease patients. J Adv Nurs. 1986;11:561–7.

20. Schwarz SP, Blanchard EB. Evaluation of a psychological treatment for inflammatory bowel disease. Behav Res Ther. 1991;29:167–77.

21. Hellman S, Hellman DS. Sounding board – of mice but not men, problems of the randomized clinical trial. N Engl J Med. 1991;324:1585–91.

22. Beck AT, Ward CH, Medelson M, Mock F, Erbaugh F. An inventory of measuring depression. Arch Gen Psychiatry. 1961;4:561–71.

23. Laux L, Schaffner P, Glanzmann P, Spielberger CD. Das State-Trait-Angstinventar. Theoretische Grundlagen und Handlungsanweisung. Weinheim: Beltz;1980.

24. Bullinger M et al. Münchner Lebensqualitäs Dimensionen Liste (MLDL). Weinheim: Beltz.

25. Rudolf G. Untersuchung und Befund bei Neurosen und Psychosomatischen Erkrankungen. Materialien zum 'Psychischen und Sozial-Kommunikativen Befund' (PSKB). Weinheim: Beltz;1981.

26. Malchow H, Ewe K, Brandes JW et al. European Cooperative Crohn's Disease Study (ECCDS): results of drug treatment. Gastroenterology. 1984;86:249–66.

27. Best WR, Becktel JM, Singleton JW, Kern F. Development of a Crohn's Disease Activity Index. Gastroenterology. 1976;70:439–44.

# 25
# Treatment strategy in chronic active Crohn disease (CD)

## R. MODIGLIANI

Chronic active CD encompasses three main situations: steroid resistance, steroid dependency and the need for repeated intestinal resections.

There is no universally agreed definition of steroid resistance. In our experience, 8% of patients with active CD failed to reach clinical remission after 7 weeks of treatment with oral prednisolone (1 mg kg$^{-1}$ d$^{-1}$)[1]. After surgical complications have been ruled out, therapeutic options include: increasing the steroid dose by 50%, given parenterally, artificial nutrition and surgery. The choice between these therapies depends upon the past history of the disease and its topography. It is not known whether intravenous cyclosporin is effective in this situation.

Steroid dependency is defined as a recrudescence of symptoms at repeated attempts to reduce the dose of prednisone below a given value, or as early relapses after steroid withdrawal. It occurs in 30–40% of patients treated with steroids for an attack of CD[2]. If prednisone is needed at a daily dose of 10 mg or less, and is well tolerated, it should probably be maintained. Otherwise, any effort to withdraw steroids should be made using one of the following tools:

1. Mesalazine, 4 g daily: it is probably useful in some patients and should be tried first[3];
2. Surgery should be considered whenever it is reasonable;
3. Immunosuppression is the most useful method in this setting. Azathioprine (2 mg/kg daily) and 6-mercaptopurine (1.5 mg/kg daily) are the best-established drugs in steroid-dependent CD. They are effective in 60–70% of cases, allowing a significant decrease in the dose or total withdrawal of steroids while remission is maintained. This beneficial effect is delayed by 1–9 months (mean: 3 months). Side-effects requiring interruption of the drug occur in 10–20% of cases (bone-marrow suppression, pancreatitis, hepatitis). Brain lymphoma has been reported in two patients on azathioprine/6-mercaptopurine for CD. It is not known how long these immunosuppressors should be continued once remission has been achieved and steroids withdrawn. Early interruption leads to relapse in about 40% of

patients within one year. Preliminary evidence suggests that this is not the case if the treatment is given for more than three and half years[4].

Methotrexate (25 mg intramuscularly once a week for 16 weeks) has been shown to induce significantly more remissions (clinical remission and discontinuation of steroids) than placebo (39.4% vs 19.1% respectively; $p = 0.025$) in chronic active CD[5]. Also, its effect occurs (one month) earlier than that of azathioprine. Methotrexate is, overall, well tolerated; also, it seems to be of help after failure of azathioprine.

Oral cyclosporin does not seem to help in steroid-dependent CD. Other treatments are not yet fully evaluated: anti-CD4 monoclonal antibody, budesonide (a steroid with fewer side-effects).

Patients who undergo a third or fourth small intestinal resection are at risk of short bowel syndrome. Prescription of azathioprine/6-mercaptopurine to prevent further relapse and surgery is logical but has not yet been tested in this situation. It has been shown that mesalamine, given immediately after surgery, reduces the rate of endoscopic recurrence and clinical relapse[6]. Whether this drug should be given to any patient undergoing intestinal resection for CD remains to be established.

## References


1. Modigliani R, Mary JY, Simon JF et al. and the Groupe d'Etudes Thérapeutiques des Affections Inflammatoires Digestives. Clinical, biological and endoscopic pictures of attacks of Crohn's disease. Evolution on prednisolone. Gastroenterology. 1990;98:811–18.
2. Landi B, N'Guyen Anh T, Cortot A et al. and the GETAID. Endoscopic monitoring of Crohn's disease. A prospective randomized clinical trial. Gastroenterology. 1992;102:1647–53.
3. Modigliani R, Colombel JF, Dupas JL et al. on behalf of the GETAID. Mesalamine (M) in Crohn's disease (CD) patients with prednisolone-induced remission: effect on steroid weaning and remission maintenance in the year after weaning: a placebo-controlled, multicentre double-blind trial. Gastroenterology. 1995;108:A878.
4. Lemann M, Bouhnik Y, Scemama G et al. Effect of immunosuppressive therapy withdrawal on the course of Crohn's disease (CD) in prolonged remission using azathioprine (ASP) or 6-mercaptopurine. Gastroenterology. 1994;106:A658.
5. Feagan BG, Rochon J, Fedorak RN et al. Methotrexate for the treatment of Crohn's disease. N Engl J Med. 1995;332:292–7.
6. Brignola C, Cottone M, Peña A et al. and the Italian Cooperative Study Group. Mesalamine in the prevention of endoscopic recurrence after intestinal resection for Crohn's disease. Gastroenterology. 1995;108:345–9.

# Section VI
# Standards and new developments in surgical therapy

# 26
# Surgery in ulcerative colitis

E. H. FARTHMANN, U. BAUMGARTNER, A. IMDAHL
and G. RUF

## INTRODUCTION

Ulcerative colitis is a chronic inflammatory bowel disease of unknown aetiology affecting the large bowel[1]. The disease has a wide spectrum, affecting all age groups and both sexes alike with a predominance in the young and middle aged. Symptoms are more often chronic than acute. Cardinal symptoms are diarrhoea and rectal bleeding. It is a chronic relapsing disease with periods of complete absence of symptoms between attacks. On the other hand, chronic continuous disease is seen in some patients. Extraintestinal manifestations (Table 1) may occur. Factors affecting recurrences of attacks are not completely understood[2,3].

For treatment of mild or moderate attacks, sulphasalazine is useful, as verified in clinical trials[4]. Sulphasalazine also seems to be effective for prevention of recurrence[5,6]. The pharmacological mechanism of sulphasalazine still remains unknown but some studies have shown that 5-aminosalicylic acid (5-ASA) seems to be the active moiety[7]. Corticosteroids are beneficial for the first attack, as well as in relapse and in severe attacks, but have no preventive effect[8,9]. With medical treatment, many patients with ulcerative colitis can be kept in reasonably good general health and most moderate attacks will respond to this manage-

**Table 1** Extraintestinal manifestations

- Liver disease (intermittent jaundice, primary sclerosing cholangitis, coagulation defects)
- Arthritis (often precedes onset of first symptoms)
- Ocular lesions (iritis, blurred vision, orbital pain, photophobia)
- Skin manifestations (erythema nodosum, pyoderma gangrenosum, aphthous ulceration)
- Renal disease (pyelonephritis)
- Amyloid (liver, kidney, spleen)
- Other systemic complications (thromboembolic disease, haemolytic anaemia, vasculitis, coagulation defects, hypertrophic osteoarthropathy, pericarditis, chronic pulmonary disorders)

ment. However, in a substantial number of patients, medical treatment fails and surgery becomes necessary.

## CLINICAL COURSE OF ULCERATIVE COLITIS

Ulcerative colitis may be divided into ulcerative proctitis, left-sided colitis and pancolitis. The first is considered a separate entity[10]. It rarely extends beyond the rectum or sigmoid colon. In contrast to left-sided and whole colitis, systemic symptoms, cancer and extraintestinal manifestations hardly occur. The course of ulcerative proctitis is benign in that less than 6% of patients observed for 20 years required surgery. The likelihood of disease extending to the sigmoid is less than 30% at 20 years[11].

Medically treated ulcerative colitis with substantial or total involvement of the colon has a relapse rate of nearly 100% within the first 10 years after onset of the disease. The cumulative colectomy rate for all forms of colitis over 30 years is up to 60%. When the resection rate is related to the different extent of the disease, a striking gap between pancolitis and proctitis can be observed (Figure 1)[12]. About one third of patients requiring colectomy are operated upon during the first acute attack of the disease[13].

The survival rate of patients with ulcerative colitis is inversely correlated with the severity of the first attack and the extent of the disease[14]. The causes of the excess mortality in colitic patients in comparison with the general population

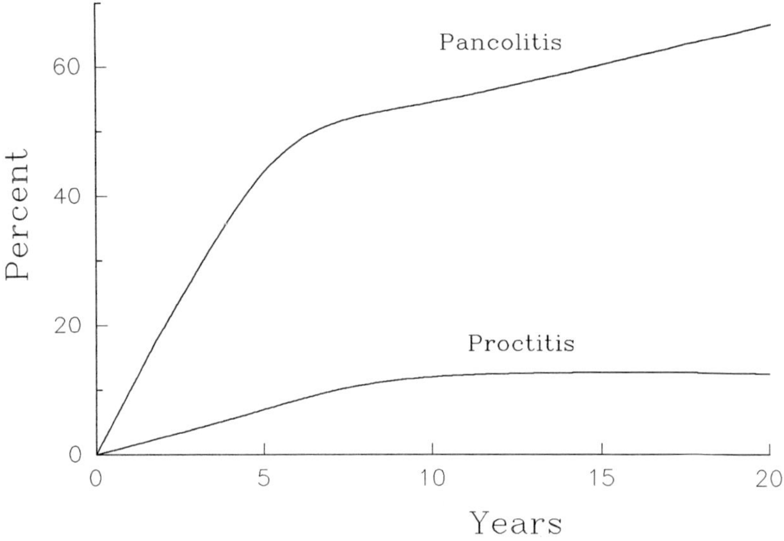


**Figure 1** Cumulative colectomy-ileostomy rates. The resection rate depends upon the extent of the disease. Patients with pancolitis at the first diagnosis have a cumulative resection rate of more than 60% at 20 years. In contrast, patients with ulcerative colitis confined to the rectum have a benign course. The resection rate stabilizes after 10 years, usually not exceeding a cumulative resection rate of 10%[12]

are: primarily, lethal outcome of an acute attack with delayed surgical intervention; and, only secondarily, cancer[15].

# CANCER AND DYSPLASIA IN ULCERATIVE COLITIS

## Cancer

The risk of ulcerative-colitis-associated carcinoma is not as great as it was supposed to be (cumulative risk of 42% at 25 years)[16]. The probability of developing a carcinoma is considerably less than assumed earlier, and even studies doubting any difference from the general population have been reported (Table 2)[17–25].

There is agreement that the risk of cancer is influenced by the extent of the colitis, age of the patient and severity of the first attack[26]. Controversy exists, however, about the malignant potential of polyps and strictures[27,28]. Explanations for the discrepancies observed between the different studies (Table 2) are: population bias (referral centre vs unselected populations), geographical differences, different criteria for entry to the study and different methods of analysis[29]. Finally, an important factor governing the risk of cancer is treatment policy. Removal of the diseased mucosa by conventional or restorative proctocolectomy within the first 10 years eliminates the risk of colitic cancer[21,30].

Probably the best cohort study of cancer risk is that of Gyde et al.[22] who studied 823 patients with ulcerative colitis from the West Midlands and Oxford regions of England and Stockholm County, Sweden. The cumulative risk of colorectal cancer in extensive colitis was 7.2% at 20 years and 16.5% at 30 years from the onset of the disease.

In contrast to earlier reports (5-year survival: 0–18.6%), the prognosis of colorectal cancer in colitic patients is no worse than that of sporadic cancer (5-year survival: 40–50%)[11].

**Table 2** Cumulative risk of colorectal cancer (%): extensive disease

| No. of patients | Years after onset | | | | Reference |
| | 15 | 20 | 25 | 30 | |
|---|---|---|---|---|---|
| 234 | 9.6 | 24.2 | 34 | – | Kewenter et al. 1978[17] |
| 267 | 7.0 | 11.0 | 20 | 30 | Greenstein et al. 1979[18] |
| 676 | – | – | 8.0* | 20* | Prior et al. 1982[19] |
| 959 | – | 5.0 | – | – | Maratka et al. 1985[20] |
| 783 | 1.1 | 1.4 | – | – | Hendriksen et al. 1985[21] |
| 823 | 3.0 | 7.2 | 11.0 | 16.5 | Gyde et al. 1988[22] |
| 401 | 3.0 | 5.0 | 9.0 | – | Lennard-Jones et al. 1990[23] |
| 1161 | – | – | 3.1** | – | Langholz et al. 1992[24] |
| 486 | – | 7.0 | – | – | Gillen et al. 1994[25] |

*Only 'interval' cancer
**No significant difference from the risk of sporadic cancer

## Dysplasia

The efficacy of surveillance programmes to detect cancer and dysplasia in ulcerative colitis has been the subject of controversy[31,32]. Up to 30% of patients who developed a carcinoma during surveillance did not show any dysplasia prior to surgery[33]. Only 75% of (procto)colectomy specimens, removed because of cancer, carried dysplastic lesions distant (> 3 cm) to the tumour[34–36].

Evidence of dysplasia as a marker of high cancer risk has been questioned since no one knows about the spontaneous regression rates of such lesions[11,37]. However, recent studies suggest that prophylactic surgery should be recommended if dysplasia is discovered during surveillance in the case of high-grade dysplasia, persistent low-grade dysplasia, dysplastic mass (broad-based elevation) and polypoid dysplastic lesion[32,36,37].

Molecular studies were designed to differentiate between sporadic and colitis-associated cancer. The reduced frequency of c-Ki-ras mutation in colitic vs sporadic carcinoma led to the hypothesis that this difference is due to different genetic defects[38–40]. However, studies on $P_{53}$ gene expression, which is the most common abnormality in sporadic colorectal cancer[41], and other genetic changes have shown no significant differences (Table 3).

**Table 3** Colon carcinoma – genetic instability

|  | Sporadic | Colitis-associated |
|---|---|---|
| Oncogen activation | Yes | Yes |
| Suppressor gene mutation/loss | Yes | Yes |
| p53 mutation | Late | Early |
| loss | Late | Late |
| c-Ki-Ras mutation | Frequent | Rare |

Although colitis-associated carcinomas share many of the changes found in their precursor dysplasias, proving their common clonal origin, no genetic alterations reliably mark the transition between dysplasia and carcinoma[42]. Therefore, molecular biology analysis does not yet contribute to the decision of surgical intervention.

## SURGERY IN ULCERATIVE COLITIS

### A bit of history

Appendicostomy for surgical treatment of ulcerative colitis was first suggested by Keetley in 1895 and first performed by Wier in 1902 at the Roosevelt Hospital in New York[43]. Through the appendicostomy, the colon was irrigated with various fluids[44]. If the appendix had been removed by a previous appendectomy, a caecostomy was used instead. However, both procedures were ineffective.

Simple ileostomy, published by Brown in 1913 with encouraging results, became widely used[45]. It was the logical step because it provided a total faecal diversion from the diseased colon. The mortality and morbidity was high and, in many cases, some or all of the large bowel had to be removed.

Colonic resection, initially performed as a limited resection, was carried out in several stages. A three-stage procedure with ileostomy, subtotal colectomy and abdominoperineal excision of the rectum became the procedure of choice[46].

Ileostomy and primary partial colectomy performed by Miller et al.[47] in 1942 became more radical and, in 1951, Gardner and Miller[48] reported on ileostomy with immediate colectomy. The one-stage proctocolectomy, with the advantage of removing all the diseased colon in one step, appreciated the pathology of the ulcerative colitis[49–51].

The Kock pouch (continent ileostomy) with creation of an internal reservoir using the terminal ileum with a nipple valve for prevention of leakage did, in 1969, overcome some disadvantages of the conventional ileostomy[52].

Sphincter-saving operations (ileosigmoid anastomosis as a three-stage procedure) were first described by Lilienthal[53] in 1901 and by Devine[54] in 1943. The ileorectal anastomosis introduced by Aylett in 1950 became the leading procedure[55].

The disadvantages with recurrent disease, cancer risk and the need for further surveillance have pushed forward the surgical approach to ileoanal anastomosis after a transanal mucosal proctocolectomy described by Ravitch and Sabiston[56] in 1947 with a straight anal anastomosis or an ileoanal pullthrough operation performed by Soave in 1964[57]. The results were promising, but other surgeons were not able to achieve the same good results.

A further advance in surgical treatment was the introduction of restorative proctocolectomy, i.e. mucosal proctectomy with pelvic pouch and ileoanal anastomosis published by Parks and Nicholls in 1978[58]. The evacuation problems with the S-shaped pouch led to changes in the pouch design. The J-pouch suggested by Utsunomiya, H-pouch favoured by Fonkalsrud and W-pouch performed by Nicholls, as well as the introduction of the double-stapling technique by Keighley, all brought about improvement in the results[59–64].

## Indications and type of surgical treatment

The indications for surgical treatment are: restoration of health in chronic disease, prevention of risk of colon cancer and saving of life during a severe attack.

## Emergency surgery

In patients presenting with a severe attack of ulcerative colitis not responding to medical treatment, surgical intervention is necessary when the disease is progressing to the stage of fulminating colitis, toxic colon dilatation (Table 4) or even perforation. In some cases, severe peranal haemorrhage may necessitate immediate surgery.

Patients admitted to hospital often have no previous history of bowel disease. Any patient presenting for the first time with bloody diarrhoea must be assumed to be suffering from acute colitis until proved otherwise[11]. Bloody diarrhoea,

**Table 4**  Features of fulminating colitis and toxic dilatation

| **Fulminating colitis*** | |
| --- | --- |
| Tachycardia | > 100/min |
| Temperature | > 38.6°C |
| Leukocytosis | > 10 500 |
| Hypoalbuminaemia | < 3.0 g/L |
| Frequency | > 9/day |
| **Toxic colon dilatation** | |
| Radiological diameter of the colon > 6 cm | |

*Fulminating colitis is diagnosed when at least two of these criteria occur together

tenesmus and abdominal colic dominate the clinical picture, accompanied by anaemia, severe dehydration, fever and tachycardia. Abdominal pain suggests impending perforation and abdominal distension may indicate the beginning of dilatation of the colon. Repeated plain abdominal radiographs and immediate sigmoidoscopy should be performed. Stool cultures must be collected urgently to exclude infective colitis.

Figure 2 illustrates the management of acute colitis: if the patient improves after medical resuscitation (hydration, antibiotics, steroids, total parenteral nutrition), surgery is not needed. Depending on the further course, long-term medication or elective surgery may be appropriate. If the condition worsens, or toxic dilatation or even perforation is evident, immediate surgery is necessary. If intensive medical treatment does not improve the condition within 24–72 h but the patient remains in a stable condition, surgery may be postponed by one or two days (urgent surgery). It is important not to delay surgical intervention because the mortality rate rises steeply when perforation has already occurred (Table 5)[65–68].

In a severe attack, one-stage-colectomy is best performed either with a closed rectum (Hartmann procedure) or formation of a sigmoid mucous fistula[11]. By

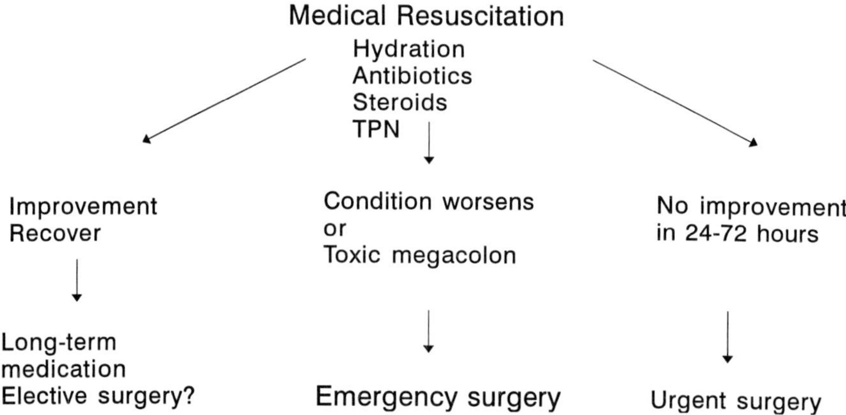


**Figure 2**  Management of acute colitis. TPN = total parenteral nutrition

**Table 5**  Emergency surgery for toxic dilatation (mortality rates)

| Reference | No perforation (%) | With perforation (%) |
|---|---|---|
| Binder et al. 1974[65] | 5 | 50 |
| Fazio 1980[66] | 5 | 29 |
| Greenstein et al. 1985[67] | 2 | 44 |
| Heppell et al. 1986[68] | NS | 20 |

this procedure, most of the diseased mucosa will be removed, at the same time preserving the possibility of secondary restorative intervention. Multiple colon fistulae (blowholes) proposed by Turnbull et al. in 1971[69] decompress the colon after toxic dilatation and avoid spontaneous perforation. However, today this procedure is obsolete as it does not influence the underlying disease and has a high mortality rate[11]. Emergency total proctocolectomy may be indicated when massive rectal haemorrhage is encountered. However, this is rarely the case. Most of the surgeons today avoid this procedure as an emergency since the mortality rate is substantially greater (15%) than after subtotal colectomy with ileostomy (6%)[70,71].

## Elective surgery

Indications for elective surgical treatment are: failure of medical treatment, chronic continuous disease, strictures, burned-out colitis, verified dysplasia of the mucosa, side-effects of corticosteroids, reconstruction after emergency surgery and verified cancer. Occasionally, surgery is needed for extraintestinal manifestations of ulcerative colitis.

Failure of medical treatment over a prolonged period results in a state of chronic morbidity for the patient[72]. The degree of this morbidity is often not appreciated prior to colectomy. Chronic continuous disease with episodes of acute attacks which do not respond adequately to medical treatment leads to destruction of the mucosa. Irreversible mucosal damage and fibrosis of the wall (burned-out colitis), similar to a third-degree burn injury of the skin, are followed by colorectal dysfunction with high-frequency diarrhoea. Colectomy, even without restoring continence, improves dramatically the general health and the quality of life of the patient.

Patients found to have a rectal carcinoma have often been considered to be unsuitable for restorative proctocolectomy. However, as long as the principles of cancer surgery can be followed, pelvic pouch need not be contraindicated. It is important, however, that the mid- and/or lower rectum are not involved by advanced carcinoma.

Frequent treatment of acute attacks of ulcerative colitis or severe extraintestinal manifestations need high doses of corticosteroids to obtain remission[73]. Side-effects like corticosteroid-induced osteoporosis, even with spontaneous fractures of vertebrae, can be seen especially in younger patients. Morbidity induced by the disease or by long-term medical treatment should be compared with that of a proposed surgical intervention.

## Surgical options in elective surgery

The current principle of surgical treatment in ulcerative colitis is removal of most of the diseased mucosa. This can be achieved by proctocolectomy with ileostomy (Brooke or Kock ileostomy), by colectomy with ileorectal anastomosis and by restorative proctocolectomy with ileum pouch–anal anastomosis.

Total proctocolectomy with either conservative or intersphincteric proctectomy and a Brooke everted end-ileostomy remain satisfactory procedures for inflammatory bowel disease. The advantage is the removal of all diseased mucosa. The disadvantages are the permanent ileostomy, unhealing perineal wounds (17–85%), sexual complications (0–30%), bladder dysfunction and (very important) the finality of the procedure. Therefore, today, it may only be indicated when a pelvic pouch operation or an ileorectal anastomosis is not possible because of poor function of the anal sphincter or a destroyed rectum.

Continent ileostomy (Kock pouch) is considered to be cosmetically superior to an end-ileostomy. However, if the patient has to choose between a Brooke ileostomy and a Kock pouch, he or she should be informed about the high reoperation rate of the latter with revision of the nipple valve (approximately 50%), pouchitis (10%), fistula formation and stoma stricture[11].

Ileorectal anastomosis can be considered a safe conservative operation in selected patients with ulcerative colitis. It has certain advantages over some of the alternative sphincter-saving procedures, like avoidance of intraoperative pelvic nerve disruption and presacral vein haemorrhage. Functional results are comparable to those of the pelvic pouch procedures[74,75]. On the other hand, disease is left in place and recurrence of inflammation and also the long-term risk of cancer developing in the rectal stump can be a serious problem. During surveillance, more than half of patients require subsequent rectal excision (Table 6)[13,76–82]. If an ileorectal anastomosis is to be considered, absence of severe proctitis and dysplasia, full continence and a compliant rectum are preconditions.

Restorative proctocolectomy combines the radicality of proctocolectomy with the functional outcome of ileorectal anastomosis[74]. Ileum pouch–anal anastomosis, performed either by proctomucosectomy and handsewn anastomosis or by the double-stapling technique, in the transitional zone (as a one-stage or two-stage procedure with or without a temporary ileostomy) is a safe surgical

**Table 6** Mortality, morbidity and failure of ileorectal anastomoses

| Reference | No. of cases | Mortality (%) | Leakage (%) | Failure[*] |
|---|---|---|---|---|
| Aylett 1966[76] | 300 | 6 | 12 | 5 |
| Fazio et al. 1975[77] | 157 | 2 | 1 | – |
| Gruner et al. 1975[78] | 57 | 7 | 10 | – |
| Oakley et al. 1985[79] | 145 | 0 | 2 | 24 |
| Khubchandani et al. 1985[80] | 110 | 0 | 2 | 10 |
| Backer et al. 1988[81] | 59 | 0 | 0 | 22 |
| Parc et al. 1989[82] | 197 | – | – | 25 |
| Leijonmarck et al. 1990[13] | 60 | 4 | 2 | 57 |

[*]Failure is defined as the necessity for a permanent ileostomy. (Modified from Reference 83)

method and currently the first choice for the treatment of ulcerative colitis[114]. The morbidity of these techniques is now as low as 10% with no mortality[85,61]. But it is generally accepted that enthusiasm for this method of sphincter preservation should alter neither the indications for nor the thresholds to surgery unless we know more about the long-term outcome and the nature of pouchitis, the major complication after restorative proctocolectomy.

## QUALITY OF LIFE AFTER SURGERY

Quality of life is a difficult concept to define in objective terms. In any single case, the question has to be raised whether the quality of life can be improved by surgical intervention in ulcerative colitis. Several studies have addressed this issue regarding functional, social and psychological aspects. Although it is difficult to compare the results of these studies, it has become apparent that surgery is beneficial when it is used carefully, irrespective of the surgical procedure employed[86–90].

## References


1. Jewell DP, Lowes JR. Aetiology and pathogenesis of ulcerative colitis and Crohn's disease. Triangle. 1988;27:137–41.
2. Mee AS, Jewell DP. Factors inducing relapse in inflammatory bowel disease. Br Med J. 1978;2:801–2.
3. Rampton DS, McNeil NI, Sarner M. Analgesic ingestion and other factors preceding relapse in ulcerative colitis. Gut. 1983;24:187–9.
4. Baron JH, Connell AM, Lennard-Jones JE, Avery Jones F. Sulphasalazine and salicylazosulfadimidine in ulcerative colitis. Lancet. 1965;1:1094–6.
5. Järenot G. New salicylates as maintenance in ulcerative colitis. Gut. 1994;35:1155–8.
6. Lichtenstein GR. Medical therapies for inflammatory bowel disease. Curr Opin Gastroenterol. 1994;10:390–403.
7. Jewell DP, Truelove SC. The first international symposium on sulfasalazine in the treatment of ulcerative colitis. Scand J Gastroenterol. 1988;23(suppl):148.
8. Lennard-Jones JE, Misiewicz JJ, Connell AM, Baron JH, Avery Jones F. Prednisone as maintenance treatment for ulcerative colitis in remission. Lancet. 1965;1:188–9.
9. Truelove SC, Witts LJ. Cortisone and corticotropin in ulcerative colitis. Br Med J. 1959;1:387–94.
10. Juby LD, Long DE, Dixon MF, Axon ATR. Prognostic indicators and clinical course in proctosigmoiditis. Int J Colorectal Dis. 1990;5:177–80.
11. Keighley MRB, Williams NS. Surgery of the anus, rectum and colon. 2nd edn. London: WB Saunders; 1993.
12. Farmer RG, Easley KA, Rankin GB. Clinical pattern, natural history, and progression of ulcerative colitis. A long-term follow-up of 1116 patients. Dig Dis Sci. 1993;38:1137–46.
13. Leijonmarck CE, Persson PG, Hellers G. Factors affecting colostomy rate in ulcerative colitis: an epidemiologic study. Gut. 1990;31:329–33.
14. Edwards FC, Truelove SC. The course and prognosis of ulcerative colitis. Parts I and II: Short-term and long-term prognosis. Gut. 1963;4:299–315.
15. Devlin BH, Datta D, Dellipiani AW. The incidence and prevalence of inflammatory bowel disease in North Tees Health District. World J Surg. 1980;4:183–93.
16. DeDombal FT, Watts JM, Watkinson G, Goligher JC. Local complications of ulcerative colitis: structure, pseudopolyposis and carcinoma of the colon and rectum. Br Med J. 1966;1:1442–7.
17. Kewenter J, Ahlman H, Hulten L. Cancer risk in ulcerative colitis. Ann Surg. 1978;15:824–8.
18. Greenstein AJ, Sachar DB, Smith H et al. Cancer in universal and left-sided ulcerative colitis: factors determining risk. Gastroenterology. 1979;77:290–4.

19. Prior P, Gyde SN, Macartney JC, Thompson H, Waterhouse JAH, Allan RN. Cancer morbidity in ulcerative colitis. Gut. 1982;23:490–7.
20. Maratka Z, Nedbal J, Kocianova J, Hevelka J, Kudrmann J, Hendl J. Incidence of colorectal cancer in proctocolitis: a retrospective study of 959 cases over 40 years. Gut. 1985;26:43–9.
21. Hendriksen C, Kreiner S, Binder V. Long term prognosis in ulcerative colitis – based on results from a regional patient group from the county of Copenhagen. Gut. 1985;26:158–63.
22. Gyde SN, Prior P, Allan RN et al. Colorectal cancer in ulcerative colitis: a cohort study of primary referrals from three centers. Gut. 1988;29:206–17.
23. Lenard-Jones JE, Melville DM, Morson BC, Williams CB. Precancer and cancer in extensive ulcerative colitis: findings among 401 patients over 22 years. Gut. 1990;31:800–6.
24. Langholz E, Munkholm P, Davidsen M, Binder V. Colorectal cancer risk and mortality in patients with ulcerative colitis. Gastroenterology. 1992;103:1444–51.
25. Gillen CD, Walmsley RS, Prior P, Andrews HA, Allan RN. Ulcerative colitis and Crohn's disease: a comparison of the colorectal cancer in extensive colitis. Gut. 1994;35:1590–2.
26. Ohman U. Colorectal carcinoma in patients with ulcerative colitis. Am J Surg. 1982;144:344–9.
27. Morson BC, Dawson IMP. Gastrointestinal pathology. 2nd edn. Oxford: Blackwell Scientific; 1979.
28. Gumaste V, Sachar DB, Greenstein AJ. Benign and malignant colorectal strictures in ulcerative colitis. Gut. 1992;33:938–41.
29. Katzka I, Brody RS, Morris E, Katz S. Assessment of colorectal cancer risk in patients with ulcerative colitis: experience from a private praxis. Gastroenterology. 1983;85:22–9.
30. Ritchie JK, Powell-Tuck J, Lennard-Jones JE. Clinical outcome of the first ten years of ulcerative colitis and proctitis. Lancet. 1978;1:1140–3.
31. Axon ATR. Cancer surveillance in ulcerative colitis – a time for reappraisal. Gut. 1994;35:587–9.
32. Bernstein CN, Shanahan F, Weinstein WM. Are we telling patients the truth about surveillance colonoscopy in ulcerative colitis? Lancet. 1994;343:71–4.
33. Connell WR, Talbot IC, Harpaz N et al. Clinicopathological characteristics of colorectal carcinoma complicating ulcerative colitis. Gut. 1994;35:1419–23.
34. Ransohoff DF, Riddell RH, Levin B. Ulcerative colitis and colonic cancer: problems in assessing the diagnostic usefulness of mucosal dysplasia. Dis Colon Rectum. 1985;28:383–8.
35. Taylor BA, Pemberton JH, Carpenter HA. Dysplasia in chronic ulcerative colitis: implications for colonoscopic surveillance. Dis Colon Rectum. 1992;35:950–6.
36. Connell WR, Lennard-Jones JE, Williams CB, Talbot IC, Price AB, Wilkinson KH. Factors affecting the outcome of endoscopic surveillance for cancer in ulcerative colitis. Gastroenterology. 1994;107:934–44.
37. Vemulapalli R, Lancet P. Cancer surveillance in ulcerative colitis: More of the same or progress? Gastroenterology. 1994;107:1196–9.
38. Bell SM, Kelly SA, Hoyle SA et al. CK$_1$-ras mutations in dysplasias and carcinoma complicating ulcerative colitis. Br J Cancer 1991;64:174–8.
39. Melzer SJ, Mane SM, Wood PK et al. Activation of C-K$_i$-ras in human gastrointestinal dysplasias determined by direct sequencing of polymerase chain reaction products. Cancer Res. 1990;50:3627–30.
40. Burmer GC, Levine DS, Kulander BG et al. CK$_i$-ras mutations in chronic ulcerative colitis and sporadic colon carcinoma. Gastroenterology. 1990;99:416–20.
41. Taylor HW, Boyle M, Smith SC, Bustin S, Williams NS. Expression of p53 in colorectal cancer and dysplasia complicating ulcerative colitis. Br J Surg. 1993;80:442–4.
42. Kern SE, Redston M, Seymour AB. Molecular genetic profiles of colitis-associated neoplasms. Gastroenterology. 1994;107:420–8.
43. Corbett RS. A review of the surgical treatment of chronic ulcerative colitis. Proc R Soc Med. 1945;38:277–90.
44. Lockhart-Mummery JP. Diseases of the rectum and colon. 2nd edn. London: Bailliere;1934.
45. Brown JY. The value of complete physiological rest of large bowel in the treatment of certain ulcerative and obstructive lesions with description of operative technique and report of a case. Surg Gynecol Obstet. 1913;16:610–13.
46. Castell RB. Surgical treatment of ulcerative colitis. Gastroenterology. 1948;10:63–7.
47. Miller CG, Gardner C, Ripstein CB. Primary resection of the colon in ulcerative colitis. J Can Med Assoc. 1949;60:584–5.
48. Gardner C, Miller CG. Total colectomy for ulcerative colitis. Arch Surg. 1952;63:370–2.

49. Brooke BN. The management of an ileostomy including its complications. Lancet. 1952;2:102–4.
50. Goligher JC. Primary excisional surgery in the treatment of ulcerative colitis. Ann R Coll Surg Engl. 1954;15:316–25.
51. Ripstein CB, Miller CG, Gardner C. Results of the surgical treatment of ulcerative colitis. Ann Surg. 1952;135:14–18.
52. Kock NG. Intra-abdominal reservoir in patients with permanent ileostomy. Arch Surg. 1969;99:223–31.
53. Lilienthal H. Hyperplastic colitis: extirpation of the entire colon, upper sigmoid and four inches of ileum. Ann Med. 1901;1:164–5.
54. Devine H. Method of colectomy for desperate cases of ulcerative colitis. Surg Gynecol Obstet. 1943;76:136–8.
55. Aylett SO. Ileorectal anastomosis: Review 1952–1968. Proc R Soc Med. 1971;64:967–73.
56. Ravitch MM, Sabiston DC. Anal ileostomy with preservation of the sphincter. Surg Gynecol Obstet. 1947;84:1095–9.
57. Soave F. A new technique for treatment of Hirschsprung's disease. Surgery. 1964;56:1007–14.
58. Parks AG, Nicholls RJ. Proctocolectomy without ileostomy for ulcerative colitis. Br Med J. 1978;2:85–8.
59. Fonkalsrud EW. Update on clinical experience with different surgical techniques of the endorectal pull-through operation for colitis and polyposis. Surg Gynecol Obstet. 1987;165:309–16.
60. Harms BA, Pahl AC, Starling JR. Comparison of clinical and compliance characteristics between S and W ileal reservoirs. Am J Surg. 1990;159:34–40.
61. Keighley MRB, Winslet MC, Yoshioka K, Lightwood R. Discrimination is not impaired by excision of the anal transition zone after restorative proctocolectomy. Br J Surg. 1987;74:1118–21.
62. Nicholls RJ, Pezim ME. Restorative proctocolectomy with ileal reservoir for ulcerative colitis and familial adenomatous polyposis. A comparison of three reservoir designs. Br J Surg. 1985;72:470–5.
63. O'Connell PR, Pemberton JH, Brown ML, Kelly KA. Determinants of stool frequency after ileal pouch-anal anastomosis. Am J Surg. 1987;153:157–62.
64. Utsunomiya J, Iwama T, Matsuo M, Sawai S, Yaegashi K, Hirayama R. Total colectomy, mucosal proctectomy and ileoanal anastomosis. Dis Colon Rectum. 1980;23:459–66.
65. Binder SC, Patterson JF, Glotzer DJ. Toxic megacolon in ulcerative colitis. Gastroenterology. 1974;66:909–15.
66. Fazio VW. Toxic megacolon in ulcerative colitis and Crohn's colitis. Clin Gastroenterol. 1980;9:389–407.
67. Greenstein AJ, Sachar DB, Gibas A et al. Outcome of toxic dilatation in ulcerative and Crohn's colitis. J Clin Gastroenterol. 1985;7:137–44.
68. Heppell J, Farkouh C, Dube S, Peloquin A, Morgan S, Bewrnard D. Toxic megacolon: an analysis of 70 cases. Dis Colon Rectum. 1986;28:789–92.
69. Turnbull RB Jr, Hawk WA, Weakley FL. Surgical treatment of toxic megacolon: ileostomy and colostomy to prepare patient for colectomy. Am J Surg. 1971;122:325–31.
70. Block GE, Moossa AR, Simonowitz D, Hassan SZ. Emergency colectomy for inflammatory bowel disease. Surgery. 1977;82:531–6.
71. Hosking SW, Kane SP, Cour-Palais IJ. Reducing the surgical mortality of acute colitis. A district hospital experience. J R Coll Surg Edinburgh. 1985;30:255–7.
72. Truelove SC. Medical treatment of ulcerative colitis and indications for colectomy. World J Surg. 1989;12:142–7.
73. Jewell DP. Medical management of severe ulcerative colitis. Int J Colon Dis. 1988;3:186–9.
74. Pemberton JF, Kelly KA, Beart RA, Dozois RR, Wolff BG, Ilstrup P. Ileal pouch-anal anastomosis for chronic ulcerative colitis long-term results. Ann Surg. 1987;206:504–13.
75. Wexner SD, Jensen L, Tothemnberger DA, Wong WD, Goldberg SM. Long-term functional analysis of the ileal reservoir. Dis Colon Rectum. 1989;32:275–81.
76. Aylett SO. Three hundred cases of diffuse ulcerative colitis treated by total colectomy and ileorectal anastomosis. BMJ. 1966;1:1001–5.
77. Fazio VW, Turnbull RB Jr, Goldsmith MG. Ileorectal anastomosis: a safe surgical technique. Dis Colon Rectum. 1975;18:107–14.
78. Gruner OP, Flatmansk A, Naas R et al. Ileorectal anastomosis and ulcerative colitis. Scand J Gastroenterol. 1975;10:641–6.

79. Oakley JR, Jagelman DG, Fazio VW et al. Complications and quality of life after ileorectal anastomosis for ulcerative colitis. Am J Surg. 1985;149:23–30.
80. Khubchandani IT, Sandfort MR, Rosen L, Sheets JA, Stasik JJ, Riether RD. Current status of ileorectal anastomosis for inflammatory bowel disease. Dis Colon Rectum. 1985;32:400–3.
81. Backer O, Hjortrup A, Kjaergaard AM. Evaluation of ileorectal anastomosis for the treatment of ulcerative proctitis. J R Soc Med. 1988;81:210–11.
82. Parc R, Legrand M, Frileux P et al. Comparative clinical results of ileal-pouch anal anastomosis and ileorectal anastomosis in ulcerative colitis. Hepatogastroenterology. 1989;36:235–9.
83. Binderow SR, Wexner SD. Current surgical therapy for mucosal ulcerative colitis. Dis Colon Rectum. 1994;37:610–24.
84. Järvinen HJ, Luukkonen P. Comparison of restorative proctocolectomy with and without covering ileostomy in ulcerative colitis. Br J Surg. 1991;78:323–5.
85. Heald RJ, Allen DR. Stapled ileo-anal anastomosis: a technique to avoid mucosal proctectomy in the ileal pouch operation. Br J Surg. 1986;73:571–2.
86. McLeod RS, Fazio VW. Quality of life with the continent ileostomy. World J Surg. 1984;8:90–5.
87. Pemberton JH, Phillips SF, Ready RR, Zinsmeister AR, Beahrs OH. Quality of life after Brooke ileostomy and ileal pouch-anal anastomosis. Comparison of performance status. Ann Surg. 1989;209:620–6.
88. McLeod RS, Lavery IC, Leatherman JR. Factors affecting quality of life with a conventional ileostomy. World J Surg. 1986;10:474–80.
89. Sagar PM, Lewis W, Holdsworth PJ, Johnston D, Mitchell C, Macfie J. Quality of life after restorative proctocolectomy with a pelvic ileal reservoir compares favorably with that of patients with medically treated colitis. Dis Colon Rectum. 1993;36:584–92.
90. McLeod RS, Churchill DN, Lock AM, Vanderburgh S, Cohen Z. Quality of life with ulcerative colitis preoperatively and postoperatively. Gastroenterology. 1991;101:1307–13.

# 27
# Pros and cons of the ileoanal pouch

## J. STERN, U.A. HEUSCHEN and C. HERFARTH

The surgical treatment of ulcerative colitis requires total proctocolectomy since partial resection of the colon has not proved useful in the surgical treatment of this chronic inflammatory bowel disease. The so-called restorative proctocolectomy or ileoanal pouch operation (IAP) is now performed in most cases world wide. A series of critical aspects is inherent to this challenging surgical technique. As alternatives, the ileorectal anastomosis and the conventional proctocolectomy with terminal ileostomy are also used. A comparison of the different surgical procedures has to take into account the respective complication rates, metabolic effects and potential functional consequences. Moreover, there are special indications in which the ileoanal pouch operation is superior to the alternatives. At least, there are several methodological variations which are tailored to solve particular problems. To evaluate the application of the restorative proctocolectomy comprehensively, a comparison between the treatment results in ulcerative colitis and in familial polyposis is necessary.

## PRINCIPLES OF THE ILEOANAL POUCH OPERATION

In the first operative phase, a colectomy is performed. This can, in most cases, be performed close to the bowel wall. In the presence of an obvious colorectal carcinoma, the involved bowel segments have to be removed using surgical oncological techniques. In the pelvic region and in the absence of malignancy, the operation can be performed close to the bowel wall. In the lower rectum, two techniques are possible in principle. One requires complete removal of the diseased mucosa, which can usually be achieved by a transanal proctomucosectomy over approximately 3 cm. A less-radical technique leaves a residual portion of the mucosa, and the rectum is transsected between 2 and 4 cm proximally in a transmural manner. The fundamental aim of the restorative proctocolectomy is to both maintain the natural continence and avoid a permanent stoma. A basic requirement in order to achieve these aims involves the creation of a neoreservoir.

In the second phase, the reconstruction is achieved by folding the terminal ileum, forming a pouch. The pouch will then be anastomosed at the dentate line by pulling it through the muscular rectal cuff or by creating a distal pouch rectal anastomosis. In order to perform the anastomosis deep with the pelvis, sufficient mobilization of the ileum is mandatory. Most surgeons prefer the preservation of the ileocolic artery as a general rule in order to be able to ligate a hindering arch of the superior mesenteric artery without impairing blood flow to the pouch[2,8].

In the ileorectostomy, the preparation of the rectum is not fully completed and the small bowel is anastomosed to the rectum in an end-to-end fashion after colectomy. In the standard coloproctectomy, the rectum and, in most cases, the anal sphincter is completely removed since the small bowel is used to create a permanent terminal ileostomy. For the ileoanal pouch procedure, most study groups perform a protective loop ileostomy for about 3 months combined with a pouch anal anastomosis. However, the operation can be performed in a single step without the protective ileostomy.

## SELECTION OF PATIENTS

Between 1982 and December 1994, 443 patients with ulcerative colitis were treated surgically at the Department of Surgery, University of Heidelberg (Figure 1). Three hundred and four patients (68%) were treated by an ileoanal pouch operation. Within the same period, 112 patients with familial polyposis were treated surgically in a similar fashion; an ileoanal pouch operation was performed in 93 patients (83%). The overwhelming majority of the patients with ulcerative colitis were treated secondary to severe colitis which was refractory to conservative treatment. An emergency situation was present in 9.2% of patients. In 30 patients, a simultaneously occurring colitis associated with carcinoma was present, 2% of patients were treated due merely to dysplasia in the colon on

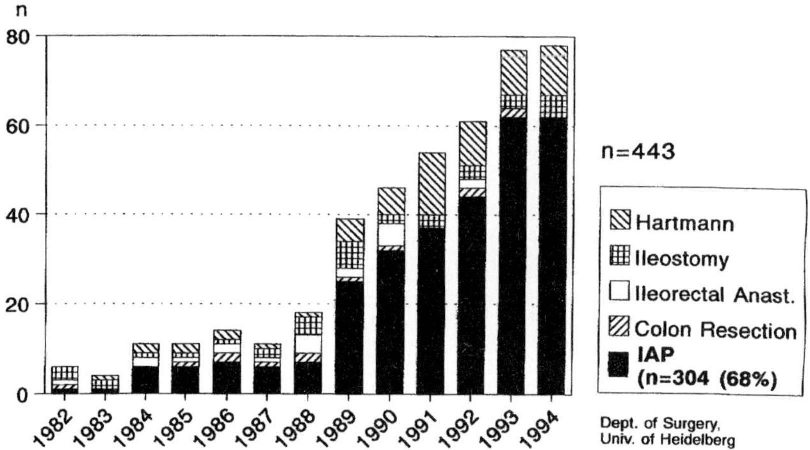


**Figure 1** Surgical therapy of ulcerative colitis. Over the years, the ileoanal pouch procedure (IAP) has become the treatment of choice

coloscopy with the prophylactic intention of preventing the occurrence of secondary carcinoma.

## COMPARISON OF DIFFERENT PROCTOCOLECTOMY PROCEDURES

### Perioperative morbidity

A total of 4 complications should be mentioned specifically in conjunction with the ileoanal pouch operation. We may be confronted with: postoperative ileus; local septic complications in the small pelvis, specifically in the area of the anal pouch anastomosis; inflammation of the pouch, the so-called pouchitis; and the development of stenosis in the area of the anal pouch anastomosis. A comprehensive analysis of the published data (2800 pouches, 24 publications) shows general agreement with our own experience (Figure 2). With a separate analysis of the data according to the underlying diseases, ulcerative colitis or familial polyposis, it becomes obvious that the incidence of these complications is not simply due to the operative technique. Postoperative ileus is observed with the same frequency as for other large abdominal operations. Local septic complications are almost 3 times more frequent if the underlying disease is ulcerative colitis rather than familial polyposis. Pouchitis after familial polyposis is exceptionally rare while it represents a frequent problem in ulcerative colitis. An increased rate of anal pouch stenosis in the presence of ulcerative colitis is probably due to the increased incidence of local septic complications in these cases (Figure 3).

Local septic complications are the most frequent cause of a definitive loss of the pouch unless it is possible to manage this problem surgically. Besides the

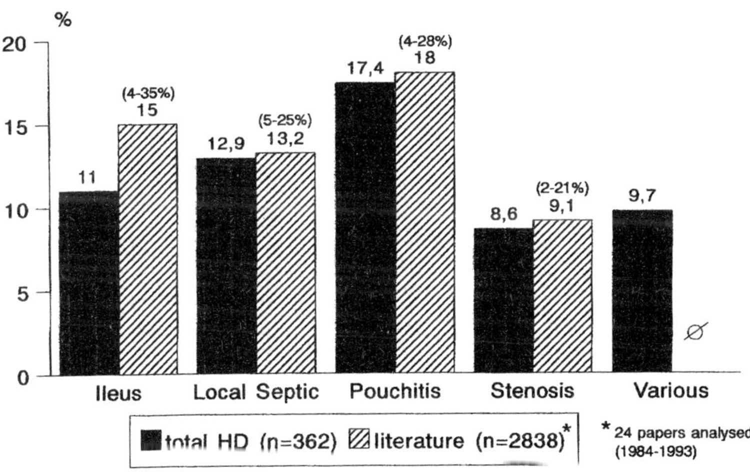


**Figure 2** Complication rates after IAP are considerable. This diagram shows our own experience in comparison with data from the literature

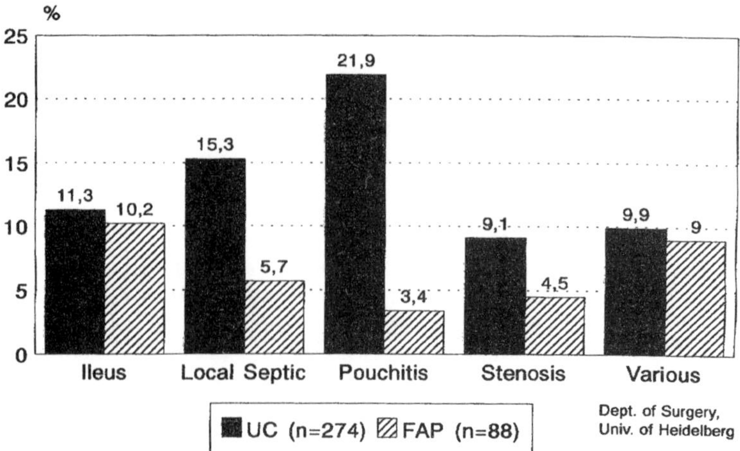


**Figure 3** The underlying disease is related to major complications after IAP. UC = ulcerative colitis; FAP = familial adenomatous polyposis

underlying disease, risk factors include: high-dose cortisol-therapy at the time of operation; age greater than 40 y at operation; perirectal fistulae; and increased body weight; as well as active proctitis which is typical for ulcerative colitis in contrast to familial polyposis.

The ileorectal anastomosis and conventional proctocolectomy are not free from complications. According to an analysis in the literature, the incidence of postoperative ileus after ileorectal anastomosis is 12%. Additionally, rectal carcinoma was observed in 2.8% and a secondary proctectomy was necessary in 26%. The postoperative morbidity after a conventional proctocolectomy ranged between 30% and 37%, an ileus between 6% and 21%. Between 7% and 24% of patients suffer problems which stem from the ileostomy. The continent ileostomy (so-called Kock pouch) also carries a considerable postoperative morbidity similar to the problems occurring after ileoanal pouch operation[3–5,13,15,19]. If the postoperative complication rate of the individual operative procedures is evaluated in a critical manner, it is apparent that secondary operations (so-called re-do-operations) necessary after ileoanal pouch are usually successful[2,26]. Only 3% of neoreservoirs had to be removed in our own patient population. This compares favourably with a review of the pertinent literature in which rates between 3% and 14% have been reported. Similarly, the so-called relative non-responder carrying a protective ileostomy for more than 2 years is found in less than 3.9% (in the literature: 2–19%; Table 1).

## Functional results

It is frequently mentioned that the frequency of bowel movements, averaging 6.5 stools per 24 h, and a partially reduced continence (night-time incontinence in the form of uncontrolled stool smearing in 40% of cases), as well as long-term medication with a propulsive medication, represent criticisms of the ileoanal pouch operation[8,9,22,26]. In these cases, usually, the lower daily stool fre-

**Table 1** Extirpation of the pouch and long-term loop ileostomy

| | Dept. of Surgery, Univ. of Heidelberg | | | Literature* |
| --- | --- | --- | --- | --- |
| | UC<br>(*n* = 274) | FAP<br>(*n* = 88) | Total<br>(*n* = 362) | Total<br>(*n* = 2838) |
| Extirpation of pouch | 10 (3.6%) | 1 (1.1%) | 11 (3.0%) | 7.6%<br>(3–14%) |
| Loop ileostomy<br>(> 2 years) | 12 (4.3%) | 2 (2.2%) | 14 (3.8%) | 8.5%<br>(2–19%) |

*Analysis of 24 papers, 1984–1993. UC: ulcerative colitis; FAP: familial adenomatous polyposis

quency and better continence after ileorectal anastomosis is compared. It has to be mentioned, however, that restorative proctocolectomy is a radical procedure which cures the disease while ileorectal anastomosis does not remove the diseased organ entirely. Moreover, a slight increase in the frequency of bowel motions is not usually perceived as a severe reduction in quality of life by most patients[13,19,21]. Also, terminal ileostomy does not appear to be a better solution for this problem. It is necessary to change the stool bag 4–6 times per day and sanitary conditions are even more important than after continence-preserving operations. Another aspect is the high cost of the life-long supply of stoma bags. The stool frequency is, to a large extent, influenced by the high stool volume after proctocolectomy[18,22]. This is usually caused by a reduced back resorption of sodium ions from the stool. The small bowel is not able, in this respect, to replace the lost colorectum entirely. The increased salt and water loss has to be regulated by the kidneys so the total volume loss remains constant compared with controls. In this regard, the different operative procedures of proctocolectomy do not differ very much from each other. The same is true for the increased faecal loss of bile salts and the change in the spectrum of specific bile acids.

According to our own experience, the indicators of quality of life, such as social contact and professional rehabilitation, were consistently superior after ileoanal pouch operation compared with ileoanal anastomosis and conventional proctocolectomy. This is essentially confirmed by other investigators. There is no doubt that the degree of patient satisfaction with this operative procedure is in most cases very high.

## INDICATORY VIEW POINTS

A clear contraindication for restorative proctocolectomy is Crohn disease[2,9]. The possibility of recurrent disease in the small bowel pouch with limited therapeutic benefits and the potential consequence of substantial small bowel loss during potentially necessary operative reintervention, as well as the increased risk of fistula formation, are clear contraindications for the application of the ileoanal pouch operation in these cases. In approximately 10% of cases of a chronic inflammatory bowel disease, it is not possible, either histopathologically or clinically, to make a diagnosis of Crohn disease or ulcerative colitis. In cases of a so-called indeterminate colitis, we proceed surgically in the same way as with ulcerative colitis. In the presence of an uncertain diagnosis or when the patient is in a poor general condition, such as in an emergency or when there are significant signs of cortical steroid side-effects, it is advisable to perform the procedure in a multistep fashion. In the first operation, a subtotal colectomy only is performed, and the re-establishment of continuity, in the form of an ileoanal pouch operation, can be performed after establishing the correct diagnosis or after the general condition has stabilized[2,23].

In the case of colitis-associated colorectal carcinoma, there is no principal contraindication for continuity-maintaining restorative proctocolectomy[2]. However, it is important to guarantee general surgical oncological criteria during the operation. In these cases, an oncological curative operation is more important than maintaining function. In advanced tumour stages, as well as in cases of very distal rectal carcinoma, restorative proctocolectomy should not be performed because potential problems, such as remanifestation of the malignancy in the small pelvis or development of peritoneal carcinomatosis, can be very difficult consequences of ileoanal anastomosis (Table 2).

**Table 2**  Restorative proctocolectomy in patients with associated colorectal carcinoma

| Patients with carcinoma ($n$) | IAP performed in: |
| --- | --- |
| UC ($n$ = 403) | |
|   Colon 21 | 8/21 (38%) |
|   Rectum 10 | 2/10 (20%) |
|   Total 31 | |
| FAP ($n$ = 112) | |
|   Colon 23 | 12/23 (56%) |
|   Rectum 6 | 2/6 (33%) |
|   Total 29 | |

Experience of the Dept. of Surgery, Univ. of Heidelberg. UC: ulcerative colitis; FAP: familial adenomatous polyposis

A compromised anal sphincter system, as well as manifest perirectal fistulae, are contraindications for the ileoanal pouch operation. There are, however, some specific exceptions to this rule: in the presence of a surgically reparable localized defect of the sphincter (for example post-traumatic), it is, in principle, possible to operate while maintaining continuity. Because sphincter reconstruction in the presence of manifest inflammation of the rectum is problematic, we conduct, as a first step, the ileoanal pouch operation with the creation of a protective ileostomy. In a subsequent step, the reconstruction of the anal sphincter is performed and a functional training period follows. If an improved sphincter function is diagnosed, the ileostomy is closed at the last step. We have, in this way, obtained satisfactory results in two cases.

One special situation of the perirectal fistula system is a manifest rectovaginal fistula. Usually, in these cases, there is no important inflammation of the pelvic floor region and therefore the ileoanal anastomosis is, in fact, a very good treatment of the fistula disease (Table 3).

**Table 3** Perirectal fistula is a contraindication for IAP. The exception is rectovaginal fistula

| | |
|---|---|
| Retrovaginal fistula occurrence in UC | 10/403 (2.4%) |
| IAP performed | 7/10 (70%) |
| Remanifestation of fistula | 3/7 (43%) |
| Final success | 7/7 (100%) |

From the Dept. of Surgery, Univ. of Heidelberg.
UC: ulcerative colitis

## PROTECTIVE ILEOSTOMY IN THE ILEOANAL POUCH OPERATION

The majority of authors favours the temporary placement of a protective ileostomy while performing the ileoanal pouch operation. By contrast, a number of study groups have published successful results after a single-step operation[27]. The most important argument in favour of protective ileostomy is the protection of the large anastomoses during the healing phase, as well as the good control of potential complications. Personal experience of treating the artificial stoma by the patients appears to be of lower priority.

## TECHNICAL ASPECTS

Special care must be taken to obtain functional results, with regard to a low frequency of bowel movements and good continence, which are as good as possible. Further aims are the sufficient treatment of the underlying disease as well as a very low postoperative morbidity. A number of modifications of the Parks and Nicholls procedure have been tested in the past[7,10,14,16,17,20,24,28]. Postoperative function and the size of the reservoir correlate well, as many studies have shown. Surgeons have tried to obtain the optimal size of reservoir by different folding of the small bowel, for example the J, S and W reservoirs. Other popular configurations include the Kock pouch and the lateral reservoir according to Fonkalsrud. However, comparative studies have shown that the pouch design is of secondary importance (Table 4). It is not clear whether a primarily very large constructed reservoir is of functional advantage in the long-term.

**Table 4** Evaluation of different pouch designs: clinical trials

| Design | Reference | Year |
|---|---|---|
| W > S > J | Nicholls and Pezim[17] | 1985 |
| S > J | Nasmyth et al.[16] | 1986 |
| S > J | Tuckson and Fazio[28] | 1991 |
| J = S | McHugh et al.[14] | 1987 |
| J = S | Pescatori et al.[24] | 1988 |
| J = W | Keighley et al.[10] | 1988 |
| S = W | Harms et al.[7] | 1990 |
| J = K | Öresland et al.[20] | 1990 |

W = 4 loops, S = 3 loops; J = 2 loops, K = Kock pouch

It is important for good function to obtain a secure means to empty the reservoir. This can be achieved by a side-to-end anastomosis (J or W pouch) or by a very short outlet (for example, a modified S pouch). Maintenance of the deep rectum and the transitional zone are considered advantages. This has led surgeons to favour performance of the technically less-demanding so-called double-stapling technique[1,27]. Some studies, however, have not shown any advantages and have demonstrated that persisting residual rectal mucosa can cause substantial problems[6]. Handsewn and staple techniques are both possible. They each have their own advantages and disadvantages which are of secondary importance.

Several comparative investigations of the individual opinions of patients have demonstrated clearly the high level of acceptance of the ileoanal pouch operation as a mode of treatment despite the accompanying problems[11,12,15,24]. Careful preoperative selection of patients, a situation-adapted approach, as well as a corresponding operative technique, in conjunction with competent postoperative follow-up, have made ileoanal pouch operation, overall, the best surgical option. Restorative proctocolectomy continues to replace conventional proctocolectomy and terminal ileostomy worldwide.

## References


1. Braun J, Schumpelick V. Die direkte ileumpouchanale Anastomose. Chirurg. 1993;64:614–21.
2. Buhr HJ, Heuschen U, Stern J, Herfarth Ch. Kontinenzerhaltende Operaton nach Proktocolektomie. Indikation, Technik und Ergebnisse. Chirurg. 1993;64:601–13.
3. Berry AR, de Campos R, Lee EC. Perianal and pelvic morbidity following perimuscular excision of the rectum for inflammatory bowel disease. Br J Surg. 1986;73:675–7.
4. Bokey EL, Dent OF, Zubrzycki J, Chapuis PH, Dunn DW. Surgical morbidity after ileostomy in New South Wales. Med J Aust. 1984;141:494–5.
5. Calstedt A, Fasth S, Hultén L, Nordgren S, Palselius I. Long-term ileostomy complications in patients with ulcerative colitis and Crohn's disease. Int J Colorectal Dis. 1987;2:22–5.
6. Choen S, Tsunoda A, Nicholls RJ. Prospective randomized trial comparing anal function after hand sewn ileoanal anastomosis with mucosectomy versus stapled ileoanal anastomosis without mucosectomy in restorative proctocolectomy. Br J Surg. 1991;78:430–4.
7. Harms BA, Pahl AC, Starling JR. Comparison of clinical and compliance characteristics between S and W ileal reservoirs. Am J Surg. 1990;159:34–9.
8. Herfarth Ch, Stern J. Colitis ulcerosa – Adenopatosis coli. Funktionserhaltende Therapie. Berlin, Heidelberg, New York: Springer; 1990.
9. Herfarth Ch, Stern J. Ileum-Pouch: Indikationen, Techniken, Langzeitergebnisse. Dtsch Med Wochenschrift. 1991;116:1485–90.
10. Keighley MR, Yoshioka K, Kmiot W. Prospective randomized trial to compare the stapled double lumen pouch and the sutured quadruple pouch for restorative proctocolectomy. Br J Surg. 1988;75:1008–11. Comment in: Br J Surg. 1989;6:989.
11. Köhler LN, Pemberton JH, Zinsmeister AR, Kelly KA. Quality of life after proctocolectomy. A comparison of Brooke ileostomy, Kock pouch and ileal pouch–anal anastomosis. Gastroenterology. 1991;101:679–84.
12. Köhler LN, Pemberton JH, Hodge DO, Zinsmeister AR, Kelly KA. Long-term functional results and quality of life after ileal pouch–anal anastomosis and cholecystectomy. World J Surg. 1992;16:1126–32.
13. Leijonmarck CE, Lofberg R, Ost A, Hellers G. Long-term results of ileorectal anastomosis in ulcerative colitits in Stockholm County. Dis Colon Rectum. 1990;33:195–200.
14. McHugh SM, Diamant NE, Mc Leod R, Cohen Z. S-pouches vs. J-pouches. A comparison of functional outcomes. Dis Colon Rectum. 1987;30:671–7.
15. Meister R, Gall FP. Ileorectostomie versus ileo-anale Anastomose mit Reservoir bei Colitis ulcerosa und Adenomatosis coli. Langenbecks Arch Chir. 1987;372:401–6.

16. Nasmyth DG, Williams NS, Johnston D. Comparison of the function of triplicated and duplicated pelvic ileal reservoirs after mucosal proctectomy and ileo-anal anastomosis for ulcerative colitis and adenomatous polyposis. Br J Surg. 1986;73:361–6.
17. Nicholls RJ, Pezim ME. Restorative proctocolectomy with ileal reservoir for ulcerative colitis and familial adenomatous polyposis: a comparison of three reservoir designs. Br J Surg. 1985;72:470–4.
18. O'Connell PR, Pemberton JH, Brown ML, Kelly KA. Determinants of stool frequency after ileal pouch–anal anastomosis. Am J Surg. 1987;153:157–64.
19. Oakley JR, Jagelman DG, Fazio VW et al. Complications and quality of life after ileorectal anastomosis for ulcerative colitis. Am J Surg. 1985;149:23–30.
20. Öresland T, Fasth S, Nordgren S, Hallgren T, Hultén L. A prospective randomized comparison of two different pelvic pouch designs. Scand J Gastroenterol. 1990;25:986–96.
21. Pemperton JH, Kelly KA. Achieving enteric continence: principles and applications. Mayo Clin Proc. 1986;61:586–99.
22. Pemperton JH. Neorectum and assessment of anorectal function following surgery. In: Kumar D, Waldron DJ, Wiliams NS, eds. Clinical measurement in coloproctology. Berlin, Heidelberg, New York: Springer; 1991.
23. Penna C, Dande F, Parc R et al. Previous subtotal colectomy with ileostomy and sigmoidostomy improves the morbidity and early functional results after ileal pouch–anal anastomosis in ulcerative colitis. Dis Colon Rectum. 1993;36:343–8.
24. Pescatori M, Mattana C, Castagnet M. Clinical and functional results after restorative proctocolectomy. Br J Surg. 1988;75:321–4.
25. Santavirta J, Mattila J, Kokki M, Poyhonen L, Matikainen M. Absorption of bile acids after ileoanal anastomosis. Ann Chir Gynaecol. 1990;79:134–8.
26. Setti-Carraro P, Ritchie JK, Wilkinson KH, Nicholls RJ, Hawley PR. The first 10 years' experience of restorative proctocolectomy for ulcerative colitis. Gut. 1994;35:1070–5.
27. Sugerman HJ, Newsome HH, Decosta G, Zfass AM. Stapled ileoanal anastomosis for ulcerative colitis without a temporary diverting ileostomy. Ann Surg. 1991;213:606.
28. Tuckson WB, Fazio VW. Functional comparsion between double and triple ileal loop pouches. Dis Colon Rectum. 1991;23:17–21.

# 28
# Current standards in surgery for Crohn disease

M. STARLINGER

Crohn disease is a pan-intestinal disorder which is, at the present time, incurable by either drug treatment or surgery. Although the initial manifestations may affect many different regions of the intestine (small bowel, ileocaecal region, colon), spread of the disease to previously unaffected intestinal segments is possible, both distally and proximally, in an unpredictable manner. Endoscopically and microscopically detectable changes are often seen at sites quite remote from the macroscopic changes[1]. Because of its characteristic pattern of transmural inflammation, the disease gives rise to the typical complications of stenotic scarring and fistula and abscess formation. It is these complications, together with extension of the inflammation (particularly to the colon), unresponsive to therapy, and giving rise to anaemia, hypoalbuminaemia, impaired performance, and a requirement for long-term steroid therapy, that constitute the major indications for surgery. Practically all patients with this disorder need to undergo at least one operation during the course of their disease[2]. The timing of surgery is determined by symptoms and by the nature of the complications. In other words, the purely endoscopic or radiological demonstration of stenosis in an asymptomatic patient is not an indication for surgery. Bland fistulae between neighbouring bowel segments, or cutaneous fistulae that are asymptomatic (i.e. with a small volume of leakage) also do not constitute an indication for urgent surgery. However, if a fistula leads to functional bypassing of large segments of intestine (e.g. an ileo-sigmoid fistula), or if an enterocutaneous fistula causes symptoms from maceration of the skin and a high volume of leakage, surgical therapy by resection of the fistulous bowel segment must be considered. Similarly, associated abscesses represent an indication for surgical treatment of the bowel segment responsible. Emergency surgery for overt ileus or free perforation, however, is rare.

The above considerations demonstrate that the indications for surgery in an individual case can only be assessed by close co-operation between the gastroenterologist and the surgeon. Such co-operation is particularly important in cases where a widespread inflammatory process, e.g. in the colon, cannot be satisfactorily controlled, or can only be controlled at the cost of significant side effects of drug (cortisone) therapy, but where surgery entails the placing of a temporary or permanent stoma.

The variety of possible clinical pictures, and hence of therapeutic strategies, makes it extraordinarily difficult to draw up a systematic scheme of generally applicable rules. Nevertheless, in the following I will present, firstly, the principles of the surgical techniques used, and then the basic indications for surgery in typical clinical situations.

## PRINCIPLES OF SURGICAL TREATMENT

Surgery for Crohn disease differs radically from other surgical procedures, particularly cancer surgery, with respect to purely technical aspects, such as routes of access and techniques of resection and anastomosis. The fundamental principles are summarized in Table 1.

In order to satisfy these requirements, the current extent of disease and the nature of the complication necessitating surgery should be well understood and defined preoperatively. This generally requires colonoscopy and investigation of the small bowel as described by Sellink. When there is a suspicion of abscess formation, this should be demonstrated by CT (and drained), or excluded. The main reason for this is that the preliminary drainage of abscesses and appropriate antibiotic therapy converts the abscess into an bland fistula (usually over 10–14 days), significantly simplifying the operative procedure and avoiding intraoperative spillage of organisms leading to postoperative abscess formation.

Careful preoperative demonstration of the current problem makes it possible to work out the operative strategy in consultation with the gastroenterologist and the patient, and provides protection from unexpected intraoperative surprises which would inevitably lead to over-hasty and therefore frequently wrong decisions. In addition, it is precisely in the large bowel that the current extent of disease is hard to determine before the bowel is opened, and the intra-abdominal relationships are unpredictable due to inflammatory or postoperative adhesions.

**Table 1**  Principles of surgical techniques in Crohn disease

| | |
|---|---|
| Route of access | – No incisions in areas that might subsequently need to be used as a stoma site |
| Tactics | – Only treat the disease complication that constituted the indication for surgery. Exception: stenoses distal to an anastomosis<br>– Preliminary drainage of accessible abscesses (CT or ultrasound guided) |
| Resection | – Bowel-sparing. No safety margins to be left beyond macroscopically recognizable extension of disease; no systematic lymph node dissection<br>– No resection of short stretches of stenotic strictures; use strictureplasty<br>– No resection of loops of bowel not affected by Crohn disease, but secondarily affected by entero-enteral fistulae. These should be freed and the fistulous opening oversewn<br>– No bypass operations<br>– Use of omental plugs to close parietal abscess cavities or fistulous tracks |
| Drainage | – Drainage only to preformed abscess cavities |

The systematic application of these principles has significantly increased the safety of surgical procedures in Crohn disease.

As recently as 15 years ago, the perioperative mortality and postoperative complication rates (abscesses, anastomotic insufficiency, ileus, sepsis) for surgery for Crohn disease were significantly higher than in comparable patients without chronic inflammatory bowel disease[3–5]. Perforating complications, such as fistulae or abscesses, preoperative steroid therapy, or multiple prior operations, are associated with a significantly higher risk of postoperative complications[3,6] (Figure 1). In an analysis of 621 abdominal operations during the period 1980–1992 at the Surgical Clinic in Tübingen, there was no significant difference between the complication rates for first and subsequent operations (5.4% vs 8.2%). Over this period, the complication rate fell continuously from an initial 19% to 5% at the present time (Figure 2). At the same time, mortality fell from 0.6% in the early 1980s to 0% at the present time, with an annual average of 80–100 abdominal operations over the last five years.

Over this whole period of observation, an increased risk of postoperative complications was only seen for preoperatively pre-existing abscesses, but not for septic complications (abscesses, fistulae, free perforations) overall. Since the introduction of preliminary drainage (1989), this difference has also ceased to be apparent.

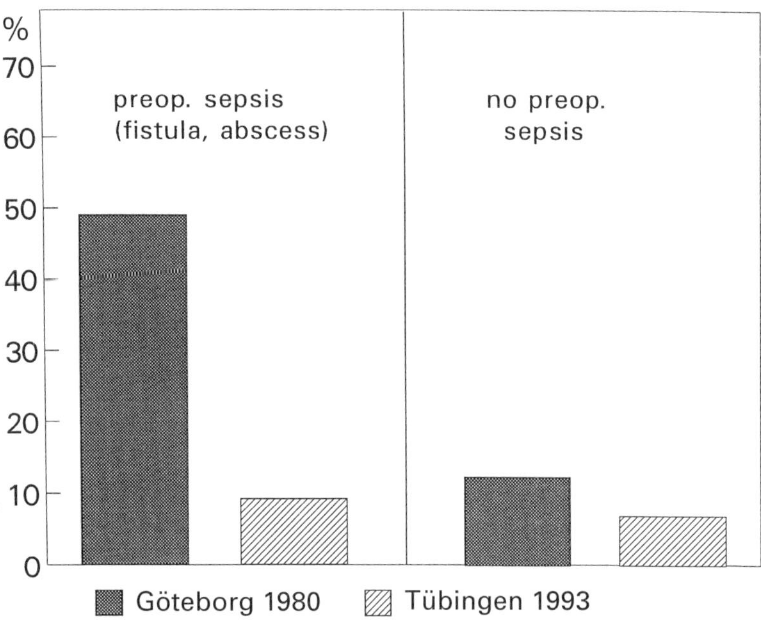


**Figure 1** Comparison of postoperative complication rates after abdominal operations for septic complications of Crohn disease (preoperative sepsis, fistula, abscess, free perforation) and purely obstructive complications or treatment resistance (no preoperative sepsis). Göteborg: Fasth et al. 1980[3], period 1969–1977, $n = 153$. Tübingen: period 1979–1993, $n = 621$

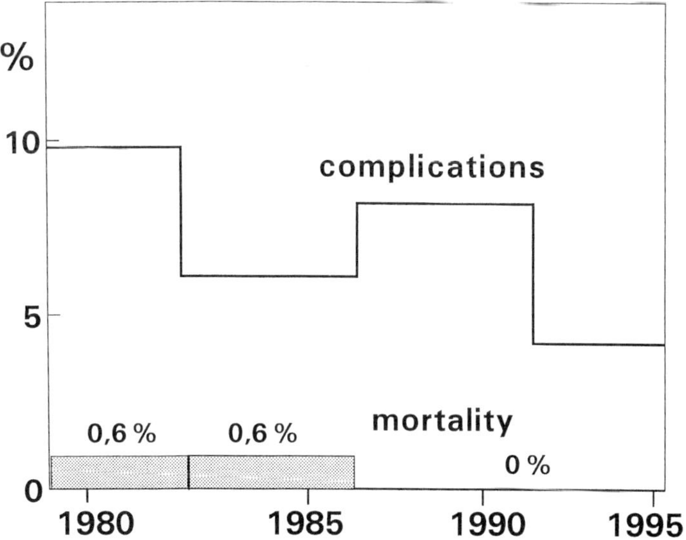


**Figure 2** Change in complication rates (re-laparotomy, anastomotic insufficiency, delayed haemorrhage, postoperative ileus, sepsis, intra-abdominal abscess, postoperative fistulae) and mortality after abdominal operations since 1979 (Tübingen University Surgical Clinic). Percentages shown are complication rates or mortality over successive four-year periods

## INDICATIONS FOR SURGERY

In addition to the very welcome observation that surgery for Crohn disease has become very safe, with a low complication rate – a consideration that might have led to the mistaken adoption of wider indications for surgery – additional factors must also be taken into consideration in deciding for or against surgery for a particular problem in a particular patient. As initially mentioned, the condition is incurable, and relapses are frequent after both medical[7] and surgical[8–11] treatment. In addition to the purely technical elimination of a complication, therefore, it is essential to consider the question of which operation will ensure a particularly low relapse rate, while simultaneously achieving the lowest possible incidence of postoperative sequelae, such as diarrhoea, after extensive bowel resection, or the need for a stoma.

In this context, there are major differences from one case to another, depending not so much on the nature of the complication leading to surgery (stenosis, fistula, refractoriness to treatment) as on the localization of disease in the bowel. It would therefore seem useful to discuss the different types of localization that can occur.

### Small bowel

Isolated extensive involvement of the small bowel is rare (4% in the Tübingen series)[12]. Such disease generally has a relatively benign course, i.e. perforating complications are rare. Surgical treatment only becomes necessary at the stage of stenotic scarring, since resection of extensive inflammatory changes is associated with significant loss of small bowel and the danger of the short-gut syndrome. Plastic operations to widen areas of stenotic scarring are indicated if diagnostic techniques can exclude acute inflammatory change and if the symptoms have not responded to preoperative medical therapy.

## Ileocaecal region

About one half of all patients present with primary ileocaecal involvement, of relatively limited extent. In such situations, the need for surgery should nowadays be considered early in the presence of suspected perforating complications (fistulae, abscesses), failure to respond to medical treatment, or short-lived remissions and frequent relapses of symptoms[13,14]. The relapse rate after surgery is undoubtedly lower than after medical treatment[15]. Numerous studies over the past few years have demonstrated that, after surgical resection in this region, only approximately half of patients are likely to suffer renewed symptoms over the following 10 years, and only around one third will require further surgery[8–10,14]. The consequences of surgery are not severe, provided this has been carried out in a bowel-sparing manner and less than 50 cm of the terminal ileum and, at most, the ascending colon are involved[16].

## Colon

In around 50% of cases, the large intestine is involved as well as the small intestine at the time of diagnosis, and, in 25% of cases, the disease presents as isolated colitis without involvement of the small bowel. Much more important than this global observation that involvement of the colon is common with and without involvement of the small intestine, is the fact that approximately half of all patients suffer more or less continuous involvement of the whole large intestine, implying a need for colectomy if surgery is carried out. In contrast, primarily segmental involvement, i.e. discontinuous disease with the possibility of segmental resection for complications, is rare (Table 2).

The rectum is involved in approximately half of all patients, particularly those with left-sided colitis. These patients, like those with extensive perianal fistulae, will sooner or later have to put up with a permanent stoma. For this reason alone, surgery for left-sided and total colitis is often deferred, and often refused by the patient despite many years' steroid dependence and significant impairment of quality of life. Here too, it is up to the gastroenterologist treating the patient, possibly in collaboration with other patients from a self-help group, to

**Table 2**  Extent of Crohn colitis ($n = 323$) at initial diagnosis and end of follow-up (mean follow-up 9.4 years)

|  | Initial diagnosis | End of follow-up |
| --- | --- | --- |
| Total colitis | 48.6% | 69.3% |
| Right-sided colitis | 24.8% | 16.7% |
| Left-sided colitis | 17.3% | 6.5% |
| Segmental colitis | 9.3% | 7.4% |
| Involvement of rectum | 39.9% | 60% |

advise patients and bring home to them the significant gain in performance achievable after colectomy and ileostomy. Studies over the past few years have demonstrated the excellent quality of life achieved by patients with chronic inflammatory bowel disease after ileostomy[17].

Despite this essentially positive attitude to removal of the whole large intestine and placement of an ileostomy, we in Tübingen have also tried over the past few years to maintain bowel continuity.

At 15 years, the risk of loss of the colon in Crohn colitis was 18% and the risk of proctectomy was 10%. A temporary stoma had been placed in 22% of patients and a permanent one in 12% (Figure 3). In over half these patients, the indication was treatment-resistant perianal fistulae.

In the colon, in particular, the extent of the surgical procedure is determined by the nature of the complication necessitating surgery. Segmental stenoses or perforating complications can often be treated by segmental resection if the residual colon is currently free from inflammation, and if the simultaneous presence of active proctitis or marked perianal fistulae has not created the need for an ileostomy to eliminate perianal symptoms.

The justification for such a bowel-sparing procedure in the colon is the observation that the risk of a symptomatic relapse or a renewed need for surgery, even in patients with primary pancolitis, is no higher than after colectomy. The risk at 10 years is 60% (symptoms) and 32% (surgery), respectively. The justification for more widespread use of plastic procedures to widen the colon, as recently proposed by Dürig[18], cannot yet be assessed due to lack of adequate experience.

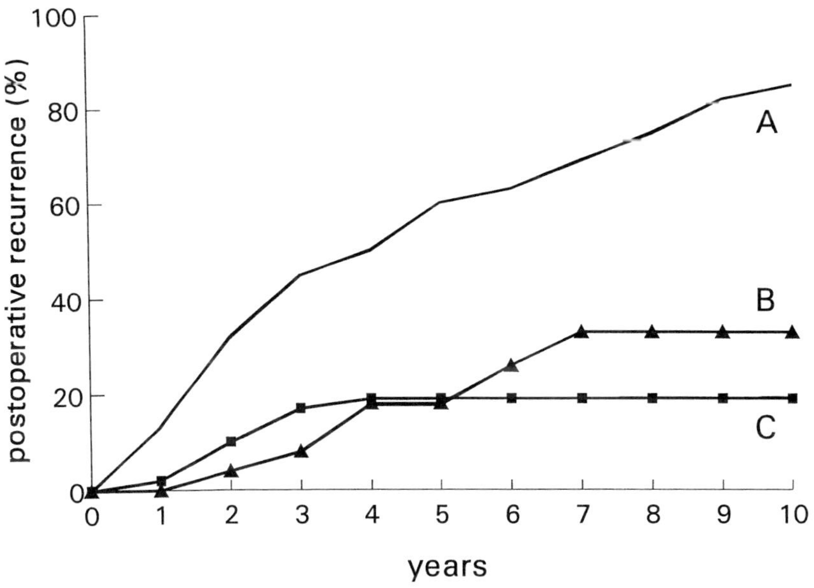


**Figure 3**   Risk of postoperative relapse after surgery for complications of total colitis (*n* = 82). **A**: symptomatic relapse; **B**: risk of relapse surgery following colectomy (*n* = 26); **C**: risk of relapse surgery following segmental resection (*n* = 56)

However, in the presence of widespread inflammation refractory to treatment, complete resection of the diseased bowel segment, perhaps with placement of a permanent stoma, is essential.

Simultaneous excision of the rectum is only required in exceptional circumstances. It is particularly in the presence of extensive perianal fistulae that bypassing of the rectum with proximal closure leads to rapid symptomatic improvement. In about 60% of cases, the stoma can be closed once again after the fistulae have healed. Primary proctectomy is also contraindicated by the high risk of perianal healing by secondary intention, often with the formation of a persistent perineal sinus, if the procedure is carried out during the florid stage of perianal fistulous disease with abscess formation.

## POSTOPERATIVE RELAPSES

After removal of an affected intestinal segment, endoscopic relapse is demonstrable in almost all patients only weeks after surgery. These endoscopic changes, in the form of aphthae or ulcers, are characteristically found very close to the anastomosis, and their severity has prognostic significance[19]. In other words, the earlier these changes occur and the more extensive they are, the sooner they lead to symptoms that necessitate further treatment, sometimes even repeated surgery.

In all, a symptomatic relapse rate of some 5–6% per year must be expected[8]. The relapse rate is highest (10% per year) in patients with extensive involvement of both the small and large bowel, who have often received primary treatment with multiple segmental resections[9]; and it is lowest in colitis treated at the onset by total colectomy and ileostomy[20].

In addition, the nature of the primary complication (stenosis or fistula/abscess) leading to the initial operation undoubtedly has prognostic significance. Although retrospective studies have led to differing outcomes, prospective studies have confirmed this fundamental division into relatively bland (stenosing) patterns of disease and disease complicated by fistulae and abscesses; this subdivision also demonstrates different frequencies of symptomatic flare-ups and different frequencies of surgical operations[11]. These prognostic considerations do not provide us with any new approaches to surgical treatment deviating from the concept outlined above. Symptomatic relapses are also only treated surgically if the cause of the symptoms (stenotic scarring or inflammation with fistula and abscess formation) cannot be treated medically. The fact that such relapses mostly develop at the ileocolic anastomosis and are therefore endoscopically accessible, ought to lead to consideration of endoscopic dilatation for purely stenotic changes, before further surgery is undertaken. Initial experience shows that balloon dilatation is a low-risk procedure which can postpone the need for further surgery, for some years at least, in the majority of patients[21,22].

## SUMMARY

Almost all patients with Crohn disease are obliged to undergo surgery at least once during the course of their disease. Soon after surgical removal of a diseased bowel segment, specific changes of Crohn disease can again be demonstrated endoscopically. Repeated operations are therefore not rare. For this reason, procedures achieving maximum bowel sparing and limited to eradication of the complication necessitating surgery are nowadays the standard approach. Careful preoperative diagnostic investigation of the extent of involvement and the nature of the complication is essential. Abscesses are, if possible, treated by preliminary drainage, and the associated sepsis treated by antibiotics. Fistulae opening into uninvolved bowel segments are merely excised and oversewn. Only the origin of the fistulae, in bowel affected by Crohn disease, must be excised. Bland stenotic strictures can be dilated by strictureplasty. In the colon too, bowel-sparing procedures are possible, since segmental resection of the bowel segment responsible for the current complication (fistula, stenosis or abscess) does not carry a higher risk than primary colectomy with ileorectal anastomosis.

Only steroid-resistant pancolitis is treated by colectomy. The use of such a procedure allows a permanent stoma to be avoided for many years, even in Crohn colitis (the risk of a permanent stoma in Crohn colitis being around 10% over fifteen years). Careful planning of the operative procedure has significantly reduced the perioperative risk. Mortality should be less than 1% and the rate of severe complications, such as anastomotic insufficiency, abscesses, or peritonitis, is also less than 5% nowadays. This means that, in some cases, the indications for surgery can be extended. Hitherto, the only indications for surgery have been treatment-resistant symptoms of stenosis, the development of septic complications, such as fistulae or abscesses, and steroid-resistant colitis. Patients with limited involvement of the terminal ileum and frequent symptomatic inflammatory relapses undoubtedly benefit from early surgery even in the absence of a complication, since the chance of a long-lasting symptom-free interval following surgery is much lower (around 50% symptomatic relapses at 10 years) than after purely medical treatment.

## References


1. Lescut D, Vanco D, Bonniere P et al. Perioperative endoscopy of the whole small bowel in Crohn's disease. Gut. 1993;34:647–9.
2. Makowiec F, Starlinger M, Jenss H, Jehle E, Becker H-D. Prognostische Faktoren bei Morbus Crohn. Ist die Wahrscheinlichkeit einer späteren Operation bei Erstdiagnose abschätzbar? Dtsch Med Wschr. 1991;116:961–7.
3. Fasth S, Hellberg R, Hulten L, Magnusson O. Early complications after surgical treatment for Crohn's disease with particular reference to factors affecting their development. Acta Chir Scand. 1980;146:519–26.
4. Kessler H, Gall FP. Chirurgische Therapie des Morbus Crohn – Entwicklungen und Ergebnisse der letzten zwei Jahrzehnte. Chir Gastroenterol. 1993;9:278–85.
5. Lorenz D, Lorenz U, Hagmüller E, Saeger HD. Morbus Crohn: Resektionstherapie im Verlauf von zwei Jahrzehnten. Zentralbl Chir. 1993;118:127–34.
6. Post S, Betzler M, von Ditfurth B, Schürmann G, Küppers P, Herfarth C. Risks of intestinal anastomoses in Crohn's disease. Ann Surg. 1991;213:37–42.
7. Salomon P, Kornbluth A, Aisenberg J, Janowitz HD. How effective are current drugs for Crohn's disease? J Clin Gastroenterol. 1992;14:211–15.
8. Williams JG, Wong WD, Rothenberger DA, Goldberg SM. Recurrence of Crohn's disease after resection. Br J Surg. 1991;78:10–19.
9. Michelassi F, Balestracci T, Chappel R, Block GE. Primary and recurrent Crohn's disease. Ann Surg. 1991;214:230–40.

10. Makowiec F, Köveker G, Weber P, Jenss H, Starlinger M. Morbus Crohn: Krankheitsaktivität und Rezidiv nach Operation. Dtsch Med Wschr. 1990;115:1659–64.
11. Rutgeerts P, Geboes K, Vantrappen G, Beyls J, Kerremans R, Hiele M. Predictability of the postoperative course of Crohn's disease. Gastroenterology. 1990;99:956–63.
12. Tan WC, Allan RN. Diffuse jejunoileitis of Crohn's disease. Gut. 1993;34:1374–8.
13. Andrews HA, Keighley MRB, Alexander-Williams J, Allan RN. Strategy for management of distal ileal Crohn's disease. Br J Surg. 1991;78:679–82.
14. Scott NA, Hughes LE. Timing of ileocolonic resection for symptomatic Crohn's disease – the patient's view. Gut. 1994;35:656–7.
15. Dirks E, Goebell H, Schaarschmidt K, Körster S, Quebe-Fehling E, Eigler FW. Clinical relapse of Crohn's disease under standardized conservative treatment and after excisional surgery. Dig Dis Sci. 1989;34:1832–40.
16. Hulten L. Surgical treatment of Crohn's disease of the small bowel or ileocecum. World J Surg. 1988;12:180–5.
17. Award RW, El-Gohary TM, Skilton JS, Elder JB. Life quality and psychological morbidity with an ileostomy. Br J Surg. 1993;80:252–3.
18. Dürig M. Chirurgisches Therapiekonzept bei Morbus Crohn. Dtsch Med Wschr. 1994;119:843–6.
19. Rutgeerts PJ. Prevention of early recurrence of Crohn's disease after ileal resection with ileo-colonic anastomosis. Eur J Gastroenterol Hepatol. 1994;6:113–16.
20. Andrews HA, Lewis P, Allan RN. Prognosis after surgery for colonic Crohn's disease. Br J Surg. 1989;76:1184–90.
21. Blomberg B, Rolny P, Järnerot G. Endoscopic treatment of anastomotic strictures in Crohn's disease. Endoscopy. 1991;23:195–8.
22. Breysem Y, Janssens JF, Coremans G, Vantrappen G, Hendrickx G, Rutgeerts P. Endoscopic balloon dilation of colonic and ileo-colonic Crohn's strictures: long-term results. Gastrointest Endosc. 1992;38:142–7.

# 29
# Non-resective surgery for Crohn disease

## M. R. B. KEIGHLEY

## INTRODUCTION

Crohn disease is a disorder of unknown aetiology causing strictures, abscesses, fistulae, colitis and severe anorectal disease. The standard surgical treatment for patients with complications of disease – obstruction, abscess, fistula, destructive anal disease, malignant change and colitis – is to resect the affected segment of bowel. Resection of anorectal disease results in a permanent stoma which, for some patients, is unacceptable. Resection of small bowel disease is often associated with recurrence and, for patients who have had four or five previous resections, there is a danger that ablative surgical treatment may result in the short bowel syndrome and severe malabsorption. Thus, there are a number of situations where non-resective surgery is playing a greater role in the management of Crohn disease than was the case 10 or 20 years ago.

## STRICTUREPLASTY

When Crohn and his colleagues first described regional ileitis, resection was the preferred surgical option. In the ensuing years, resection was replaced by bypass operation, largely due to the high mortality and morbidity which at that time attended resection.[1] Bypass operations usually involved a side-to-side anastomosis or an exclusion bypass, leaving the Crohn segment out of circuit. The bypass was used both as a means of conserving bowel and as an attempt to maintain low morbidity. Unfortunately, side-to-side bypass was attended by high rates of recurrence, serious metabolic sequelae, persistent local sepsis and, in some instances, malignancy in the bypassed segment[2]. Furthermore, when bypass procedures were compared with resection, the curative recurrence rates were higher with a shorter disease free interval after bypass operation than after resection (Figure 1). Thus, bypass operations fell into disrepute and were largely abandoned by most surgeons.

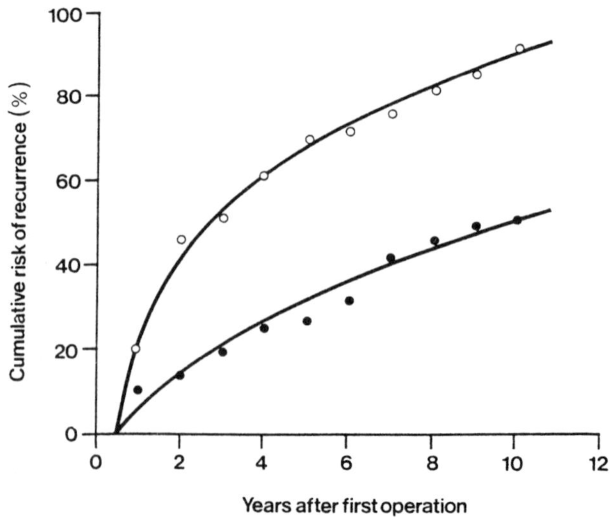

**Figure 1** The cumulative risk of recurrence: bypass compared with excision. The chance of requiring a second definitive operation each year after the primary procedure. ○ Bypass; ● excision (Reprinted from Keighley and Williams. Surgery of Anus, Rectum and Colon. London: Saunders)

## The birth of strictureplasty

The idea of overcoming an inactive stricture by non-resectional surgery originated in the Indian subcontinent where enteroplasty was proposed for the treatment of inactive tubercular strictures of the terminal ileum[3]. This idea was explored in Crohn disease and pioneered in the United Kingdom by the late Emanuel Lee of Oxford[4,5]. In fact, it is quite possible that Bryan Brooke performed the first successful strictureplasty for Crohn disease in Birmingham in 1961 but this case was not reported in the literature. The principle of strictureplasty was to divide the bowel at the site of the stricture longitudinally and to close it transversely in the same manner as a Heineke–Mikulicz pyloroplasty (Figures 2–4).

## Birmingham experience of strictureplasty

We have used the principle of strictureplasty since 1976 and analysed the results of 265 strictureplasties in 61 patients (Table 1); 2.4 strictureplasties were performed on average per patient; the mean length of the strictureplasties was 10.5 cm; associated resections were performed at 24 of the 89 operations. The indications for strictureplasty were: obstruction in 81, enterocutaneous fistulae in 7 and ileostomy bleeding in 1. Twenty-nine patients had a single strictureplasty and 32 had multiple strictures.

Twenty-four of 46 patients followed up for more than five years have required further operations, usually for recurrent strictures. However, it has been difficult to know whether recurrences are at the same site as the strictureplasty or have occurred in previously uninvolved segments of gut. Three patients requiring reoperation were found to have small bowel carcinomas but it was impossible to

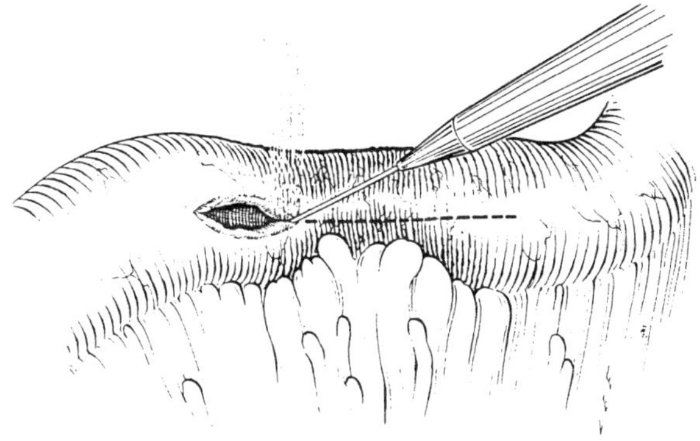

**Figure 2** Short strictureplasty. A longitudinal incision is made over the strictured segments of the small bowel. The aim is to open the entire stenotic segment and enter thin-walled dilated segments proximal and distal to the area of stenosis (Reprinted from Keighley and Williams. Surgery of Anus, Rectum and Colon. London: Saunders)

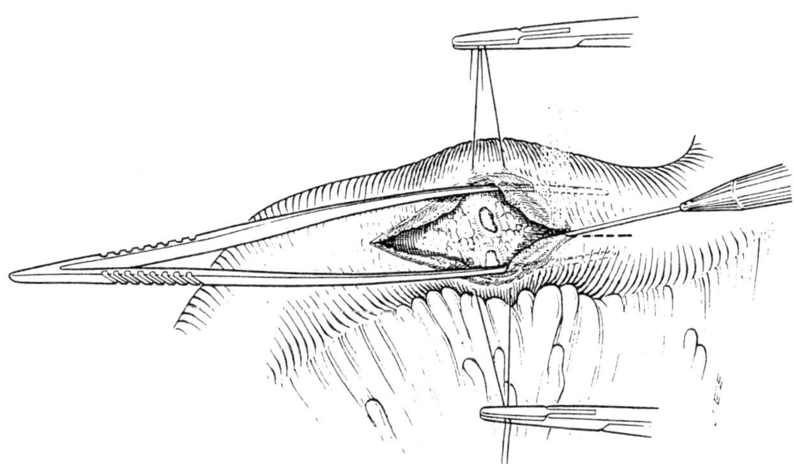

**Figure 3** Non-toothed forceps help to complete the enterotomy (Reprinted from Keighley and Williams. Surgery of Anus, Rectum and Colon. London: Saunders)

be certain whether these tumours developed from a previous strictureplasty site.

Strictureplasty in our experience was associated with a low rate of complications (Table 2). Seven patients developed enterocutaneous fistulae, five of whom had coexisting sepsis or fistula at the time of operation. Thus, we no longer advise an unprotected strictureplasty in the presence of co-existing sepsis or an enterocutaneous fistula.

Eighty per cent of patients were completely asymptomatic six months after operation; most had gained weight and there was a significant rise in serum albumin. Recurrence after strictureplasty is higher than after small bowel resection. On the other hand, strictureplasty tends to be used for patients with multi

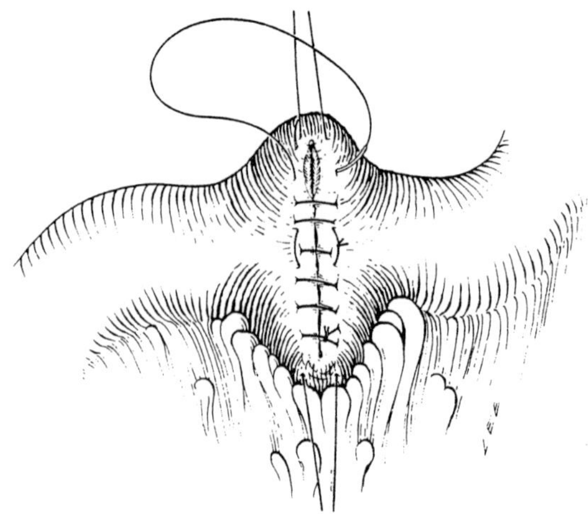

**Figure 4** The enterotomy is closed transversely as a single-layer extramucosal technique using either a continuous or an interrupted suture technique  (Reprinted from Keighley and Williams. Surgery of Anus, Rectum and Colon. London: Saunders)

**Table 1**  Sites of strictureplasty: data from Birmingham

| | |
|---|---|
| Number of patients | 61 |
| Total number of operations | 89 |
| Number of patients having previous resection | 47 |
| Total number of strictureplasties | 265 |
| Sites: | |
|    Duodenum | 9 |
|    Jejunum | 89 |
|    Ileum | 147 |
|    Ileocaecal | 20 |
|    Ileorectal | 10 |

**Table 2**  Complications of 265 strictureplasties: data from Birmingham

| | |
|---|---|
| Wound sepsis | 9 |
| Bleeding | 1 |
| Abscess | 2 |
| Thromboembolism | 2 |
| Postoperative enterocutaneous fistula | 7 |

focal disease or for those in whom bowel must be preserved for fear of developing short-gut syndrome. It is hardly surprising that recurrence rates are significantly greater when an operation is used to treat multifocal disease rather than when pathology is localized to one segment of the bowel. Thus, when we compared 41 patients treated by strictureplasty with 41 who had undergone a conventional resection, the surgery-free interval was only 2.9 years after strictureplasty compared with 7.9 after resection (Table 3). These findings do not negate the value of strictureplasty; merely, they serve to underline that stricture-

**Table 3**  Comparison between resection and strictureplasty

|  | Resection ($n = 41$) | Strictureplasty ($n = 41$) |
|---|---|---|
| Number of operations | 221 | 130 |
| Duration of follow up (years) | 17.2 | 15.2 |
| Surgery-free interval (years) | 7.9 | 2.9 |

From Sayfan et al.[17]

plasty tends to be performed for a different group of patients with more aggressive disease than does resection.

## Experience from other centres

The overall experience amongst surgeons in other centres has been compared with our own (Table 4). By and large, the operation of strictureplasty is safe; it successfully controls the symptoms attributable to obstruction, nutrition is improved and complication rates are low. Nevertheless, there is a slightly higher incidence of recurrent disease than has been reported after resection.

**Table 4**  Experience with strictureplasty in various centres

| Author | Number | % Recurrence | Follow-up (months) | % Complications |
|---|---|---|---|---|
| Kendall[18] | 5 | 100 | 6 | 20 |
| Dehn[19] | 24 | 46 | 40 | 7 |
| Fazio[20] | 50 | 22 | 8 | 16 |
| Pritchard | 13 | 69 | 24 | 15 |
| Spencer | 35 | 20 | 24 | 14 |
| Alexander-Williams[21] | 64 | 39 | 24 | 30 |

## FAECAL DIVERSION ALONE

The concept of faecal diversion alone also emanated from Oxford. Emanuel Lee explored the role of faecal diversion as an alternative to conventional surgical resection with three objectives in mind:

1. To achieve colonic healing and allow intestinal continuity subsequently to be restored without resection where disease was diffuse but not severe enough to warrant a proctocolectomy.

2. To facilitate major resection in those with poor health.

3. To limit resection in patients with diffuse disease[6,7].

These indications have subsequently been expanded to include the avoidance of growth retardation in children, to protect or avoid a primary anastomosis and to delay or prevent rectal excision. More recently, faecal diversion has been explored in the management of refractory perianal disease, particularly to allow perianal and rectovaginal fistulae to heal spontaneously or to facilitate their repair. Faecal diversion has been used both to allow perianal disease to resolve and to facilitate reconstructive procedures without the risk of sepsis[8,9]. Others argue, however, that faecal diversion has no impact on perianal disease[10,11]. Some have even demonstrated that faecal diversion alone may in fact exacerbate rectal disease by precipitating diversion proctocolitis[12,13].

Faecal diversion has an undeniable role in protecting an intestinal anastomosis after resection for Crohn disease and its role in this regard is not disputed. The main source of controversy is in the use of faecal diversion alone in an attempt to improve ileocolitis or to achieve resolution of perianal disease.

## Methods of faecal diversion

When the concept of faecal diversion was first developed, the fashion was to divide the ileum in a manner termed split ileostomy. In this way, the terminal ileum was delivered as an everted ileostomy and the proximal end of the divided ileum was brought out as a mucous fistula. This arrangement allowed the introduction of medication down the distal limb into the colon whilst the proximal everted bud acted as a normal ileostomy. Unfortunately, patients find mucous fistulae difficult to tolerate. Furthermore, closure of a split ileostomy involves laparotomy.

The alternative method of faecal diversion is by loop ileostomy. This can be constructed through a small trephine at the ileostomy site and it does not require a laparotomy for closure. Provided the proximal limb of the loop ileostomy is adequately everted, loop ileostomy achieves satisfactory defunction of the bowel. However, there is a tendency with loop ileostomy for retraction, particularly if the loop is not delivered over a rod in the early postoperative period.

## Results of faecal diversion

We and others have demonstrated that faecal diversion allows mucosal regeneration and healing of Crohn ulcers[14]. We analysed the results of faecal diversion alone in 44 patients and reported immediate remission in 82% and sustained remission for more than 12 months in 70%. Unfortunately, restoration of intestinal continuity was only achieved in 6 (14%) of these patients and many remained defunctioned (Table 5).

Faecal diversion has also been used to allow spontaneous healing of perianal lesions and for surgical excision of fistulae or, at the time of reconstruction, for rectovaginal fistulae. Zelas and Jagelman[8] reported improvement of perianal disease after loop ileostomy alone in 22 out of 23 patients. Unfortunately, these

**Table 5**   Results of faecal diversion: Birmingham ($n = 44$)

| | |
|---|---|
| Immediate remission | 36 (82%) |
| Sustained remission (12 months) | 31 (70%) |
| Steroids (before:after) | 30 : 9 |
| Restoration of intestinal continuity | 6 (14%) |
| Remained defunctioned | 21 (47%) |
| Proctocolectomy | 17 (39%) |

spectacular results have not been reproduced in all centres, and, in certain cases, faecal diversion has been associated with progression of perianal disease[15]. We are currently analysing our results to determine those factors which are associated with sustained improvement of perianal disease following faecal diversion alone. At the moment, we seem unable to predict the outcome from clinical parameters alone. The main drawback to faecal diversion is defunction proctitis which, although rare, may masquerade as severe inflammatory disease in the bypassed colon[16]. Sometimes, it is extremely difficult to distinguish continued inflammatory bowel disease from defunction proctitis. Faecal challenge may not always distinguish the two conditions.

## OTHER FORMS OF NON-RESECTIONAL SURGERY

### Enterocutaneous fistula

Postoperative enterocutaneous fistula can often be managed by conservative measures alone, using total parenteral nutrition and drainage of abscess, provided there is no distal obstruction and provided there is no evidence of residual Crohn disease.

### Anorectal disease

Anorectal disease is often managed by non-resectional surgery. Abscesses are drained. Perianal fistulae may be laid open if they are very superficial but we prefer the policy of Seton fistulotomy for trans-sphincteric fistulae. High or complex fistulae require a combination of faecal diversion, drainage and Seton fistulotomy.

Rectovaginal fistulae may be managed by mucosal advancement flaps, provided there is no evidence of rectal disease but case selection is crucial and some of these patients may require faecal diversion.

Anorectal strictures may be managed by repeated dilatation and fissures may be controlled by local injection of steroids or by very gentle anal dilatation.

### References


1. Garlock JH, Crohn BB, Klein SH, Yarnis H. An appraisal of long term results of surgical treatment of regional ileitis. Gastroenterology. 1951;19:414–23.
2. Greenstein AJ, Sachar D, Puccilo A et al. Cancer in Crohn's disease after diversionary surgery. Am J Surg. 1978;135:86–90.
3. Katariya RN, Sood S, Rao PG et al. Strictureplasty for tubercular strictures of the gastrointestinal tract. Br J Surg. 1977;64:496–8.
4. Lee ECG, Papaioannou N. Recurrences following surgery for Crohn's disease. Clin Gastroenterol. 1980;9:419–38.
5. Lee ECG, Papaioannou N. Minimal surgery for chronic obstruction in patients with extensive or universal Crohn's disease. Ann R Coll Surg Engl. 1982;64:229–34.
6. Harper PH, Kettlewell MGW, Lee ECG. The effect of split ileostomy on perianal Crohn's disease. Br J Surg. 1982;69:608–10.
7. Harper PH, Truelove SC, Lee ECG, Kettlewell MGW, Jewell DP. Split ileostomy and ileocolostomy for Crohn's disease of the colon and ulcerative colitis: a 20 year survey. Gut. 1983;24:106–13.
8. Zelas P, Jagelman DG. Loop ileostomy in the management of Crohn's colitis in the debilitated patient. Ann Surg. 1980;191:164–8.

9. Hellers G, Bergstrand O, Ewerth S et al. Occurrence and outcome after primary treatment of anal fistulae in Crohn's disease. Gut. 1980;21:525–7.
10. Oberhelman HA. The effect of intestinal diversion by ileostomy on Crohn's disease of the colon. In: Weterman IT, Pena AS, Booth CC, eds. The management of Crohn's disease. Amsterdam: Excerpta Medica; 19??:216–19.
11. Ritchie JK, Lennard-Jones JE. Crohn's disease of the distal large bowel. Scand J Gastroenterol. 1976;11:433–6.
12. Glotzer DJ, Glick ME, Goldman H. Proctitis and colitis following diversion of the fecal stream. Gastroenterology. 1981;80:438–41.
13. Roediger WEW. The starved colon – diminished mucosal nutrition, diminished absorption and colitis. Dis Colon Rectum. 1990;33:858–62.
14. Winslet MC, Keighley MRB. Defunctioned proctitis: A diagnostic dilemma. Gut. 1988;29:A1454.
15. Hywel-Jones J, Lennard-Jones JE, Lockhart-Mummery HE. Experience in the treatment of Crohn's disease of the large intestine. Gut. 1966;7:448–52.
16. Korelitz BI, Cheskin LJ, Sohn N, Sommers SC. The fact of the rectal segment after diversion of the fecal stream in Crohn's disease: its implications for surgical management. J Clin Gastroenterol. 1985;7:37–43.
17. Sayfan J, Wilsdon DAL, Allan A, Andrews H, Alexander-Williams J. Recurrence after strictureplasty or resection for Crohn's disease. Br J Surg. 1989;76:335–8.
18. Kendall GP, Hawley PR, Nicholls RJ, Lennard-Jones JE. Strictureplasty: a good operation for small bowel Crohn's disease? Dis Colon Rectum. 1986;29:312–16.
19. Dehn TCB, Kettlewell MGW, Mortensen MJM, Lee ECG, Jewell DP. Ten year experience of strictureplasty for obstructive Crohn's disease. Br J Surg. 1989;76:339–41.
20. Fazio VW, Tjandra JJ. Strictureplasty for Crohn's disease with multiple long strictures. Dis Colon Rectum. 1993;36:71–2.
21. Alexander-Williams J, Haynes IG. Conservative operations for Crohn's disease of the small bowel. World J Surg. 1985;9:945–51.

# 30
# Optimized treatment of fistulae in Crohn disease

W. D. WONG, C. BELMONTE and J. PEREZ

## INTRODUCTION

Crohn disease has a wide spectrum of manifestations and complications that often present a formidable challenge to even the most experienced and skilled clinician. Not the least of these is the propensity to fistula formation that is so often present in patients with this difficult disease. Fistulae can be broadly classified as either internal or external and, depending on their location and severity, can present very serious nutritional and metabolic consequences and incapacity to the patient. Fistulae are reported to occur in 20–60% of patients with Crohn disease[1-4] and are seen much more commonly in small bowel disease than with Crohn colitis[5]. External fistulae have been reported with a fre quency of 9–21%[3,6,7]. External fistulae can be classified into high volume (greater than 500 ml/24 h) or low volume (less than 500 ml/24 h). Internal fistulae are reported to be present in 16–35% of patients with this disease[6,8-11]. Fistulae occur in Crohn disease as a result of full-thickness or transmural inflammation and disease that ruptures into an adjacent organ, usually another hollow viscus, or alternatively through the anterior abdominal wall, most commonly at the site of a previous incision or drain site. Although stenosis and partial obstruction have been considered to be significant factors in fistula formation, Kahn et al.[12] have shown that fistulae frequently develop independently of stenosis and concluded that inflammation rather than increased intraluminal pressure was the primary factor. Full-thickness fissure formation is thought to be a major factor. An abscess may have been present as Steinberg et al.[13] noted that 7 of 10 patients in their series had an abscess associated with the development of an internal fistula. Patients usually present with signs and symptoms of sepsis with fever, increased pain, diarrhoea or evidence of obstruction. Recent drainage from a new external opening is evident if the fistula is external. The patient will probably relate a worsening of their Crohn disease status associated with anorexia, fatigue and progressive weight loss. Serious metabolic consequences may be apparent. Fistulous complications in Crohn disease, whether internal or external, present a significant management challenge with associated mortality rates of up to 10%.

## OVERVIEW

The management of patients with fistulae related to Crohn disease depends on a number of defining features. Many fistulae, because of their location and severity, have minimal impact on treatment needs. For example, an ileocolic fistula between the terminal ileum and the caecum would have little adverse effect on the patient's clinical status above and beyond that which is directly attributable to the primary disease focus as a fistula in this location is not likely to have any physiological consequences. On the other hand, a large-diameter fistula between the jejunum and the colon might have significant metabolic consequences. A scenario of even greater consequence is the high-volume proximal enterocutaneous fistula in the presence of life-threatening sepsis, fluid and electrolyte imbalance and nutritional deficit in a Crohn patient who has been experiencing a severe flare-up of disease. The management of patients with severe life-threatening fistulae and sepsis can be very challenging and requires a team approach that should include the gastroenterologist, the surgeon, skilled nurses and paramedical staff. Treatment can be divided into four phases: stabilization, investigation, conservative supportive treatment and definitive medical or surgical treatment[14].

## Phase 1: Stabilization

The combination of third-space losses from inflammation and fistula effluent rapidly depletes the patient's intravascular volume. The first priority is to re-establish adequate volume status to ensure adequate tissue perfusion and urine output. Any associated septic focus must be sought and adequately drained. Sometimes, this may require an emergency operation, although, nowadays, with the advent of advanced imaging techniques, the septic focus can usually be drained percutaneously, thus avoiding emergency surgery with its attendant risks. Antibiotics should be reserved for patients who are septic. If the fistula is external and of high volume, every attempt should be made to diminish intestinal output. This not only makes fluid and electrolyte management simpler, but also makes skin and wound care easier.

## Phase 2: Investigation

Once the patient has been stabilized and the sepsis has been controlled, the fistula should be investigated to determine the course and origin of the fistula tract, the presence of any persistent abscess, the extent of active Crohn disease and the presence or absence of distal obstruction. A fistulogram is the best method of defining an external fistula tract. Once its origin has been determined, a contrast study of the gastrointestinal tract is indicated to further define the extent of diseased bowel. The site of the fistula will determine whether a barium enema or an upper intestinal series is likely to be most informative. In many instances, both studies will be required. Endoscopic procedures are used to complement radiographic studies. The role of CT scanning in the initial evaluation of a fistula tract is limited to the identification of an associated abscess, as well as defining the extent, nature and location of the underlying disease.

## Phase 3: Conservative supportive treatment

Total parenteral nutrition (TPN) should be started early, after volume and electrolyte deficits have been corrected and sepsis is under control. TPN has been a major advance in the management of patients with major fistulous complications of Crohn disease. TPN can reduce the volume of external fistula effluent; however, its effect on spontaneous closure of Crohn-related fistulae is not established. As stated by Reber et al.[15] the greatest contribution TPN has made is the simplification of nutritional management for patients with enterocutaneous fistulae that allows for better timing of surgery if needed and improved nutritional status of patients undergoing re-operation and increased rate of postoperative recovery.

Enteral nutrition can supply complete nutritional support for selected patients with nutritional deficits related to fistulous disease in Crohn disease. In most cases, TPN is initially necessary to stabilize the patient and to establish positive nitrogen balance. Once this is achieved, patients with distal small bowel or colonic fistulae are candidates for enteral feeding. Unfortunately, patients with gastroduodenal and upper small bowel fistulae are not candidates unless the diet can be delivered to the bowel distal to the fistula.

Somatostatin analogue has been shown to be effective in non-Crohn disease high-output external fistulae in reducing fistula output and shortening the time to spontaneous closure. However, it has no effect on fistulae that are anatomically incapable of closure and does not appear to be effective in the treatment of fistulae related to intrinsic intestinal disease, such as Crohn disease[16].

## Phase 4: Definitive treatment

External fistulae occurring in patients with Crohn disease can be subdivided into two types according to aetiology. Those fistulae secondary to spontaneous extension of active disease have a very low rate of spontaneous closure (10%), whereas those occurring secondary to leakage of an anastomosis usually close with conservative management (86%)[17]. Internal fistulae are almost invariably due to active Crohn disease. Treatment needs will be determined by fistula location, fistula-related symptoms and effect, and disease activity. Medical therapy may effect fistula closure in properly selected patients; however, the majority of symptomatic fistulae will probably require surgical intervention.

### Medical treatment

The occurrence of fistulous disease in Crohn patients generally parallels the disease severity. As disease activity subsides, either spontaneously or as a response to conventional medical therapy, some fistulae may heal. However, this is the exception rather than the rule. In general, fistulae in Crohn disease are refractory to steroids and/or sulphasalazine. Any drug that could reliably and safely result in fistula closure would be a welcome addition to the treatment armamentarium for this difficult problem. Recently, some of the immunosuppressive agents have been shown to promote fistula closure on a limited basis. Their role has yet to be fully determined but the initial results show some potential promise.

In 1980, Present et al.[18] reported that, in a double-blind study, 6-mercaptopurine (6-MP) was more effective than placebo in closing fistulae related to Crohn disease (31% vs 6%). In a follow-up study reported in 1985, the authors documented closure in 13 of 34 (38%) fistulae with improvement in an additional 9 patients (26%) with the use of 6-MP[19]. No improvement was noted in 35%. The mean time of response was fairly protracted at 3.1 months. Although all types of fistulae responded, the best results were noted in fistulae involving the abdominal wall and entero–entero fistulae. If 6-MP was maintained, long-term response was satisfactory; however, recurrence occurred in all eight patients in whom the drug was discontinued. They concluded that 6-MP is an effective drug for the treatment of fistulae in severe refractory Crohn disease.

Another immunosuppressant, cyclosporin A, has been widely used in organ transplantation. Several studies in recent years have reported efficacy with the oral administration of this drug in treating Crohn fistulae. However, patient numbers have been very limited with variable response and relapse rates. Peltekian et al.[20] reported a response in two of four fistulae within 4 weeks; however, one recurred while still on the medication while the other recurred after cessation. Strange et al.[21] reported that all five patients treated with oral cyclosporin A responded; disease recurred in one patient while on the drug and two further patients after the drug was stopped. More recently, continuous intravenous infusion of cyclosporin A has been demonstrated to produce a more rapid response in improvement and closure of fistulae in Crohn patients. Hanauer and Smith[22] reported complete closure in 10 of 12 fistulae in five patients with this disease after a mean of 7.9 days. Five of the 10 fistulae recurred (range 3 weeks to 7 months), two of them after the initial dose was lowered. While side-effects were minor, one patient developed a mycotic aneurysm after 7 months of treatment. Present and Lichtiger in 1994 reported a long-term 64% significant improvement of closure rate in 16 patients with active fistula who were treated initially with intravenous cyclosporin A and later switched to oral administration[23]. They concluded that intravenous cyclosporin is effective treatment for a variety of Crohn-related fistulae and that its future role awaits controlled trials as well as determination of the risk–benefit ratio.

### Surgical treatment

Fistula remains one of the commonest indications for surgical intervention although certainly not all fistulae require operative repair. Farmer et al. showed that patients with ileocolic Crohn disease and fistula required surgical intervention in 86% of cases whereas only 69% of all patients ultimately came to surgery[24]. In another study, Greenstein et al.[25] reported that 52 of 63 (82%) patients with fistula ultimately required surgery compared with only 48 of 97 (49%) of patients with fistulae. Spontaneous closure of external fistulae secondary to active Crohn disease is unlikely. Driscoll and Rosenberg[26] noted that 10 of 11 patients with active Crohn disease who had enterocutaneous fistulae required surgical treatment. In an initial report by the Birmingham group[17] who reported on 39 Crohn external fistulae, nine postoperative fistulae involving no active disease closed spontaneously with medical treatment. In contrast, all 30 patients with active Crohn disease required surgical resection. In a subsequent report, this group found that only 7 of 24 postoperative fistulae closed spontaneously, and they concluded that surgical resection and anastomosis is the best option when surgery is required[27]. Attempts at simple closure of the fistula in four patients resulted in abscesses in three. Of three patients treated with strictureplasty, two developed leaks. Of 20 patients with Crohn disease and spontaneously occurring fistulae, spontaneous closure occurred in only one. Therefore, surgical resection is almost always advised for significant external fistulae associated with active Crohn's disease. In most situations anastomosis can be done primarily, although, in some patients with extensive concomitant intra-abdominal sepsis, the creation of a proximal stoma may be prudent. Results of strictureplasty in active Crohn disease with enterocutaneous fistulae were poor as only one of three was successful.

Michelassi et al.[11] have outlined the indication of surgery in patients with fistulae in Crohn disease as follows: when drainage was a matter of personal embarrassment, such as with an enterovaginal fistula; when the fistula communicated with the genitourinary tract; and when the fistula produced functional or anatomic bypass of a major segment of intestine with consequent malabsorption and/or profuse diarrhoea.

Not all fistulae require immediate surgery. In a review of 83 internal fistulae in 59 patients with Crohn disease, Glass et al.[28] concluded that the presence of an internal fistula, even when it involves the bladder, is not an absolute indication for immediate surgery and advocated a treatment policy that is dictated by the severity of the symptoms.

Surgical management of specific types and locations of fistulae will be discussed under the two broad categories of internal and external fistulae individually.


## INTERNAL FISTULAE

### Gastric and duodenal fistulae

Gastrocolic and duodenal colic fistulae in Crohn disease are very rare. Pichney et al.[29] reviewed only 83 reported cases in the literature. Feculent emesis is the hallmark of the clinical diagnosis but was present in only 33% of gastrocolic and 2% of duodenal colic fistulae. Barium enema is the best method of establishing the diagnosis as it is more sensitive than barium swallow[29]. Of 14 enterocolic–gastroduodenal fistulae reported by Michelassi et al.[11], one was diagnosed by history and physical examination, 11 by radiological or endoscopic studies and three intraoperatively. Fistulae to the stomach and duodenum almost invariably arise secondary to Crohn ileitis or colitis and only very rarely from primary gastroduodenal Crohn disease[29–31]. However, in Pichney et al.'s collective review of the literature[29], they found five reported cases of fistulae arising from primary gastric Crohn disease and one fistula arising from primary duodenal Crohn disease.

Since gastroduodenal Crohn fistulae almost invariably arise from ileal or colonic disease, surgical intervention for the symptomatic fistula should be directed at the primary disease organ. Ileal and/or colonic resection with simple closure of the stomach or duodenum is safe and effective in most instances. This is usually accompanied by a simple debridement or cuff excision in the case of the duodenum or similar debridement or wedge excision in the case of the stomach[28–31]. Rarely, the duodenal opening is not suitable for primary closure and, in these instances, a serosal patch utilizing a loop of jejunum can be used or, alternatively, a duodenal jejunostomy or a Roux-en-Y[32,33]. An omental patch is another useful adjunct and, in all cases, temporary decompression of the duodenum by nasogastric, duodenal or retrograde jejunostomy intubation should be performed[11].

## Entero–enteric fistulae

Fistulae between matted loops of small bowel in close proximity and at a similar level are generally asymptomatic and often do not require treatment for their own sake. Surgical intervention, therefore, is dependent on the status of the primary disease. At the University of Chicago, in a review of 639 Crohn-associated fistulae, Michelassi et al.[11] reported on 51 enteric fistulae which came to surgical resection. Forty-one (80%) were completely resected with the diseased bowel. However, in ten cases, a non-diseased distant loop of small intestine was the site of fistula. In these instances, the uninvolved intestine was detached and oversewn and the diseased bowel only was resected.

## Ileocaecal fistulae

Ileocaecal fistulae are generally incidental findings at the time of ileocaecal resection or on small bowel contrast studies. They are generally asymptomatic and treated by ileocaecal resection when indications are present for surgical treatment of the primary disease[10,11].

## Ileosigmoid fistulae

Another very common internal fistula occurring in Crohn disease is the ileosigmoid fistula. Surgical management is controversial. There is no debate regarding the need for resection of the diseased ileal segment; however, management of the sigmoid is the crux of the controversy. Fazio et al.[34] favour a double-resection approach, citing a significant complication rate with leakage and colocutaneous fistula formation following simple sigmoid closure. Other authors, however, consider it rare that the sigmoid colon is significantly affected by Crohn disease and advocate simple closure of the sigmoid if careful examination reveals no evidence of significant disease[10,11,35]. Block and Schraut[35] reported 48 cases treated by simple sigmoid closure when minimal disease was present with no incidence of postoperative complications. Our approach at the University of Minnesota is to perform a double resection only if significant inflammation, induration and disease of the sigmoid is confirmed on gross inspection, palpation and intraoperative endoscopic examination. Thus, in cases where minimal disease is apparent, simple debridement with suture closure of the sigmoid with resection of the ileal segment is performed.

## Enterovesical fistulae

Enterovesical fistulae occur in approximately 5% of patients with Crohn disease[11]. At the University of Chicago, a clinical diagnosis of enterovesical fistula was suspected in 25 of 36 patients with this disorder. A fistula was demonstrated by small bowel contrast studies in only three patients, barium enema in six, and cystoscopy in 15[11]. The presence of an enterovesical fistula is not necessarily an absolute indication for surgery. Many of these young patients have minimal urinary symptoms and recurrent urinary tract infections are often not a problem[28]. They occur more commonly in men (71%) probably due to the protective effect of the uterus and vagina in women[6]. Symptomatic enterovesical fistulae are treated by surgical resection. The involved bowel can be pinched off from the bladder. If an opening in the bladder is evident, suture closure is indicated. In many instances, however, the actual fistula tract will not be readily apparent, in which case catheter drainage of the bladder for 7–10 days with confirmation of closure by cystography prior to removal is usually all that is required. Commonly associated with enterovesical fistula is a concomitant fistula into the sigmoid; if the sigmoid colon is significantly diseased, it should be resected as well as the ileal segment. However, if minimal sigmoid disease is present, simple suture closure is adequate. The Cleveland Clinic reported their experience with 63 patients with enterovesical fistula treated by surgical resection. Thirty-four per cent had an associated intra-abdominal abscess. Only one of the 61 surgically treated fistulae recurred. An enterocutaneous fistula developed in 6.4%. They concluded that surgical treatment of enterovesical fistula in Crohn disease is safe and effective[36]. Many of these enterovesical fistulae can be managed by non-operative means. The group at Birmingham, UK identified 19 enterovesical fistulae in 799 patients with Crohn disease (2.4%). Four of these were treated conservatively and all remained asymptomatic. They advise resection of the affected segment of bowel with primary anastomosis if persistent symptomatic fistulae are identified[37].

## Enterovaginal fistulae

Enterovaginal fistulae are a relatively rare occurrence in Crohn disease. The diagnosis can usually be made by speculum examination of the vagina or visualization of the fistula with a flexible fibre optic scope. The treatment is generally surgical with resection of the diseased ileum with primary anastomosis. The opening in the vagina is usually very small and does not require any repair. Most patients who present with enterovaginal fistula have had a previous hysterectomy[11].

## EXTERNAL FISTULAE

## Enterocutaneous fistulae

As discussed earlier, enterocutaneous fistula in association with active Crohn disease is unlikely to heal spontaneously and surgical intervention is usually necessary. Any associated sepsis must be controlled. Once the patient is in a stable state, definitive surgical intervention can be undertaken. If the fistula was associated with a large abscess that was percutaneously drained, or if it resulted following previous surgery, it is preferable to have a minimum waiting period of 6–8 weeks prior to surgical correction of the fistula. However, in some instances, there will be associated sepsis that will require exploratory laparotomy and, in such instances, drainage of the sepsis with resection of diseased bowel is performed. Primary anastomosis can be considered if both ends of the bowel to be anastomosed are soft, pliable and without significant inflammation. In some instances, however, there is such severe septic process that resection of the diseased segment with creation of a temporary stoma is more prudent. The chronic enterocutaneous fistula in a stable patient is best treated by resection of the diseased segment of bowel with primary anastomosis. The tract in the abdominal wall can be curetted and left open.

## Colocutaneous fistulae

In general, colocutaneous fistulae are low volume and associated with few nutritional and metabolic consequences. A colocutaneous fistula from an isolated area of segmental colitis can be treated by segmental resection and primary anastomosis. However, a colocutaneous fistula in the presence of considerable colon involvement may be best treated by either subtotal colectomy and ileorectal anastomosis or total proctocolectomy with ileostomy if the disease process extensively involves the rectum and/or perianal region as well as the colon.

## Paraileostomy fistulae

Paraileostomy fistulae are extremely rare. Greenstein[6] reported 15 cases in a series of over 1000 patients with Crohn disease. Such fistulae are almost invariably due to recurrent disease at or just proximal to the ileostomy. The presence of a fistula creates significant problems with pouching of the stoma and requires surgical correction. The diseased segment of bowel is resected and the stoma is recreated on the contralateral side of the abdomen.

## Rectovaginal fistulae

Rectovaginal fistula in Crohn disease was reported to occur in 90 of 886 female patients with Crohn disease evaluated at St. Mark's Hospital[38]. This disease can be a devastating problem for the Crohn patient and can be a challenge for the treating clinician. Some patients have relatively minimal symptoms and symptomatic treatment in these instances is often the most appropriate therapy. Surgical treatment has been viewed with considerable pessimism in the past. However, recently, there has been a trend to more aggressive surgical management of selected patients with this disease. Recent favourable results support this more-aggressive approach to rectovaginal fistula in Crohn disease. Vaginal fistulae can be classified as either anovaginal or rectovaginal depending on the relationship of the tract to the anal canal. Of 80 classifiable vaginal fistulae in Crohn disease in the St. Mark's series[38], 36 were either extrasphincteric or suprasphincteric, 42 were trans-sphincteric and 2 were superficial. Of these, medical treatment and local surgical repair were successful in one third of the patients. Proctectomy was required in 38 of the patients because of extensive colonic involvement, rectal disease or associated anal lesions. Interestingly, only in 10 was a rectovaginal fistula listed as the significant indication for proctectomy. They concluded from this large series that either medical therapy or local surgical repair should be considered whenever feasible. Sher et al.[39] reported on 14 patients with Crohn disease who underwent surgical repair of rectovaginal fistula using a transvaginal approach. All patients had a proximal diverting loop ileostomy. The fistula healed with surgical management in 13 of the 14 treated patients; mean follow-up was 55 months. They advocate the transvaginal method as a preferred surgical approach because of the ease of raising a vaginal flap. Morrison et al.[40] reported the Ochsner Clinic results in 12 patients with rectovaginal fistula, 10 of whom had large bowel disease. Four patients had a primary repair of the fistula, four patients had staged repair with faecal diversion and four patients had such extensive colonic and anorectal disease that proctocolectomy was performed in the first instance. Healing occurred in six of the eight patients undergoing repair. Success correlated with quiescent intestinal disease and absence of rectal involvement. Three of the patients with no rectal involvement healed with surgical treatment whereas only one of six patients with rectal involvement healed with surgical management. Cohen et al.[41] reported a similar experience with local repair in seven patients with symptomatic Crohn rectovaginal fistula. They advocate either one of two operative approaches. The first involves division of the rectovaginal septum with layered repair. The second approach is an endorectal advancement flap. They concluded that, in the setting of quiescent rectal disease, a local repair of rectovaginal fistula has a reasonable chance of success. Anovaginal fistulae can be repaired with a lay-open technique if very superficial[38,42]. Another approach involves fistulectomy with anocutaneous flap as reported by Hesterberg et al.[43]. There is no consensus as to whether faecal diversion is necessary in association with rectovaginal fistula repair in Crohn disease. There are many instances of successful repair without diversion, indicating that this can be accomplished in properly selected patients.

## Rectourethral fistulae

Rectourethral fistula is a very unusual complication of Crohn disease. Treatment is best accomplished by a direct repair utilizing a transanal approach or a transperineal approach. The Yorke–Mason trans-sphincteric approach is another consideration. Fazio et al. reported good results using a rectal advancement flap performed transanally[44]. A more complex variant is a rectourethral perineal fistula. Stamler et al.[45] reported such a case treated successfully by an abdominal perineal approach.

## Perianal fistulae

Perianal fistulous disease occurs in approximately 20% of Crohn patients[46]. Most fistulae are relatively asymptomatic and follow a benign course, often with spontaneous healing. When an associated abscess is present, the sepsis must be adequately drained. Once an established fistula is present, treatment will depend on the severity of the symptoms. Many have minimal symptoms and may be treated conservatively. Only a few fistulae will require surgical intervention, generally those that are symptomatic and have failed medical therapy.

Medical measures that are helpful in perianal Crohn fistulae include: the control of diarrhoea that causes additional perianal irritation, warm sitz baths for hygiene and relief of discomfort and the use of proprietary creams. Metronidazole has been advocated for the management of perianal Crohn disease, including fistulous disease[47,48]. Although initial reports suggested a very significant response rate, this benefit has not been as dramatic as was once hoped. Results are variable and difficult to measure although many clinicians continue to advocate its use in this setting.

A variety of surgical approaches have been directed at this manifestation of Crohn disease. Keighley and Allan[49] reported that, of 12 patients with low fistula in ano and Crohn disease treated by simple fistulotomy, only one healed and six patients became incontinent. Because of these disturbing results, the authors advocated a very conservative approach to this disease.

However, in more recent years, a more aggressive approach has been justified by the results of other authors writing on this subject. Morrison et al.[50] documented healing in 30 of 32 fistulae treated by fistulotomy. They emphasized that the success of surgery is greatly enhanced if the rectum is not involved and if disease is quiescent elsewhere in the gastrointestinal tract. Levien et al.[51] reported a similar correlation as 18 of 21 patients with anal fistula with no rectal involvement healed with fistulotomy. Of their entire group of 47 patients, 37 achieved complete healing after fistulotomy and, although five patients ultimately required proctectomy, none were caused by the surgical treatment of the fistula. This more-aggressive approach is supported by many other authors who report very acceptable results in properly selected patients for fistulotomy[52–58].

Fry et al.[53] treated three anterior fistulae with an endorectal advancement flap and documented healing in all three. However, only two of six fistulae treated by Jones et al.[59] using this technique healed. The use of a draining seton for fistulae that involve a considerable amount of muscle is a very useful adjunct in the surgical management of perianal Crohn fistula. Williams et al.[60] reviewed our experience at the University of Minnesota with the use of non-cutting seton for fistulae that involve more than one third of the external sphincter. Twenty-two patients underwent placement of a silicone elastomer tubing to act as a stent to promote adequate drainage for a prolonged period of time. Eight remained fully continent, five had minor incontinence to liquids, four had occasional incontinence to stool and five required proctectomy. It was concluded that the use of seton for high trans-sphincteric fistulae can limit recurrent suppuration and preserve sphincter function. Other authors have also reported on the benefits of seton use in complex fistulae related to Crohn disease[58,61–63].

Faecal diversion may temporarily improve symptoms from severe anorectal Crohn disease; however, the diversion did not alter the long-term course of the disease in the University of Toronto's experience[64]. Sher et al.[65] advocate a low Hartmann procedure for severe perianal Crohn disease and report 60% of 25 patients achieving complete healing of their fistulae. The other 10 patients showed improvement, although the disease persisted despite the faecal diversion. In a series of paediatric–aged patients, faecal diversion did not alter the course of their disease[66]. Proctectomy remains a reasonable solution for some cases that are refractory to all treatment measures. However, there is a significant incidence of unhealed perineal sinus following this procedure. In a review, by Sher et al., the incidence in the literature ranged from 12% to 80%[65].

## University of Minnesota series

Seventy patients with Crohn disease who underwent anal fistula surgery between 1988 and 1992 were reviewed. There were 43 women and 27 men with a mean age of 41 years (range 18–87 y). Mean duration of disease was 13 y (range 6 months–28 y). Mean follow-up was 23 months (range 1–124 months). The site of disease was: perianal only in 9 patients (12%); colon and rectum 26 patients (37%); ileocolic 25 patients (35%); small bowel only in 10 patients (14%). Fifty-eight patients accounted for 79 fistulae: 33 intersphincteric, 41 trans-sphincteric, 4 suprasphincteric and 1 extrasphincteric. The other 12 patients had 3 or more fistulae. Thirty patients underwent successful fistulotomy of 26 intersphincteric and 8 low trans-sphincteric fistulae. Thirty-four patients with 33 high trans-sphincteric, 4 suprasphincteric and 1 extrasphincteric fistulae required the use of 62 setons of which 28 setons in 23 patients were removed: 19 were removed without recurrence, 6 failed and required further surgery and 3 were exchanged for a new seton. Twenty-eight setons are still in place. Six setons had spontaneous muscle division with good outcome in 5. Silastic tubes were used for 50 setons (80%); suture material for 10 (16%); and rubber band for 2 (4%). Thirteen patients underwent proctectomy: factors with a strong association for proctectomy were: 3 or more fistulae (8 of 12 patients); rectal involvement (10 of 18 patients); both 3 or more fistulae and rectal involvement (7 of 7 patients). Continence status was reviewed in 54 patients by questionnaire. Sixteen of 28 patients (57%) who underwent fistulotomy were fully continent. Twenty-three of 28 (82%) undergoing seton placement had total continence. We conclude that fistula in the anus in Crohn disease can be successfully managed by fistulotomy for simple fistula and by seton placement for complex fistula.


## SUMMARY

Fistulae in Crohn disease are a challenging problem for the clinician. While many such fistulae are totally asymptomatic and do not require any treatment, others cause severe nutritional, metabolic and wound-care problems that demand corrective measures. Some will respond to a variety of medical measures while the majority of symptomatic fistulae will require surgical intervention. The principles outlined in this chapter can very often result in the successful management of this difficult problem.


## References


1. Veloso FT, Cardoso V, Fraga J, Carvalho J, Dias LM. Spontaneous umbilical fistula in Crohn's disease. J Clin Gastroenterol. 1989;11(2):197–200.
2. Pettit SH, Irving MH. The operative management of fistulous Crohn's disease. Surg Gynecol Obstet. 1988;167:223–8.
3. Hill GL, Bourchier RG, Witney GB. Surgical and metabolic management of patients with external fistulas of the small intestine associated with Crohn's disease. World J Surg. 1988;12:191–7.

4. Schraut WH, Abraham VS. A comparison of complications following ileocolonic resection for Crohn's disease and for non-inflammatory bowel disease. Colo-proctology. 1987;9:289–95.
5. Schofield PF. Natural history and treatment of Crohn's disease. Ann R Coll Surg Engl. 1968;36:258–79.
6. Greenstein AJ. Surgery for Crohn's disease. Surg Clin N Am. 1987;67:573–96.
7. Burchell MC. Spontaneous umbilical fistula in Crohn's disease. Dis Colon Rectum. 1989;32:621–3.
8. Rankin JB, Watts DH, Melknyk CS, Kelly ML. National Cooperative Crohn's disease study: extraintestinal manifestations and perianal complications. Gastroenterology. 1979;77:914–20.
9. Koelbel G, Schmiedl U, Majer MC et al. Diagnosis of fistulae and sinus tracts in patients with Crohn's disease. Value of MR imaging. AJR. 1989;152:999–1003.
10. Annibali R, Pietri P. Fistulous complications of Crohn's disease. Int Surg. 1992;77:19–27.
11. Michelassi F, Stella M, Balestracci T, Giuliante F, Marogna P, Block GE. Incidence, diagnosis, and treatment of enteric and colorectal fistulae in patients with Crohn's disease. Ann Surg. 1993;218(5):660–6.
12. Kahn E, Markowitz J, Blomquist K, Daum F. The morphologic relationship of sinus and fistula formation to intestinal stenoses in children with Crohn's disease. Am J Gastroenterol. 1993;88(9):1395–8.
13. Steinberg DM, Cooke WT, Alexander-Williams J. Abscess and fistulae in Crohn's disease. Gut. 1973;14:865–9.
14. Wong WD, Buie WD. The management of intestinal fistulas. In: MacKeigan JM, Cataldo PA, eds. Intestinal stomas. St. Louis: Quality Medical Publishing, Inc.; 1993:307–28.
15. Reber HA, Roberts C, Way LW, Dunphy JE. Management of gastrointestinal fistulas. Ann Surg. 1978;188:460–7.
16. Hild P, Dobroschke J, Henneking K, Rieck B. Treatment of enterocutaneous fistulas with somatostatin. Lancet. 1986;2:626.
17. Hawker PC, Givel JC, Keighley MRB, Alexander-Williams J, Allan RN. Management of enterocutaneous fistulae in Crohn's disease. Gut. 1983;24:284–7.
18. Present DH, Korelitz BI, Wisch N, Glass JL, Sachar DB, Pasternak BS. Treatment of Crohn's disease with 6-mercaptopurine. N Engl J Med. 1980;302:981–7.
19. Korelitz BI, Present DH. Favorable effect of 6-mercaptopurine on fistulae of Crohn's disease. Dig Dis Sci. 1985;30(1):58–64.
20. Peltekian KM, Williams CN, MacDonald AS et al. Open trial of cyclosporin in patients with severe active Crohn's disease refractory to conventional therapy. Can J Gastroenterol. 1988;2:5–11.
21. Strange EF, Fleig WE, Rehklau E et al. Cyclosporin A treatment in inflammatory bowel disease. Dig Dis Sci. 1989;34:1387–92.
22. Hanauer SB, Smith MB. Rapid closure of Crohn's disease fistulas with continuous intravenous Cyclosporin A. Am J Gastroenterol. 1993;88(5):646–9.
23. Present DH, Lichtiger S. Efficacy of cyclosporine in treatment of fistula in Crohn's disease. Dig Dis Sci. 1994;39(2):374–80.
24. Farmer RG, Hawk WA, Turnbull RB Jr. Indications for surgery in Crohn's disease. Gastroenterology. 1976;71:245–50.
25. Greenstein AJ, Kark AE, Dreiling DA. Crohn's disease of the colon. 1. Fistula in Crohn's disease of the colon: classification, presenting features and management in 63 patients. Am J Gastroenterol. 1974;62:419–29.
26. Driscoll RH, Rosenberg IH. Total parenteral nutrition in inflammatory bowel disease. Med Clin N Am. 1978;62:185–201.
27. Keighley MRB, Heyen F, Winslet MC. Enterocutaneous fistulas and Crohn's disease. Acta Gastroenterol Belg. 1987;50:580–600.
28. Glass RE, Ritchie JK, Lennard-Jones JE, Hawley PR, Todd IP. Internal fistulas in Crohn's disease. Dis Colon Rectum. 1985;28:557–61.
29. Pichney LS, Fantry GT, Graham SM. Gastrocolic and duodenocolic fistulas in Crohn's disease. J Clin Gastroenterol. 1992;15(3):205–11.
30. Greenstein AJ, Present DH, Sachar DB et al. Gastric fistulas in Crohn's disease. Report of cases. Dis Colon Rectum. 1989;32:888–92.
31. Jacobson IM, Schapiro RH, Warshaw AL. Gastric and duodenal fistulas in Crohn's disease, Gastroenterology. 1985;89;1347–52.

32. Pettit SH, Irving MH. The operative management of fistulous Crohn's disease. Surg Obstet Gynecol. 1988;167:223–8.

33. Wilk PJ, Fazio VJ, Turnbull RB Jr. The dilemma of Crohn's disease: ileoduodenal fistula complicating Crohn's disease. Dis Colon Rectum. 1977;20:387–92.

34. Fazio VW, Wilk P, Turnbull RB Jr, Jagelman DG. The dilemma of Crohn's disease: ileosigmoidal fistula complicating Crohn's disease. Dis Colon Rectum. 1977;20:381–6.

35. Block GW, Schraut WH. The operative treatment of Crohn's enteritis complicated by ileosigmoid fistula. Ann Surg. 1982;196:356–60.

36. McNamara MJ, Fazio VW, Lavery IC, Weakley FL, Farmer RG. Surgical treatment of enterovesical fistulas in Crohn's disease. Dis Colon Rectum. 1990;33:271–6.

37. Heyen F, Ambrose NS, Allan RN, Dykes PW, Alexander-Williams J, Keighley MRB. Enterovesical fistulas in Crohn's disease. Ann R Col Rectum Engl. 1989;71:101–4.

38. Radcliffe AG, Ritchie JK, Hawley PR, Lennard-Jones JE, Northover JMA. Anovaginal and rectovaginal fistulas in Crohn's disease. Dis Colon Rectum. 1988;31:94–9.

39. Sher ME, Bauer JJ, Gelernt I. Surgical repair of rectovaginal fistulas in patients with Crohn's disease: transvaginal approach. Dis Colon Rectum. 1991;34:641–8.

40. Morrison JG, Gathright JB Jr, Ray JE, Ferrari BT, Hicks TC, Timmcke AE. Results of operation for rectovaginal fistula in Crohn's disease. Dis Colon Rectum. 1989;32:497–9.

41. Cohen JL, Stricker JW, Schoetz DJ Jr, Coller JA, Veidenheimer MC. Rectovaginal fistula in Crohn's disease. Dis Colon Rectum. 1989;32:825–8.

42. Francois Y, Descos L, Vignal J. Conservative treatment of low rectovaginal fistula in Crohn's disease. Int J Colorect Dis. 1990;5:12–14.

43. Hesterberg R, Schmidt WU, Müller F, Röher HD. Treatment of anovaginal fistulas with an anocutaneous flap in patients with Crohn's disease. Int J Colorect Dis. 1993;8:51–4.

44. Fazio VW, Jones IT, Jagelman DG, Weakley FL. Rectourethral fistulas in Crohn's disease. Surg Gynecol Obstet. 1987;164(2):148–50.

45. Stamler JS, Bauer JJ, Janowitz HD. Rectourethroperineal fistula in Crohn's disease. Am J Gastroenterol. 1985;80(2):111–12.

46. Wilton PB, Goldberg SM. Perianal disease: surgical management. In: Current management of inflammatory bowel disease. Bayless TM, ed. Burlington, Ontario, Canada: BC Decker; 1989:298–304.

47. Bernstein LH, Frank MS, Brandt LJ, Boley SJ. Healing of perineal Crohn's disease with metronidazole. Gastroenterology. 1980;79:357–65.

48. Brandt LJ, Bernstein JH, Boley SJ, Frank MS. Metronidazole therapy for perineal Crohn's disease: a follow-up study. Gastroenterology. 1982;83:383–7.

49. Keighley MRB, Allan RN. Current status and influence of operation on perianal Crohn's disease. Int J Colorect Dis. 1986;1:104–7.

50. Morrison JG, Gathright JB Jr, Ray JE, Ferrari BT, Hicks TC, Timmcke AE. Surgical management of anorectal fistulas in Crohn's disease. Dis Colon Rectum. 1989;32:492–6.

51. Levien DH, Surrell J, Mazier WP. Surgical treatment of anorectal fistula in patients with Crohn's disease. Surg Gynecol Obstet. 1989;169:133–6.

52. Fuhrman G, Larach SW. Experience with perirectal fistulas in patients with Crohn's disease. Dis Colon Rectum. 1989;32:847–8.

53. Fry RD, Shemesh EI, Kodner IJ, Timmcke A. Techniques and results in the management of anal and perianal Crohn's disease. Surg Gynecol Obstet. 1989;168(1):42–8.

54. Marks CG. Anal lesions in Crohn's disease. Ann R Col Surg Engl. 1990;72:158–9.

55. Nordgren S, Fasth S, Hultén L. Anal fistulas in Crohn's disease: incidence and outcome of surgical treatment. Int J Colorect Dis. 1992;7:214–18.

56. Bayer I, Gordon PH. Selected operative management of fistula-in-ano in Crohn's disease. Dis Colon Rectum. 1994;37:760–5.

57. van Dongen LM, Lubbers E-JC. Perianal fistulas in patients with Crohn's disease. Arch Surg. 1986;121:1187–90.

58. Bernard D, Morgan S, Tassé D. Selective surgical management of Crohn's disease of the anus. Can J Surg. 1986;29(5):318–21.

59. Jones IT, Fazio VW, Jagelman DG. The use of transanal rectal advancement flaps in the management of fistulas involving the anorectum. Dis Colon Rectum 1987;30;919–23.

60. Williams JG, Rothenberger DA, Nemer FD, Goldberg SM. Fistula-in-ano in Crohn's disease. Results of aggressive surgical treatment. Dis Colon Rectum 1991;34;378–84.

61. Morrison JG, Gathright JB, Ray JE, Ferrari BT, Hicks TC, Timmcke AE. Surgical management of anorectal fistulas in Crohn's disease. Dis Colon Rectum. 1989;32:492–6.
62. White RA, Eisentat TE, Rubin RJ, Salvati EP. Seton management of complex anorectal fistulas in patients with Crohn's disease. Dis Colon Rectum. 1990;33:587–9.
63. Williams JG, MacLeod CA, Rothenberger DA, Goldberg SM. Seton treatment of high anal fistulae. Br J Surg. 1991;78:1159–61.
64. Grant DR, Cohen Z, McLeod RS. Loop ileostomy for anorectal Crohn's disease. Can J Surg. 1986;29(1):32–5.
65. Sher ME, Bauer JJ, Gorphine S, Gelernt I. Low Hartmann's procedure for severe anorectal Crohn's disease. Dis Colon Rectum. 1992;35:975–80.
66. Orkin BA, Telander RI. The effect of intra-abdominal resection or fecal diversion on perianal disease in pediatric Crohn's disease. J Pediatr Surg. 1985;20(4):343–7.

# 31
# Medical treatment for prevention of postoperative recurrence of Crohn disease?

W. E. FLEIG

Unlike ulcerative colitis, Crohn disease cannot be cured by resection of the involved intestine. Postoperative recurrence is the rule rather than an exception. Therefore, the development of strategies to prevent or, at least, delay recurrence of the disease is one of the most challenging issues at present. To this end, it is necessary to:

1. Define the meaning of 'postoperative recurrence',
2. Recognize the probability, pattern and natural course of postoperative recurrence,
3. Identify eventual early prognostic indicators, and
4. Evaluate effective preventive medical treatment.

## POSTOPERATIVE RECURRENCE

The spectrum of definitions of postoperative recurrence of Crohn disease ranges from the reappearance of endoscopic lesions, preferably at the site of the anastomosis[1], to the reappearance of clinical symptoms of the disease[2] and, finally, as the most severe type of recurrence, the need for repeated surgery[3]. Some of the recent and still-ongoing clinical trials have used endoscopic recurrence as an end point. However, since treatment of Crohn disease is, at present, directed to the signs, symptoms and complications rather than to endoscopic lesions, the reappearance of clinical 'activity' of the disease appears to be the definition of recurrence which should be used in clinical trials of prevention.

## PROBABILITY, PATTERN AND NATURAL COURSE OF POSTOPERATIVE RECURRENCE

Endoscopic lesions recur in the vast majority of resected patients within a short period of time. In a prospective study by Rutgeerts et al.[4], endoscopic recurrence was detected by routine colonoscopy in 72% within 1 year of the operation and in 87% within 3 years[5]. Similar proportions of endoscopic recurrence were reported in a small cohort prospectively followed by Gabbert and coworkers[6]. In a recent study from Sweden, 22 of 30 patients (73%) resected for Crohn disease showed preanastomotic ileal ulceration as early as 3 months after the operation, compared with 93% at 1 year and 100% at 3 years[7]. In the still-ongoing European Cooperative Crohn's Disease Study VI, comparing mesalazine with placebo for the prevention of postoperative recurrence, 65 of 117 patients (55.5%) had endoscopic lesions at the site of the anastomosis as early as 6 weeks after the operation, compared with 30%, 15.5% and 13.6% of the patients when the neoterminal ileum, the rectum and the sigmoid colon were considered, respectively, and less than 10% in the remaining parts of the colon (Fleig, Lochs, Maier, et al., unpublished data).

Clinical symptoms occurred less frequently: 33% at 3 months, 37% at 1 year and 86% at 3 years in the Swedish trial[7] compared with about 10% per year in the other studies. Reoperation is required at a rate of about 25–30% after 5, and 40–50% after 20, postoperative years[8,9]. As demonstrated in an elegant study by Rutgeerts et al.[5], the probability of clinical recurrence is clearly linked to the severity of the endoscopic lesions observed after 3 months. When lesions were graded into 5 categories (Table 1)[5], only 8% of the patients with no or minimal lesions developed symptoms within 6 years, while 43% of the patients with grade 2 and more than 84% of those with grade 3 lesions became symptomatic within the same period of time. All patients with grade 4 lesions had relapsed with clinical symptoms after 4 years.

**Table 1**   Grading of postoperative endoscopic findings

| Grade | Endoscopic finding |
| --- | --- |
| 0 | No lesions |
| 1 | < 5 aphthous lesions |
| 2 | > 5 aphthous lesions within normal mucosa, or a few skip areas of larger lesions, or lesions within 1 cm of the ileocolonic anastomosis |
| 3 | Diffuse aphthous ileitis |
| 4 | Diffuse inflammation with large ulcers, nodules and/or narrowing |

According to Rutgeerts et al., 1990[5]

## RISK FACTORS AND PROGNOSTIC INDICATORS

Several clinical parameters may affect the risk of postoperative recurrence. The impact of the preoperative location of the disease is controversial. While colonic disease appears to have the lowest rate of recurrence, it is unclear whether a strictly ileal or an ileocolonic pattern of the disease is more prone to relapse[10,11]. The continuity of the faecal stream is an important prerequisite for the development of recurrent disease[12]. The length of the preoperatively involved ileal segment correlates with the length of the segment with postoperative recurrence[13]. Several other demographic and clinical factors, such as age and duration of disease or the fistulizing, fibrostenotic or inflammatory types of disease, have been reported as risk factors but there is substantial discussion as to the clinical relevance of these findings.

Non-specific parameters of systemic inflammation, including C-reactive protein and orosomucoid have been combined to produce an index and have been described as reliable indicators of recurrence in patients with quiescent disease[14]. In fact, patients identified as prone to relapse and treated with steroids did better than similar patients on placebo[14]. It is, however, unclear whether this model, the usefulness of which has not been confirmed to date, might also be applied to the postoperative situation. The value of other potential prognostic indicators is either controversial, as for neopterin[15,16], or insufficiently assessed and difficult to use as a routine test, as for diamine oxidase activity in post-heparin plasma[17,18]. Pathological findings in tests of intestinal permeability using lactulose/mannitol[19,20] have recently been reported to precede the recurrence of clinical symptoms[21]; however, the clinical value of this has to be established. Overall, there is no single parameter or combination of parameters which, with our current state of knowledge, can reliably predict recurrence of Crohn disease after resective surgery in an individual patient.

## MEDICAL TREATMENT FOR PREVENTION OF POSTOPERATIVE RECURRENCE

There are only two fully published trials of medical treatment for the prevention of recurrence of Crohn disease in patients after curative surgery. One of these trials showed some advantage of sulphasalazine over placebo; however, the study was biased by the non-randomized assignment of patients to groups with 'radical' (i.e. according to the rules of oncological bowel surgery) and non-radical (i.e. without dissection of regional lymph nodes and without major safety margins from the grossly involved intestine) resection[22]. A preliminary analysis of a second trial using oral mesalazine (2.4 g per day) has recently been published[23]. However, this trial was not blinded since the control group received no treatment at all, and, therefore, is open to bias. The end-point was endoscopic recurrence, which occured in 52% of the mesalazine-treated and 85% of the untreated patients within 2 years. During the same period of time, a significant difference between the treated and the untreated groups was also observed with regard to the rate of clinically symptomatic recurrence (18% vs 41%).

Two other trials of mesalazine have been reported in abstract form[24,25]. In the French trial[24], 106 patients were randomized to receive either 3 g/d mesalazine (54 patients) or placebo (52 patients). Treatment was started within 15 days of 'curative' resection of ileum and/or colon. The end-point of the study was endoscopic recurrence after 12 weeks of treatment. Endoscopic lesions were found in 50% of the mesalazine patients and 63% of the placebo group (difference not significant). The Canadian multicentre study included 177 patients, 14 of which, predominantly in the placebo group, were excluded from analysis for various reasons[25] This led to some imbalance, since 87 of the remaining 163 patients were on mesalazine (3 g/d also) compared with only 76 patients on placebo.

Drug treatment was started within 8 weeks after 'curative' ileal and/or colonic resection. Mesalazine significantly reduced the rate of recurrence at 3 years from 47% on placebo to 27%. The European Cooperative Crohn's Disease Study VI is still under way. Patients within 10 days after resective surgery are randomized to receive either 4 g mesalazine (Pentasa®) or placebo for a total of 18 months. The recruitment period of this trial, aiming at a total of 300 patients, is almost completed; the end-point is clinical recurrence and results will be available in the autumn of 1996.

Three recent trials of mesalazine for the maintenance of remission have included both operated and non-operated patients with quiescent disease[26–28]. Retrospective stratification of the patients in each of these trials into previously operated and non-operated patients suggested that patients after surgery may have benefited from prophylactic treatment. In a further mesalazine trial[29], patients with recent surgery were excluded from recruitment. However, this trial is of interest in that the drug prevented recurrence in patients who had achieved remission recently, no longer than 3 months, rather than in patients with long-standing remission, as in the trial of Prantera and coworkers[27]. Starting treatment as early after the operation as possible would also seem logical for the prevention of postoperative recurrence.

Finally, another trial reported in abstract form investigated the eventual preventive action of metronidazole[30]. Treatment with 20 mg/kg body weight per day of metronidazole or placebo for 3 months was started within 1 week of ileal resection. Although the number of endoscopic recurrences at 3 months was not reduced by metronidazole, the drug significantly affected the severity of the endoscopic relapses (43% of patients with severe relapses on placebo compared with 13% on metronidazole). The rate of clinical recurrence was significantly reduced at 1 but not at 3 years after surgery.

## SUMMARY AND CONCLUSIONS

Recurrence of Crohn disease after resective surgery is frequent. New endoscopic lesions are predominantly found in the neoterminal ileum and at the anastomosis, and they occur in almost every patient within about 1 year. Clinical recurrence occurs at a rate of about 10% per postoperative year, and severe endoscopic recurrence is predictive of symptomatic recurrence with the next 3–4 years. Beyond this, there is no good pre- or early postoperative marker to predict a high risk of postoperative recurrence, justifying the eventual institution of preventive therapy.

The results of studies on the prevention of endoscopic recurrence after surgery by mesalazine are controversial. There is some preliminary evidence, however, that treatment for more than 3 months at a sufficiently high dose (> 2 g/day) may have some preventive action, not only for endoscopic, but also for symptomatic recurrence. A 3-month course of metronidazole may be effective in delaying, but not preventing, clinical relapses after surgery.

Thus, although there is some evidence that mesalazine (and perhaps metronidazole) may be effective in maintaining postoperative remission in patients with Crohn disease undergoing resective surgery, data are not conclusive enough to generally recommend preventive treatment. Furthermore, even if clinically effective, medical prevention may not be cost-effective if all patients are treated without selecting for a subgroup with a high risk of recurrence. Since treatment probably has to be started as early after surgery as possible, the detection of severe endoscopic lesions may be too late to prevent symptomatic relapse by medical therapy, although this has not yet been investigated. Therefore, better pre- or immediately postoperative predictors of the individual patient's risk of recurrence are urgently needed.

## References


1. Clavedetscher P, Deyhle P. Diagnosis of Crohn's recurrence after surgery. Endoscopy. 1975;7:27–9.
2. Lennard-Jones JE, Stadler GE. Prognosis after resection of chronic regional ileitis. Gut. 1967;8:332–6.
3. Greenstein AJ, Sachar DB, Pasternack BS, Janowitz HD. Reoperation and recurrence in Crohn's colitis and ileocolitis. Crude and cumulative rates. N Engl J Med. 1975;293:685–90.
4. Rutgeerts P, Geboes K, Vantrappen G et al. Natural history of recurrent Crohn's disease at the ileocolonic anastomoses after curative surgery. Gut. 1984;25:665–72.
5. Rutgeerts P, Geboes K, Vantrappen G et al. Predictability of the postoperative course of Crohn's disease. Gastroenterology. 1990;99:956–62.
6. Gabbert HE, Ewe K, Singe CC et al. Frührezidiv des Morbus Crohn nach 'kurativer' Ileocoecalresektion. Eine prospektive endoskopische und histologische Untersuchung. Dtsch Med Wschr. 1990;115:447–51.
7. Olaison G, Smedh K, Sjödahl R. Natural course of Crohn's disease after ileocolonic resection: endoscopically visualized ileal ulcers preceding symptoms. Gut. 1992;33:331–5.
8. Lock MR, Fazio VW, Farmer RG et al. Proximal recurrence and the fate of the rectum following excisional surgery for Crohn's disease of the large bowel. Ann Surg. 1981;194:754–60.
9. Chardavoyne R, Flint GW, Pollack S, Wise L. Factors affecting recurrence following recurrence for Crohn's disease. Dis Colon Rectum. 1986;29:495–502.
10. Lock MR, Farmer RG, Fazio VW. Recurrence and reoperation for Crohn's disease. N Engl J Med. 1981;304:1586 8.
11. Himal HS, Belliveau P. Prognosis after surgical treatment for granulomatous enteritis and colitis. Am J Surg. 1981;142:347–9.
12. Rutgeerts P, Geboes K, Peeters M et al. Effect of faecal stream diversion on recurrence of Crohn's disease in the neoterminal ileum. Lancet. 1991;338:771–4.
13. D'Haens GR, Gasparaitis AE, Hanauer SB. The length of recurrent ileitis after ileocolonic resection correlates with presurgical extent of Crohn's disease. Gastroenterology. 1993;104:A692(Abstract).
14. Brignola C, Campieri M, Farrugia P et al. The possible utility of steroids in the prevention of relapses in Crohn's disease in remission. A preliminary study. J Clin Gastroenterol. 1988;10:631–4.
15. Stange EF, Fleig WE, Ditschüneit H. Neopterin serum levels in Crohn's disease. In: Goebell H, Peskar BM, Malchow H, eds. Inflammatory bowel diseases: Basic research and clinical implications. Lancaster: MTP Press; 1988:403.
16. Judmaier G, Meyersbach P, Weiss G et al. The role of neopterin in assessing disease activity in Crohn's disease: classification and regression trees. Am J Gastroenterol. 1993;88:706–11.
17. Thompson JS. Intestinal mucosa diamine oxidase activity reflects intestinal involvement in Crohn's disease. Am J Gastroenterol. 1988;83:756–60.
18. D'Agostino L. Postheparin plasma diamine oxidase values in the follow-up of patients with small bowel Crohn's disease. Gut. 1991;32:932–5.
19. Katz KD, Hollander D, Vadheim CM et al. Intestinal permeability in patients with Crohn's disease and their healthy relatives. Gastroenterology. 1989;97:927–31.
20. Peeters M, Ghoos Y, Geypens B, Hiele M, Rutgeerts P. Lactulose/mannitol permeability index is a suitable subclinical marker to identify subjects at risk in families of Crohn's patients. Gastroenterology. 1994;106:A750(Abstract).

21. Wyatt J, Vogelsang H, Hübl W, Waldhöer T, Lochs H. Intestinal permeability and the prediction of relapse in Crohn's disease. Lancet. 1993;341:1437–9.
22. Ewe K, Herfath C, Malchow H et al. Postoperative recurrence of Crohn's disease in relation of radicality of operation and sulfasalazine prophylaxis: a multicenter trial. Digestion. 1989;42:224–32.
23. Caprilli R, Andreoli A, Capurso L et al. Oral mesalazine (5-aminosalicylic acid; Asacol) for the prevention of post-operative recurrence of Crohn's disease. Gruppo Italiano per lo Studio del Colon e del Retto (GISC). Aliment Pharmacol Ther. 1994;8:35–43.
24. Florent Ch, Cortot A, Quandale P et al. Placebo-controlled trial of Claversal® (C) in the prevention of early endoscopic relapse after 'curative' resection for Crohn's disease. Gastroenterology. 1992;102:A601(Abstract).
25. McLeod RS, Wolff BG, Steinhart H et al. Delayed recurrence following surgery for Crohn's disease (CD). Gastroenterology. 1994;106:A:733(Abstract).
26. International Mesalazine Study Group. Coated oral 5-aminosalicylic acid versus placebo in maintaining remission in inactive Crohn's disease. Aliment Pharmacol Ther. 1990;4:55–64.
27. Prantera C, Pallone F, Brunetti G et al. Oral 5-aminosalicylic acid (Asacol) in the maintenance treatment of Crohn's disease. Gastroenterology. 1992;103:363–8.
28. Brignola C, Ioannone P, Pasquali S et al. Placebo-controlled trial of oral 5-ASA in relapse prevention in Crohn's disease. Dig Dis Sci. 1992;37:29–32.
29. Gendre JP, Mary JY, Florent C et al. Oral mesalamine (Pentasa) as maintenance treatment in Crohn's disease: A multicentre placebo-controlled study. Gastroenterology. 1993;104:435–9.
30. Rutgeerts P, Hiele M, Peeters M, Geboes K, Kerremans R. Prevention of clinical recurrence after ileal resection for Crohn's disease with metronidazole: A placebo controlled trial. Gastroenterology. 1994;106:A764(Abstract).

# Index